ATLAS OF
COSMETIC
DERMATOLOGY

ATLAS OF
COSMETIC
DERMATOLOGY

ZOE DIANA DRAELOS, MD

Clinical Associate Professor, Department of Dermatology
Wake Forest University School of Medicine
Winston-Salem, North Carolina

and

Principal Investigator, Dermatology Consulting Services
High Point, North Carolina

Churchill Livingstone
A Harcourt Health Sciences Company
New York   Edinburgh   London   Philadelphia

CHURCHILL LIVINGSTONE

A Harcourt Health Sciences Company

The Curtis Center
Independence Square West
Philadelphia, Pennsylvania 19106

Library of Congress Cataloging-in-Publication Data

Draelos, Zoe Kececioght
    Atlas of cosmetic dermatology / Zoe Diana Draelos.—1st ed.
        p. ; cm.
    Complement text to: Cosmetics in dermatology.
    ISBN 0-443-06548-9
    1. Skin—Care and hygiene—Atlases.   2. Cosmetics.
I. Draelos, Zoe Kececioght.   Cosmetics in dermatology.
II. Title.
    [DNLM: 1. Cosmetics—Atlases. 2. Skin Care—methods—
Atlases. WR 17 D758a 2000]
    RL87 .D73 2000
    616.5—dc21   00-025388

ATLAS OF COSMETIC DERMATOLOGY   ISBN 0-443-06548-9

Printed in the United States of America.

Last digit is the print number: 9   8   7   6   5   4   3   2   1

To my three boys—
Michael Draelos, M.D., and Mark and Matthew—
who challenge me
to constant discovery.

FOREWORD

The cosmetic industry produces hundreds of diverse products for use on the skin, hair, and nails. Recent years have seen an important change in regard to the consumers' understanding and expectations of these multifarious products. The cosmetic industry is a huge and highly competitive enterprise where innovation is rewarded by market share, while the consumer benefits by an extraordinary choice of creative products.

In times past cosmetics were designed for the specific purpose of adornment to satisfy deep-seated needs to enhance one's appearance. Throughout history attractive persons have enjoyed psychological and societal advantages throughout the life span.

Cosmetics were somewhat like the painter's palette containing an array of multicolored pigments to adorn the surface of the canvas. Traditionally cosmetics made great use of colors and pigments to camouflage physical blemishes and to enhance desirable features. The emphasis was on beautification, a mere surface change. It was commonly understood that cosmetic formulations should be biologically inert, remaining on the surface without affecting the structures below.

This concept of inertness, in fact, was written into statutory law in the 1938 Act of Congress, which explicitly stated that cosmetics must not affect either the structure or the function of skin. If such changes did occur, that cosmetic would automatically become a drug, subjected to burdensome and costly regulations regarding safety and efficacy. Circumstances are now different. In recent decades the production of cosmetics has become a science more than just an art of beautification. As a result of powerful and sophisticated tools we can now appreciate how topically applied substances, including drugs and cosmetics, can bring about subtle but important changes in the physiologic functions of skin.

This new awareness has culminated in the concept of "cosmeceuticals," which emphasizes that substances placed on the skin have measurable effects and are not biologically inert. Cosmeceuticals cover a wide spectrum of formulations along a continuum, ranging from pure cosmetics at one end to drug-like at the other end. Terms such as "bioactive" and "functional" have entered the vocabulary, acknowledging that structural and functional changes are a reality.

Modern cosmetics are exceedingly complex, ingenious mixtures containing a multitude of ingredients, many of which are biologically active and have positive beneficial effects on the skin, enhancing its ability to subserve its main function as a protective envelope.

The new status of cosmeceuticals has generated a wide range of novel claims that include anti-aging agents, moisturization, barrier creams, sunscreens, etc. Concepts such as skin wellness have been added to the repertoire of benefits.

Instead of referring to the astonishing array of hair, skin, and nail products as cosmetics, it is now more meaningful to redesignate them as "skin care" products that are intended to promote the well being of the skin. This is a greatly expanded role to which the cosmetic industry with its cadre of basic scientists has made an impressive response. Every conceivable problem affecting the hair, skin, and nails has been addressed, yielding a veritable cornucopia of high-tech, aesthetic, diverse products that meet the everyday needs of consumers.

So, is it possible for a single person in a single text to cover this enormous galaxy of products comprehensively? Dr. Zoe Draelos, a practicing dermatologist, has done just that. She has produced a magnum opus that covers every aspect of this broad-based field. *Atlas of Cosmetic Dermatology* is an impressive text, made possible by Dr. Draelos's inexhaustible energy, high intelligence, enormous enthusiasm, and zealous dedication, accompanied by a huge store of knowledge gained by exhaustive reading and a vast practical experience of patients who seek her counsel in a dermatologic practice where 16 hour stints are not unusual.

This fact-filled text is not for casual bedtime reading or for browsing. This is a comprehensive reference book for skin-care specialists of all breeds—dermatologists, plastic surgeons, aestheticians, formulators, cosmetic scientists, salon personnel, and even marketers looking for new niches.

Every product category is thoroughly covered and is accompanied by sound advice and guidance regarding claim substantiation, safety, and efficacy. Dr. Draelos has a broad-based perspective that enables her not only to present formidable technical details but also to interpret the place and impact of skin-care products in the cosmetic universe.

Toxicology receives due attention. While the cosmetic industry has an admirable safety record, every product has the possibility of causing some persons to experience adverse effects, ranging from subjective neurosensory responses such as itching, burning, and stinging to visible changes that include various rashes, contact dermatitis, breakouts, dyspigmentations, xerosis, etc. The ingredients likely to generate these adverse events are clearly identified, along with an account of the premarketing tests certifying that the manufacturer has taken the necessary steps to assure safety.

Something interesting and informative can be found in every aspect of the broad range of subjects that are the domain of the cosmetic industry, including sensitive skin, ethnic skin, gender and age differences, and problems of adolescence and senescence.

This is a seminal work that is destined to become the classic reference for decades to come. How timely that this landmark work, which actually celebrates the achievements of the cosmetic industry, should make its appearance at the start of the new millenium.

Albert Kligman, MD, PhD

PREFACE

Cosmetic dermatology is a broad subspecialty encompassing a range of topics. These include the use of colored cosmetics, camouflaging techniques, basic skin care, cosmetic fashion trends, nail manicuring practices, surgical techniques, hair care, cosmeceuticals, and allergic and irritant contact dermatitis. It is an area of great interest as it impacts important aspects of appearance for individuals of both sexes and all ages. Mastery of cosmetic dermatology can provide the dermatologist with a valuable fund of knowledge to share with patients on a daily basis, hence the development of this atlas.

This atlas attempts to provide visual images important to an understanding of cosmetic dermatology. The pictures and many tables are designed to supplement the text, providing a useful resource for the dermatologist who requires information regarding cosmetic dermatology. I have collected these photos over the past 12 years from my clinical practice, referral practice, resident teaching sessions, consulting endeavors, and industry contacts. I am grateful to all of the individuals who lent their time, talents, and efforts to this collection.

The chapters are divided into the three anatomic areas of cosmetic dermatology: skin care, hair care, and nail care. Skin care is further divided into colored cosmetics, organized according to facial area, and skin maintenance products. An attempt has been made to synthesize information regarding product formulation, use, and adverse reactions, along with new product developments and the aesthetics of cosmetic and skin care product selection. Thus, the collective knowledge base of a cosmetic chemist, cosmetologist, makeup artist, and aesthetician has been condensed and presented in a form useful to the practicing dermatologist. No understanding of cosmetic dermatology can be complete without this broad approach.

This book is intended to serve as a complementary text to my original book, entitled *Cosmetics in Dermatology,* which presents a more detailed written review of the topic. This atlas contains the pictures and tables most useful to the dermatologist on a daily basis, with an abbreviated text that touches only the most important points. The texts can be used together, as the tables of contents are similarly organized.

Cosmetic dermatology is, without a doubt, the most rapidly advancing medical technology today. This is attributable to an improved understanding of skin physiology, due to research by dermatologists, and the new formulations developed by cosmetic chemists. Dermatologists must have the background to assist in the development and use of these new advances. This atlas is intended to aid in that pursuit. Seize the challenge!

Zoe Diana Draelos, MD

ACKNOWLEDGMENTS

. . . . —

The efforts of many individuals have culminated in the publication of this atlas. I am especially grateful to my patients, who allowed me to preserve a moment in time on film to share with others. The atlas also could not have been completed without the opportunities I have had to observe and discuss topics with those in the skin care industry. I am also indebted to my husband, Michael, who provided endless hours of text editing assistance and helped with the production of many of the photographs. He has been my continuing source of inspiration throughout the project. I must also thank my sons, Mark and Matthew, for providing the frequent diversions necessary to come back to preparation of this atlas with renewed vigor.

CONTENTS

· · · · · · · · · —

PART

SKIN
CARE

Understanding Cosmetics and Skin Care Products

An understanding of cosmetics and skin care products requires a basic fund of knowledge that encompasses product formulation, efficacy testing, safety testing, delivery systems, and cutaneous effect. These topics are the first considerations whenever any new product is conceived, researched, and tested prior to consumer release. It is the advancements that have been made in these areas that contribute to the quality and safety of products on the market today.

1

Cosmetic Formulation

There are several basic ingredients common to all cosmetic and skin care products. These ingredients are listed in Table 1–1. Most liquid and cream products are combinations of water-soluble and oil-soluble ingredients. Notable exceptions are the compressed powders used on the cheeks as blush, on the eyelids as eye shadow, and on the face. The most popular products are water-based, leading to the term oil-in-water emulsion, as water is the ingredient of highest concentration. These products evaporate quickly from the skin, leaving behind a film of active agent on the application site. Less popular formulations are oil-based and are known as water-in-oil emulsions. The concept of an emulsion, in which the water-soluble and oil-soluble ingredients coexist as one continuous liquid, is important as an emulsifier is required to accomplish this feat. Emulsifiers are one of the low-concentration ingredients that are frequently overlooked by dermatologists. Preservatives, fragrance, and coloring agents also deserve a brief evaluation, as they

can be sources of dermatologic problems. Higher-concentration ingredients and active agents are discussed under the individual product headings in the remainder of the atlas.

1. Emulsifiers

From a dermatologic standpoint, emulsifiers are important because they are the most common causes of irritant contact dermatitis with use of cosmetics and skin care products. Emulsifiers are detergents, of sorts, capable of suspending the oils within the dominant water phase. Unfortunately, emulsifiers not only emulsify the oils in the product, but also the oils on the face. This emulsification of sebum, in the author's opinion, accounts for some of the irritant contact dermatitis seen with the use of facial cosmetics designed to be worn all day. This problem is especially preva-

TABLE 1–1   Basic Cosmetic and Skin Care Product Formulation

Ingredient	Function	Ingredient	Function
Water	Diluent	Preservatives	Substances that prevent spoilage from microbial and fungal contamination and growth
Water-soluble ingredients	Hydrophilic substances necessary for product function		
Oil-soluble ingredients	Lipophilic substances necessary for product function	Fragrances	Scents that provide a pleasing smell or mask an unpleasing smell
Active agents	Substances that produce a skin benefit	Coloring agents	Agents that add color to the final product appearance
Emulsifiers	Agents that allow the hydrophilic and lipophilic substances to remain as one continuous phase		

lent in dry-complected individuals or patients with eczematous dermatoses, who have minimal sebum production or a defective cutaneous barrier. Figure 1–1 demonstrates irritant contact dermatitis of the face secondary to use of an eyelid moisturizer in a patient with atopic dermatitis.

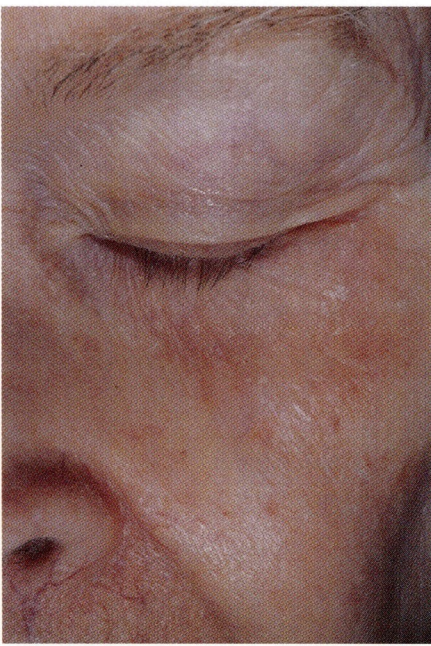

FIGURE 1–1 • Emulsifiers are used to maintain the water and oil components of a moisturizer in a single phase. This patient exhibited an irritant contact dermatitis in response to the emulsifier in an eyelid moisturizer.

2. Preservatives

The next group of ingredients, important from a dermatologic standpoint, are the preservatives. Table 1–2 lists most of the preservatives available for use in products today. This chart is valuable when reading ingredient listings and determining the function of various chemical constituents. The preservatives that are most commonly used in cosmetics and skin care products are listed in Table 1–3.[1,2] One current trend has been the development of products that claim to be "preservative-free." As a general rule, no cosmetic or skin care product can be truly preservative-free. The skin is inherently contaminated, and most products are used over a period of months with numerous openings and closings of the bottle. Organisms that frequently contaminate cosmetic and skin care products include gram-positive bacteria (*Staphylococcus aureus*, *Streptococcus* species), gram-negative bacteria (*Pseudomonas aeruginosa*, *Escherichia coli*, *Enterobacter aerogenes*), fungi (*Asperigillus niger*, *Penicillium* species, *Alternaria* species), and yeasts (*Candida* species).[3] Preservatives are necessary for product safety and stability. Their value greatly outweighs any possibility of adverse reaction.

Preservative-free products generally contain another ingredient that functions simultaneously as a preservative. For example, essential oils, such as eucalyptus, origanum, thyme, savory, and lemongrass oil, function as preservatives under the guise of a "botanical" or "all natural" additive.[4] Many alcohols and organic acids can also function as preservatives without being identified as such on the label.

TABLE 1-2   Some Preservatives Used in Cosmetics

Organic Acids

Benzoic acid	Boric acid	
Sorbic acid	Propionic acid	
Monochloroacetic acid	Sulphurous acid	
Formic acid	Citric acid	
Salicylic acid	Dehydroacetic acid	

Parabens

Methyl p-hydroxybenzoate	Butyl p-hydroxybenzoate
Ethyl p-hydroxybenzoate	Benzyl p-hydroxybenzoate
Propyl p-hydroxybenzoate	

Mercurial Compounds

Phenyl mercury acetate	Phenyl mercury nitrate
Phenyl mercury borate	

Essential Oils

Eucalyptus	Savory
Origanum	Lemongrass oil
Thyme	

Aldehydes

Formaldehyde

Alcohols

b-Phenoxyethyl alcohol	Benzyl alcohol
b-p-Chlorphenoxyethyl alcohol	Isopropyl alcohol
b-Phenoxypropyl alcohol	Ethyl alcohol

Phenolic Compounds

Phenol	Methylchlorothymol
o-Phenylphenol	Dichlorophene
Chlorothymol	Hexachlorophene

Quaternary Ammonium Compounds

Benzethonium chloride	Cetyltrimethylammonium bromide
Benzalkonium chloride	Cetylpyridinium chloride

Miscellaneous

5-Bromo-5-nitro-1,3-dioxan (Dioxin)	Trichlorsalicylanilide
2-Bromo-2-nitropropane-1,3-diol (Bronopol)	Trichlorcarbanilide
Imidazolidinyl urea (Germall 115)	5-Chloro-2-methyl-4-isothiazolin-3-one and 2-methyl-4-isothiazolin-3-one (Kathon CG)

Adapted from Wilkinson JB, Moore RJ (eds.). Harry's Cosmeticology, 7th ed. New York: Chemical Publishing, 1982, pp. 673–706.

TABLE 1-3   Comparison of Preservatives Used in Cosmetics

Preservative	Advantages	Disadvantages
Alcohols	Broad coverage, inexpensive	Volatile; high concentration required
Quaternium-15 (Dowicil 200)	Broad coverage (bacteria, yeasts, molds)	Ineffective against some *pseudomonas* species; formaldehyde releaser
Formaldehyde	Broad coverage (fungicide and bactericide)	Irritant, allergen, concentration is regulated; unpleasant odor
Quaternary ammonium compounds	Mainly gram-positive bacteria; some gram-negative bacteria	Incompatible with anionics and proteins
Parabens	Moderate coverage (fungi, gram-positive bacteria), low allergenicity, low irritancy	Poor defense against gram-negative bacteria; incompatible with nonionics and cationics; effective only at acidic pH levels
Organic mercurials	Broad coverage	High toxicity, high irritancy
Phenolics	Broad coverage; effective over a wide pH range	High irritancy, volatile
2-Bromo-2-nitropropane-1,3-diol (Bronopol)	Moderate coverage (bacteria)	Formaldehyde releaser; least effective against yeast and fungi
Methylisothiazolinone and methylchloroisothiazolinone (Kathon CG)	Broad coverage (bacteria, yeasts, fungi)	Allergenicity; irritancy; inactivated at high pH levels
Imidazolidinyl urea (Germall 115)	Moderate coverage (gram-negative bacteria)	Most effective when combined with parabens and antifungals to obtain broad coverage
Diazolidinyl urea (Germall II)	Moderate coverage (gram-negative bacteria, *Pseudomonas* species)	Most effeective when combined with parabens and antifungals to obtain broad coverage
Organic acids	Broad coverage (bacteria, yeasts)	Irritant; effective only at acidic pH levels
DMDM hydantoin (Glydant)	Broad coverage; effective over a wide pH range	Less active against yeasts

Adapted from Wilkinson JB, Moore RJ (eds.). Harry's Cosmeticology, 7th ed. New York: Chemical Publishing, 1982, pp. 673–707.

TABLE 1–4   Common Fragrance Materials

Fragrance Material	Characteristics	Fragrance Material	Characteristics
Benzyl acetate	Light floral, slightly fruity	Heliotropine	Sweet, floral, powdery
Benzyl salicylate	Warm, balsamic	Hexyl cinnamic aldehyde	Light, delicate
Iso-bornyl acetate	Fresh, piney	Indole	Floral, animalic
p-t-Butyl cyclohexyl acetate	Soft, woody	Gamma-methyl ionone	Woody, floral
Cedryl acetate	Sharp, woody	Musk ketone	Musky, animalic, warm
Citronellal	Rosy	Phenylethyl alcohol	Floral
Dihydro myrcenol	Citrus	Vanillin	Sweet, powdery, vanilla
Geraniol	Floral, rosy		

Adapted from Dallimore A. Perfumery. In Williams DF, Schmitt WH (eds.). Chemistry and Technology of the Cosmetics and Toiletries Industry. London: Blackie Academic & Professional, 1992, pp. 258–274.

3. Fragrance

Another relatively common allergen in cosmetics is the fragrance. In terms of concentration, fragrance is an extraordinarily small component of formulations, but it may be the most expensive ingredient in the product and the ingredient of greatest importance to the consumer. Fragrance imparts a mood, a feeling, an aura, and mystique to cosmetic and skin care products, which are integral parts of the application experience. Even though fragrance additives may be problematic for the dermatologist, they are essential to the consumer who may or may not purchase a product based on fragrance alone.

Fragrance additives are a complex mixture of smells, making it difficult to isolate individual substances. The average soap contains 50 to 150 fragrance ingredients; the average cosmetic contains 200 to 500 fragrance ingredients; and the average perfume contains 700 fragrance ingredients.[5] Table 1–4 lists some of the most common fragrances and their characteristic smell. These ingredients are then mixed to obtain the final scent, which is a highly prized recipe among fragrance chemists.

The concentration of fragrance ingredients also varies with fine perfumes containing 15% to 30% fragrance, colognes containing 5% to 8% fragrance, and scented cosmetics containing 0.1% to 1% fragrance. Masking fragrances, used in products claiming to be scent-free (meaning no detectable odor), have fragrance concentrations of less than 0.1%.[6] Fragrance-free products, on the other hand, have no added ingredient simply for the purpose of imparting a smell. Other additives, such as botanical extracts, may have a characteristic odor that gives fragrance to the product. Some preservatives can also double as fragrance additives without having to be listed as such. For example, phenoxyethanol smells like roses, yet it is used primarily as a preservative. Fragrance-free products may or may not have a characteristic smell.

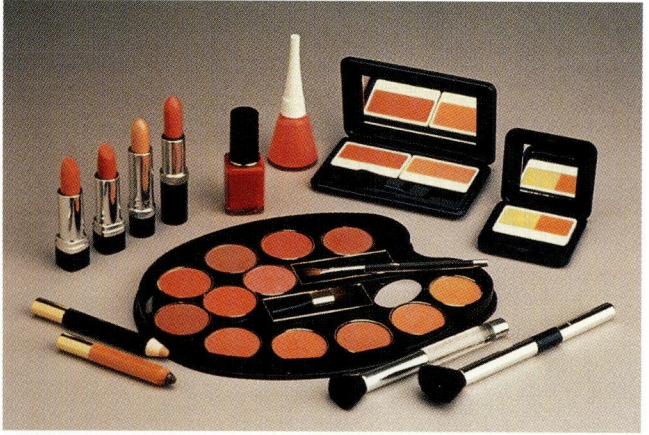

FIGURE 1–2 • Colored cosmetics are used to enhance and dramatize structures of the face and hands.

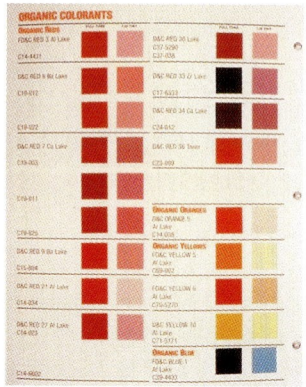

FIGURE 1–3 • Organic colorants are mixed and blended to produce fashionable colored cosmetics.

TABLE 1–5 Classification of Coloring Agents in Cosmetics and Skin Care Products in the United States

Coloring Agent Category	Permitted Use
FD & C colorants	Food, drugs, and cosmetics
D & C colorants	Drugs and cosmetics
External D & C colorants	Externally applied drugs and cosmetics, excluding those intended for the lips and mucous membranes

TABLE 1–6 Coloring Agents Used in Cosmetics

Coloring Agent Category	Coloring Agents Used in Cosmetics
FD & C colorants	FD & C Blue Nos. 1,2; FD & C Green Nos. 1,2,3; FD & C Red Nos. 2,3,4; FD & C Violet No. 1, FD & C Yellow Nos. 5,6; FD & C Red No. 3
D & C colorants	D & C Blue No. 4; D & C Green No. 5; D & C Orange Nos. 4,11,12; D & C Red Nos. 22,23,28,33; D & C Yellow Nos. 7,10; D & C Green No. 6; D & C Red Nos. 17,37; D & C Violet No. 2; D & C Yellow No. 11; D & C Orange Nos. 5,6,7,10; D & C Red Nos. 21,27; and D & C Yellow No. 7
External D & C colorants	Ext. D & C Yellow No. 7.

TABLE 1–7 Frequency of Use of Cosmetic Color Additives (in Order of Descending Frequency)

Color Additive	Effect	Color Additive	Effect
Titanium dioxide	White powder used as a base for color additives in facial foundations and powdered cosmetics	FD & C Blue No. 5	Blue pigment
		Ultramarine blue	Blue pigment
		FD & C Blue No. 1	Blue pigment
		D & C Red No. 7 Calcium Lake	Red pigment
Iron oxides	Brown pigments used in facial foundations and powdered cosmetics	Bismuth oxychloride	Light reflective material used in face powders and eyelid cosmetics
Mica	Light reflective material used in face powders and eyelid cosmetics	FD & C Red No. 4	Red pigment
		FD & C Yellow No. 6	Yellow pigment

4. Coloring Agents

The last ingredient common to cosmetic and skin care formulations is the coloring agent. Color is of utmost importance to cosmetics designed to highlight the face, cheeks, eyes, and lips (Fig. 1–2). Color is the driving force behind the fashion and allure of facial cosmetics (Fig. 1–3). Yet, color is also important for consumer acceptance of skin care products. The use of synthetic organic colors for cosmetic purposes has been regulated since 1938.[7] There are 116 permitted, certified colors available for the cosmetic chemist to combine; these are divided into three classes, listed in Table 1–5. The names of representative colorants found in cosmetics for each of the three regulated subtypes are presented in Table 1–6.[8] Table 1–7 lists the most common coloring agents in order of decreasing frequency of use in the cosmetics industry.[9] These tables are provided to help the dermatologist in reading ingredient labels and identifying coloring agents.

REFERENCES

1. Steinberg DC. Cosmetic preservation: Current international trends. Cosmet Toiletr 107:77–82, 1992.
2. Frequency of preservative use in cosmetic formulas as disclosed to the FDA—1990. Cosmet Toiletr 105:45–47, 1990.

3. Wilkinson JB, Moore RJ. Harry's Cosmeticology, 7th ed. New York: Chemical Publishing, 1982, pp. 673–706.

4. Kabara JJ. Aroma preservatives: Essential oils and fragrances as antimicrobial agents. In Kabara JJ (ed.). Cosmetic and Drug Preservation. New York: Marcel Dekker, 1984, pp. 237–270.

5. Jackson EM. Substantiating the safety of fragrances and fragranced products. Cosmet Toiletr 108:43–46, 1993.

6. Marks JG, DeLeo VA. Contact and Occupational Dermatology. St. Louis: Mosby Yearbook, 1992, pp. 145–147.

7. Berdick M. Color additives in cosmetics and toiletries. Cutis 21: 743–747, 1978.

8. Anstead DF. Cosmetic colours. In Hibbott HW (ed.). Handbook of Cosmetic Science. New York: Macmillan Company, 1963, pp. 101–118.

9. U.S. Food and Drug Administration. Cosmetic color additives: Frequency of use. Cosmet Toiletr 104:39–40, 1989.

2

Adverse Reactions to Cosmetics

The number of adverse reactions to skin care products and cosmetics is indeed small, given the tremendous popularity and widespread use of these formulations. Yet, occasionally, dermatologists are called upon to identify the cause of an allergic or irritant contact dermatitis related to product use. The incidence of irritant contact dermatitis is much higher than allergic contact dermatitis because any product can cause irritation when applied over a damaged skin barrier. Cosmetic products may also produce contact urticaria, cutaneous stinging, phototoxic reactions, and photoallergic reactions (Table 2–1). My basic approach to patients with adverse reactions to cosmetics is presented in Table 2–2.

1. Irritant Contact Dermatitis

Irritant contact dermatitis is manifested as erythematous, burning, pruritic skin that may develop microvesiculation and, later, desquamation. The dermatitis is characterized by stratum corneum damage without immunologic phenomena. The irritancy may be due to the presence of chemical factors with excessively high or low pH, or attributable to volatile vehicles that dissolve protective sebum.[6] Physical factors, including the rubbing necessary to apply cosmetics, or the abrasive particles within cosmetics, may cause irritancy. Most importantly, a damaged stratum corneum may not be able to provide a protective barrier, so that any cosmetic applied to the damaged skin will cause irritation. This is the case in patients with atopic dermatitis, xerotic eczema, or neurodermatitis. These patients frequently will describe numerous products that produce so-called allergic symptoms. In actuality, there is no immunologic basis to the dermatitis; rather, it represents an irritancy heightened by a damaged stratum corneum (Fig. 2–1).

2. Allergic Contact Dermatitis

Allergic contact dermatitis can be difficult to differentiate clinically from irritant contact dermatitis, but the distinction is important for ensuring good patient care. Both conditions may present with erythematous plaques; however, acute allergic contact dermatitis may exhibit relatively more vesiculation (Figs. 2–2 and 2–3). In some cases, late-stage allergic and irritant contact dermatitis cannot be differentiated clinically or histologically. Allergic contact dermatitis is an immunologic phenomenon requiring antigen-presenting and antigen-processing cells; as such, it is unaffected by the condition of the protective stratum corneum. Therefore, an intact stratum corneum cannot prevent development of allergic contact dermatitis in sensitized individuals. The only effective treatment course in such individuals is avoidance of the allergen.[7]

The categories of cosmetics and skin care products most likely to induce allergic contact dermatitis are listed, in order of decreasing likelihood, in Table 2–3. Those ingredients within the formulation that are most likely to cause allergic contact dermatitis are listed in Table 2–4 in order of decreasing frequency. A brief discussion of fragrances and preservatives follows, with substances specific to a given product discussed under individual product categories, later in the atlas.

a. FRAGRANCES

Fragrances, the most common causes of allergic contact dermatitis, are complex concoctions of scented materials (Fig. 2–4).[8–11] They also play an important role in the etiology of irritant contact dermatitis.[12] Table 2–5 lists the irritancy potential of some com-

TABLE 2–1 Cutaneous Reaction Patterns

Reaction Pattern	Immune System Activated	Dermatologic Appearance	Possible Causes
Irritant contact dermatitis	No	Erythema, desquamation, erosions, inflammatory papules	Soaps, detergents, strong acids, strong alkalis, solvents
Allergic contact dermatitis	Yes	Erythema, edema, vesicles, serum crusting	Poison ivy, methacrylate, formaldehyde, nickel
Nonimmunologic contact urticaria	No	Erythema, whelt	Alcohol, acetic acid, balsam of Peru, sorbic acid
Immunologic contact urticaria	Yes	Erythema, whelt	Benzoic acid, formaldehyde, menthol
Phototoxic contact dermatitis	No	Erythema	Sun, psoralens
Photoallergic contact dermatitis	Yes	Erythema, inflammatory papules, vesicles	Methylcoumarin, musk ambrette, PABA esters
Sensory irritation	No	No cutaneous findings	Lactic acid, propylene glycol, benzoyl peroxide

PABA, para-aminobenzoic acid.

mon fragrance ingredients,[13] whereas Table 2–6 lists their allergenic potential and patch test concentrations.[14]

Fragrance sensitivities can be detected by patch testing with a fragrance mixture containing the most common fragrance allergens. This mixture is included in the T. R. U. E. test kit (GlaxoWellcome, Research Triangle Park, North Carolina). The kit consists of a 2% concentration of cinnamic alcohol, cinnamic aldehyde, eugenol, isoeugenol, hydroxycitronellal, oakmoss absolute, geraniol, and alpha-amyl cinnamic alcohol in petrolatum.[15] This mixture is capable of detecting approximately 70% to 80% of fragrance sensitivities.[14] Further evaluation may require patch testing

TABLE 2–2 Draelos' Dermatologic Approach to Subject with Adverse Reactions to Cosmetics or Skin Care Products

1. Discontinue use of all topical cosmetics, over-the-counter treatment products, skin care items, cleansers, toiletries, and other such preparations. Allow the patient to use a syndet soap[1,2] and a bland moisturizer for 2 weeks.
2. Discontinue all topical prescription medications for 2 weeks, especially those that contain benzoyl peroxide, tretinoin, glycolic acid, volatile alcohols, or other drying, irritating ingredients.
3. Eliminate all sources of skin friction for 2 weeks through the use of loose, soft clothing[3] and discontinuation of sports or other activities in which repetitive skin rubbing may occur.
4. Evaluate the subject after 2 weeks to determine if any underlying dermatoses are present, such as seborrheic dermatitis, eczema, psoriasis, acne, rosacea, perioral dermatitis, etc. If a dermatosis is present, treat as appropriate for at least 2 weeks beyond visible disease resolution to allow both clinical and histologic (subclinical) resolution.
5. Conduct patch and photopatch tests on the patient to elucidate any common sources of allergic contact dermatitis. Test for contact urticaria. Determine which positive reactions are clinically relevant to the subject's sensitive skin difficulties and advise the subject appropriately.[4]
6. Perform the facial sting test on the subject by applying 10% lactic acid to the nasolabial fold or malar eminence.
7. Evaluate the subject's mental status, noting any signs of depression or other neuropsychiatric disease.
8. Allow the subject, if female, to add one facial cosmetic of low allergenic potential per week in the following order: lipstick, face powder, powder blush.[5]
9. All other cosmetics that are more common sources of difficulty in sensitive-skin subjects should be subjected to individual provocative use testing. These cosmetics should be applied nightly, for at least 5 nights, to a 2-cm area lateral to the eye. They should be tested in the following order: mascara, eyeliner, eyebrow pencil, eye shadow, facial foundation, any other colored facial cosmetics.
10. Over-the-counter treatment products and miscellaneous skin care products designed for leave-on use should be subjected to individual provocative use testing by applying them nightly, for at least 5 nights, to a 2-cm area lateral to the eye.
11. Skin care products designed to be rinsed off shortly after application should be subjected to individual use testing nightly, for at least 5 nights, in the manner recommended by the manufacturer.
12. All data, both positive and negative, should be analyzed by the dermatologist and presented to the subject in the form of products or ingredients to avoid and those appropriate for continued use.

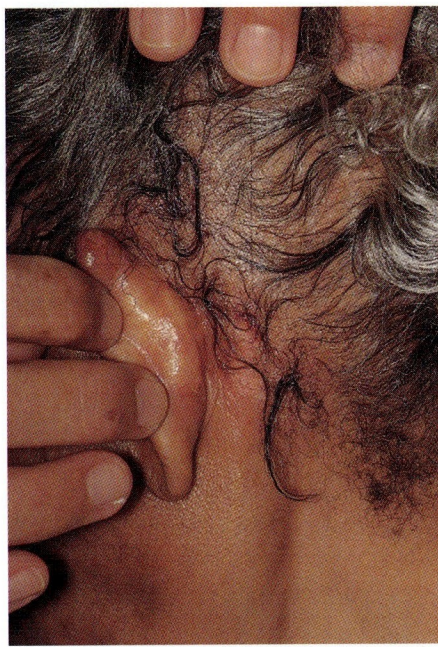

FIGURE 2–1 • Irritant contact dermatitis due to a no-lye, hair-relaxing product. Notice that the dermatitis is accentuated behind the ears, where the irritant alkali collected during the hair-straightening process.

with individual fragrances.[16] Patch testing techniques are discussed under a separate heading.

b. PRESERVATIVES

Preservatives are the next most common causes of allergic contact dermatitis. The number of adverse re-

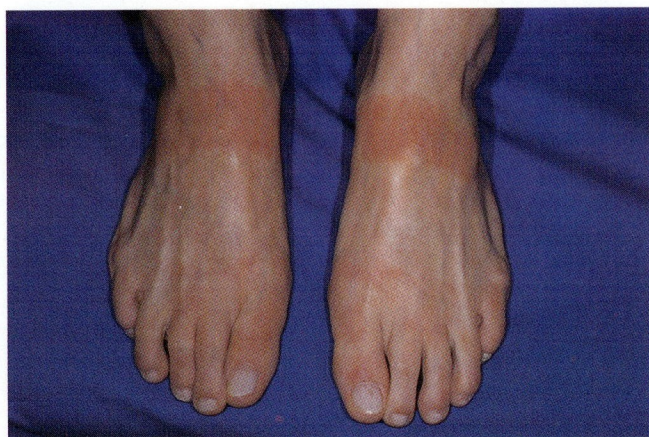

FIGURE 2–2 • Allergic contact dermatitis to a preservative contained (Kathon-CG) in a foot moisturizer. Note that the only areas affected are those where the patient perspired and experienced trauma from wearing sandals. The rubbing of the shoes, combined with the hydration of the skin, degraded the stratum corneum barrier.

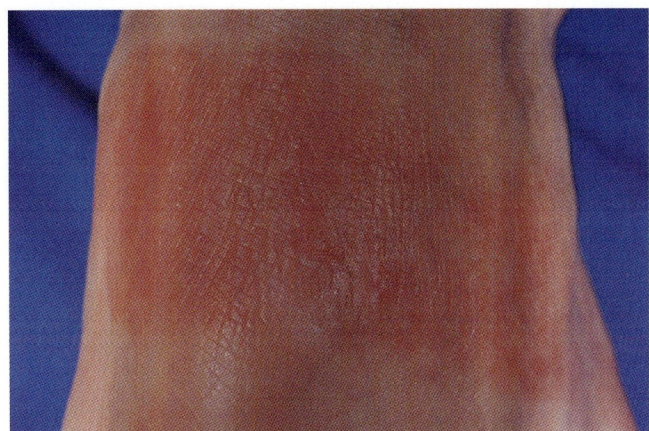

FIGURE 2–3 • A close-up of the mild allergic contact dermatitis observed in Figure 2–2.

actions to preservatives is indeed small, considering the great importance of these agents in preventing spoilage of products on the store shelf and contamination during use. Nevertheless, some patients may present with a suspected preservative allergy. Table 2–7 lists the usual concentration of the preservative in cosmetic formulations and the dilution and vehicle for patch testing, the next topic of discussion. Some of these preservatives are present on the dermatologist's standard patch test tray or T. R. U. E. Test (GlaxoWellcome, Research Triangle Park, North Carolina); others require dilution and preparation by the dermatologist.

3. Standard Dermatologic Patch Testing Techniques

Identifying a potential allergen or irritant requires both patience and skill on the part of the physician. Often,

TABLE 2–3 Causes of Allergic Contact Dermatitis

Product Category	Likelihood (%) of Allergic Contact Dermatitis
Skin care products	28
Hair care products	24
Facial cosmetics	11
Nail cosmetics	8
Fragrance products	7

Data from Adams RM, Maibach HI. A five-year study of cosmetic reactions. J Am Acad Dermatol 13:1062–1069, 1985.

TABLE 2–4 Ingredients Causing Allergic Contact Dermatitis (in Order of Decreasing Incidence)

Ingredient or Class of Ingredients	Function in Formulation
Fragrances	Provide a pleasing scent or mask an unpleasing odor
Preservatives	Prevent microbial and fungal contamination and growth
Paraphenylenediamine (PPD)	Chemical used in permanent and some semipermanent hair dyes
Lanolin	Occlusive moisturizer
Glyceryl monothioglycolate (GMTG)	Chemical found in some permanent hair waving products
Propylene glycol	A vehicle and a humectant moisturizer
Toluenesulfonamide/formaldehyde resin	Chemical used in nail polish
Sunscreens	Chemical agents that absorb ultraviolet energy on the skin

Data from Adams RM, Maibach HI. A five-year study of cosmetic reactions. J Am Acad Dermatol 13:1062–1069, 1985.

the problem clearly lies with a given cosmetic formulation, and discontinuing use of the product leads to resolution. In such cases, it may not be necessary to determine the exact allergenic ingredient. However, a situation may arise whereby the dermatitis is unremitting owing to allergy to a common ingredient found in many cosmetic and skin care products. In such cases, it is the obligation of the dermatologist to provide guidance to the patient as to the possible source of difficulty, for which patch testing is a valuable technique.

A good first step in the quest to find the allergen or irritant is to begin with the standard dermatologic patch test tray. The constituents of this tray are listed in Table 2–8. Not all of these substances are relevant to cosmetic and skin care products, however. Table 2–9 lists the relevant ingredients and in which products they are found. Once the appropriate allergens for testing have been selected, they can be applied to filter paper disks affixed to a strip of polyethylene-coated aluminum foil or placed in 8-mm chambers affixed to a nonwoven textile tape.[17] In the author's experience, the preformed chambers shown in Figure 2–5 have yielded the best results in patch testing cosmetics or skin care products. A more recent product has the allergens in hydrophilic vehicles already applied to polyester patches (T. R. U. E. Test Glaxo-Wellcome, Research Triangle, North Carolina), but this product requires application of the entire battery of tests (Fig. 2–6). The healthy skin of the upper back is selected and marked for placement of the tape strips, which are worn for 48 hours. During this time, the patient should not get the patches wet or engage in activities that induce heavy sweating. The test is initially evaluated 20 minutes after patch removal and again at 2 to 7 days.[18] Table 2–10 describes the

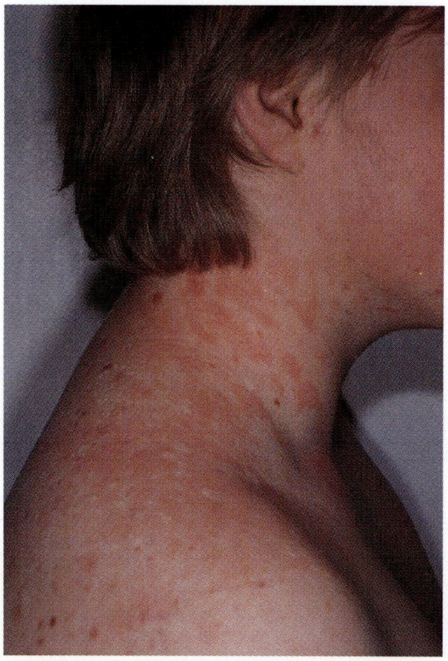

FIGURE 2–4 • Allergic contact dermatitis secondary to the fragrance in an aftershave preparation.

TABLE 2–5 Irritant Potential of Perfumes

Irritating Perfumes	Least Irritating Perfumes
Benzylidene acetone	Benzaldehyde
Methyl heptin carbonate	Benzoin resin
Methyl octin carbonate	Benzyl benzoate
Moderately Irritating Perfumes	Cinnamic acid and cinnamates
	Citrus oils
Cyclamen aldehyde	Cresol and methyl cresol
Ethyl methylphenyl glycinate	Diethyl phthalate
Eugenols gamma-nonyl lactone	Heliotropin
Balsam of Peru	Higher aliphatic aldehydes
Phenylacetaldehyde	Hydroxycitronellal
Vanillin	Menthol
	Salicylates

Adapted from Wells FV, Lubowe II. Cosmetics and the Skin. New York: Reinhold Publishing, 1964, pp. 370–374.

TABLE 2-6 Allergic Potential of Perfumes

Perfume	Allergic Potential	Patch Test Concentration (%) in Petrolatum	Perfume	Allergic Potential	Patch Test Concentration (%) in Petrolatum
Cinnamic alcohol	High	5	Geraniol	Moderate	5
Cinnamic aldehyde	High	1	Benzyl salicylate	Moderate	2
Hydroxycitronellal	High	4	Sandalwood oil	Moderate	2
Isoeugenol	High	5	Anisyl alcohol	Moderate	5
Eugenol	High	5	Benzyl alcohol	Moderate	5
Oakmoss absolute	High	5	Coumarin	Moderate	5
Alpha-amyl cinnamic alcohol	Moderate	5	Musk ambrette	Photoallergen	5

Adapted from Larsen WG. Perfume dermatitis. J Am Acad Dermatol 12:1–9, 1985.

TABLE 2-7 Preservative Use and Patch Test Concentrations

Preservative	Use Concentration	Patch Test Concentration
Quaternium-15 (Dowicil 200)	0.02%–0.3%	2% in petrolatum
Formaldehyde	0.05%–0.2%	1% aqueous
Parabens	0.1%–0.8%	3% in petrolatum if tested individually; otherwise, use 12% in petrolatum of paraben mixture*
2-Bromo-2-nitropropane-1,3-diol (Bronopol)	0.01%–0.1%	0.5% in petrolatum
Methylisothiazolinone and methylchloroisothiazolinone (Kathon CG)	3–15 ppm	100 ppm aqueous
Imidazolidinyl urea (Germall 115)	0.05%–0.5%	1% in petrolatum or aqueous
Diazolidinyl urea (Germall II)	0.1%–0.5%	1% aqueous
DMDM hydantoin (Glydant)	0.15%–0.4%	1%–3% aqueous

* Paraben mixture contains 3% each of emthyl-, ethyl-, propyl-, and butylparaben.

TABLE 2-8 Substances Included in Standard Dermatologic Patch Test Trays

Patch Test Substance	Composition	Patch Test Substance	Composition
Benzocaine	5% petrolatum	Colophony	20% petrolatum
Imidazolidinyl urea	2% aqueous	Black rubber mix	0.6% petrolatum
Thiuram mix	1% petrolatum	Ethylenediamine dihydrochloride	1% petrolatum
Lanolin alcohol	30% petrolatum	Quaternium-15	2% petrolatum
Neomycin sulfate	20% petrolatum	Mercapto mix	1% petrolatum
Paraphenylenediamine	1% petrolatum	Epoxy resin	1% petrolatum
Mercaptobenzothiazole	1% petrolatum	Balsam of Peru	25% petrolatum
p-tert-Butylphenol formaldehyde resin	1% petrolatum	Potassium dichromate	0.25% petrolatum
Formaldehyde	1% aqueous	Nickel sulfate	2.5% petrolatum
Carba mix	3% petrolatum	Cinnamic aldehyde	1% petrolatum

TABLE 2-9 Standard Patch Tray Substances and Their Relation to Cosmetics and Skin Care Products

• • • • • •

Patch Test Ingredient	Use in Cosmetics and Skin Care Products
Imidazolidinyl urea	Preservative
Lanolin alcohol	Emollient
Paraphenylenediamine	Hair dye constituent
Formaldehyde	Preservative
Colophony	Binding agent
Quaternium-15	Preservative
Balsam of Peru	Fragrance
Cinnamic aldehyde	Fragrance

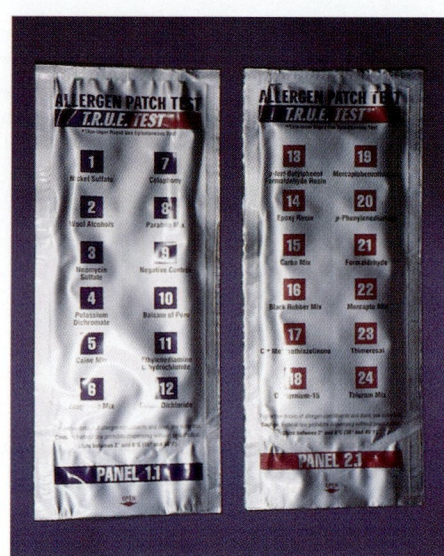

FIGURE 2–6 • An example of a patch test kit suitable for screening a large variety of allergens.

method of evaluation used by the North American Contact Dermatitis Group.

4. Customized Dermatologic Patch Testing Techniques

It is frequently necessary to patch test the patient's own cosmetics when the standard patch test tray does not contain the appropriate allergens or when the problem can be localized to one specific product. Most cosmetic preparations can be patch tested as is, meaning that the product can be directly removed from the packaging and applied to the patch test chamber. Liquid products should be allowed to dry thoroughly, however, prior to occlusion. This is espe-

cially important with mascaras, eyeliner, liquid eye shadows, and facial foundations.

Patch testing of skin care products becomes problematic, however, as distinguishing irritancy from allergenicity may be difficult (Fig. 2–7). Skin care products can be divided into those products that are intended to be left on the skin and those that are designed for a short period of contact. For example, sunscreens and facial moisturizers are intended to be worn all day, but hair shampoos and facial cleansers are designed to be rinsed shortly after application. In general, one should avoid using products intended for rinse-off application in patch tests. In any case, these products, because of their short contact time, are

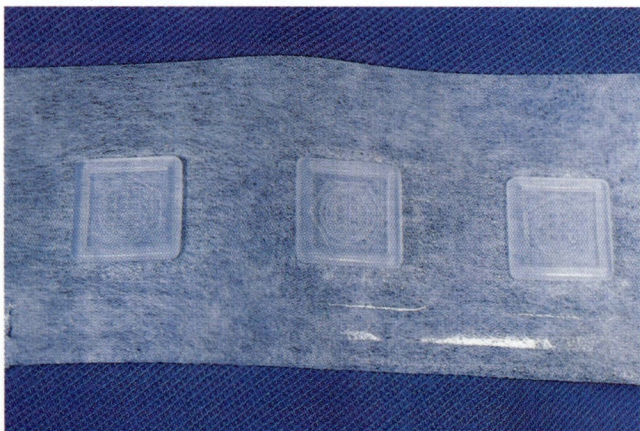

FIGURE 2–5 • These patch testing chambers, with their large wells, provide optimal exposure of the skin to the cosmetic or skin care product, allowing a reliable patch test to be performed.

TABLE 2-10 Evaluation of Patch Test Reactions

• • • • • •

Reaction Rating	Characteristics
+	Doubtful reaction, possibly caused by a weak irritant effect; only weak erythema without infiltration
+	Weak reaction; erythema with infiltration and, possibly, papules
++	Strong reaction; erythema, infiltration, papules, vesicles
+++	Extreme reaction; erythema, infiltration, papules, confluent vesicles or bullae
−	Negative reaction
IR	Irritant reaction
NT	Not patch tested

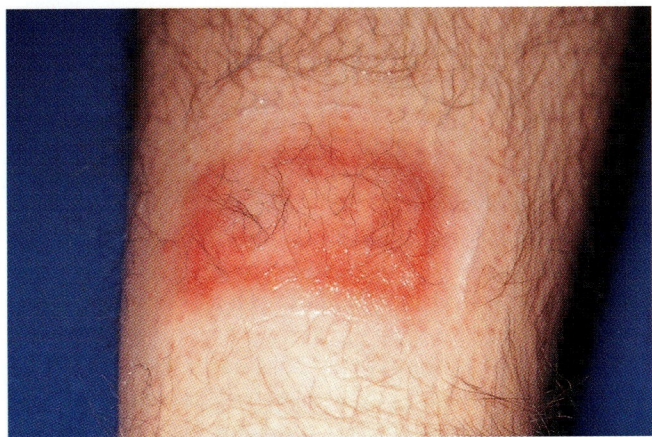

FIGURE 2–7 • This closed patch test was performed using an adhesive-containing cover. The patient experienced an allergic reaction to the adhesive, not the occluded skin care product, thereby confounding diagnosis.

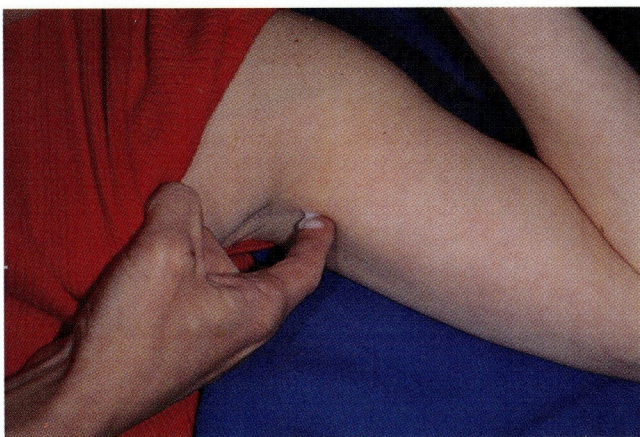

FIGURE 2–9 • Provocative use testing may be performed in an area just below the axilla.

least likely to be the source of allergic contact dermatitis.

5. Open Patch Testing Techniques

For cosmetic and skin care products that are irritants, open patch testing is the preferred technique. Open patch testing involves application of the product to the skin on the inner aspect of the arm above the elbow twice daily for 2 days or more, without occlusion or washing of the test site (Fig. 2–8). The site is then evaluated using the rating method explained in Table 2–10. This is the preferred testing technique for

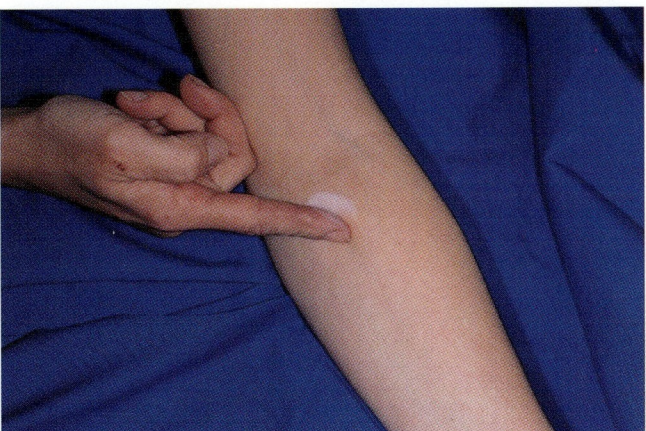

FIGURE 2–8 • The superior upper inner elbow is a suitable site for open patch testing of cosmetics and skin care products.

hair sprays and fixatives. It should be remembered, however, that false-negative results may occur with this method.

6. Provocative Use Testing Techniques

Provocative use testing is the author's favorite method of testing cosmetic and skin care products because it most closely simulates the skin site and the manner in which the product is usually applied. This method also minimizes the irritation that can arise from application of tape and patch testing chambers. Provocative use testing can be combined with patch testing, if desired. It is valuable in confirming positive reactions to cosmetic products containing ingredients that were previously found, by standard patch testing, to be sources of allergic contact dermatitis.

As originally described, provocative use testing involves twice-daily application of a product to a 3-cm patch of skin below the antecubital fossae for 1 week (Fig. 2–9). This form of skin testing is useful for leave-on skin care products, such as hand creams or body moisturizers, that are not intended to be used on the face. A modification of this test for facial cosmetics and eye cosmetics involves application of the product to the skin lateral to the eye twice daily for 1 week (Fig. 2–10). Because the skin lateral to the eye is one of the most reactive areas of the body, this is an excellent test site for leave-on facial cosmetics. Reactions to these products are evaluated in a similar manner to that described in Table 2–10.

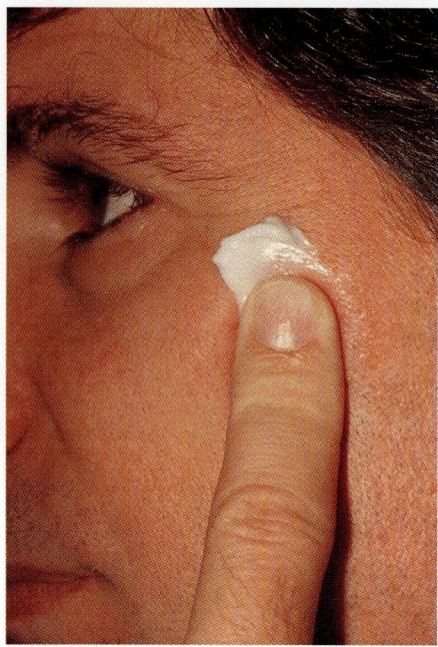

FIGURE 2–10 • A site lateral to the eye is the author's choice for provocative use testing. The skin in this location is highly reactive, increasing the chances that even low-grade irritants and allergens will be identified.

wheal-and-flare response to a topically applied chemical. The spectrum of clinical presentation ranges from itching and burning to generalized urticaria to anaphylaxis.

Nonimmunologic contact urticaria is induced by direct contactant release of histamine; thus, passive transfer is not possible. This condition is more commonly encountered than its counterpart, immunologic contact urticaria. In the latter, immunologic mechanisms are involved in histamine release; thus, the phenomenon can only be elicited in sensitized individuals, and passive transfer is possible. However, there are some chemicals that produce contact urticaria secondary to unknown mechanisms. Table 2–11 lists the nonimmunologic and immunologic causes of contact urticaria to substances encountered in cosmetics.[19] Testing for contact urticaria should be conducted under carefully controlled conditions and in an area that is convenient to resuscitation facilities, as anaphylaxis secondary to contact with topically applied chemicals has occurred in some sensitized individuals.

7. Contact Urticaria Testing

Contact urticaria is an extremely rare reaction to cosmetics and skin care products; yet it is worthy of brief mention. Contact urticaria may be an immunologic or nonimmunologic reaction to cosmetics and skin care products. It is characterized by the development of a

8. Cutaneous Stinging

Stinging is a fairly common reaction to the application of cosmetics and skin care products. This noxious stimuli can occur any time a product is applied to damaged skin with a defective barrier. However, some individuals experience a stinging or burning sensation within several minutes after applying a facial product, and the sensation intensifies over 5 to 10 minutes and

TABLE 2–11 Substances in Cosmetics That Can Cause Contact Urticaria

Nonimmunologic Contact Urticaria	Immunologic Contact Urticaria	Uncertain
Acetic acid	Acrylic monomer	Ammonium persulfate
Alcohols	Alcohols	Paraphenylenediamine
Balsam of Peru	Ammonia	
Benzoic acid	Benzoic acid	
Cinnamic acid	Benzophenone	
Cinnamic aldehyde	Diethyltoluamide	
Formaldehyde	Formaldehyde	
Sodium benzoate	Henna	
Sorbic acid	Menthol	
	Parabens	
	Polyethylene glycol	
	Polysorbate 60	
	Salicylic acid	
	Sodium sulfide	

TABLE 2–12 Substances in Cosmetics and Skin Care Products That May Induce Stinging

Slight Stinging	Moderate Stinging	Severe Stinging
Salicylic acid	Sodium carbonate	Sodium hydroxide
Phosphoric acid	Trisodium phosphate	2-Ethoxyethyl p-methoxy-cinnamate
	Propylene glycol	
	Propylene carbonate	
	Propylene glycol diacetate	
	Dimethyl phthalate	
	Benzoyl peroxide	

Adapted from Frosch PJ, Kligman AM. A method for appraising the stinging capacity of topically applied substances. J Soc Cosmet Chem 28:197–209, 1977.

resolves after 15 minutes. These patients, known as "stingers," do not tolerate certain cosmetic and skin care products, even though patch testing for allergic contact dermatitis yields negative results and no evidence of irritant contact dermatitis is present. Substances sometimes found in cosmetics that can induce stinging are listed in Table 2–12.[20] Of the ingredients listed, propylene glycol is the most common cause of cutaneous stinging in cosmetics and skin care products.

9. Photoreactions

Light-induced reactions to cosmetics and skin care products, known as phototoxic and photoallergic dermatitides, are extraordinarily rare with present-day formulations. Phototoxic reactions are based on nonimmunologic mechanisms and usually appear as a sunburn, which may be followed by hyperpigmentation and desquamation. The molecules that produce phototoxicity are generally of low molecular weight and possess highly resonant structures that readily absorb mainly ultraviolet (UVA) radiation.[21] Photoallergic dermatitis, on the other hand, is less common, is immunologically mediated, generally requires repeat exposure, and can be passively transferred. It is characterized by erythema, edema, and vesiculation. Photoallergens are generally low-molecular-weight, lipid-soluble substances that possess highly resonant structures that absorb energy over a wide range of wavelenghts, but again predominantly UVA.[22] The light energy photochemically converts the photosensitizer into its active form (Fig. 2–11).[23] Less ultraviolet radiation energy is required to elicit a photoallergic reaction compared to a phototoxic reaction.[24] Differentiating between the two may be difficult, however, especially if a severe phototoxic reaction results in vesiculation. Substances found in cosmetics and skin care products that may cause photoallergic reactions are listed in Table 2–13.[25]

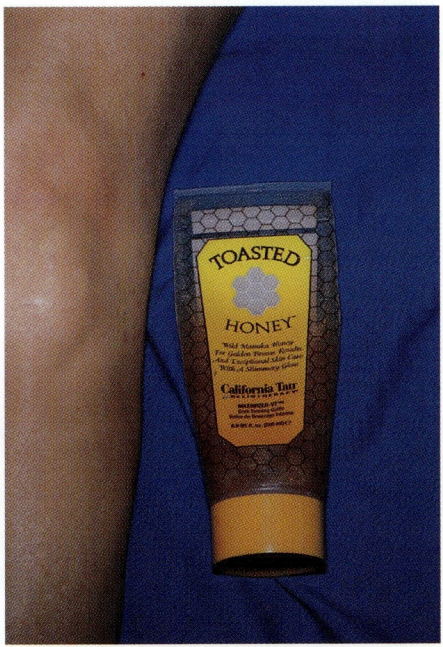

FIGURE 2–11 • This salon-dispensed tanning accelerator produced an allergic reaction on the knee following UVA radiation exposure.

TABLE 2–13 Substances in Cosmetics and Skin Care Products That May Induce Photoallergic Reactions

Ingredient	Function	Photopatch Testing Concentration (%) Formulated in Petrolatum
Methylcoumarin	Fragrance	5
Musk ambrette	Fragrance	5
PABA esters	Sunscreen	10

PABA, para-aminobenzoic acid.

Photopatch testing may be performed when a photosensitivity evaluation is required. Two patch tests are placed with the suspected chemical, one on a site to be irradiated and the other on a protected site. The patch tests are left in place on the skin for 48 hours.[26] One of the sites is subjected to ultraviolet radiation of the wavelength desired, and the test results are read within 24 to 48 hours. This process may be repeated if desired. A phototoxic reaction produces erythema and usually arises within 6 hours. By contrast, photoallergic reaction is characterized by erythema, papules, and vesicles. If only the irradiated site is positive, a diagnosis of photoallergy can be made. If both the irradiated and the protected sites are positive, a diagnosis of allergic contact dermatitis can be made. If the irradiated site shows greater positivity than the protected site, then a diagnosis of allergic contact dermatitis and photoallergy can be established.

REFERENCES

1. Bettley FR. The influence of soap on the permeability of the epidermis. Br J Dermatol 74:448–454, 1961.
2. Wilhelm KP. Effects of surfactants on skin hydration. Curr Probl Dermatol 22:72–79, 1995.
3. Pierard GE, Arrese JE, Rodriguez C, et al. Effects of softened and unsoftened fabrics on sensitive skin. Contact Dermatitis 30:286–291, 1994.
4. Amin S, Maibach HI. Cosmetic intolerance syndrome: Pathophysiology and management. Cosmet Dermatol 9(1):34–42, 1996.
5. Maibach HI, Engasser PG. Dermatitis due to cosmetics. In Fisher AA (ed.). Contact Dermatitis, 3rd ed. Philadelphia: Lea & Febiger, 1986, pp. 368–393.
6. Jackson EM. Irritation and sensitization. In Waggoner WC (ed.). Clinical Safety and Efficacy Testing of Cosmetics. New York: Marcel Dekker, 1990, pp. 23–42.
7. Baer RL. The mechanism of allergic contact hypersensitivity. In Fisher AA (ed.). Contact Dermatitis, 3rd ed. Philadelphia: Lea & Febiger, 1986, pp. 1–8.
8. Rothengorg HW, Hjorth N. Allergy to perfumes from toilet soaps and detergents in patients with dermatitis. Arch Dermatol 97:417–421, 1961.
9. Maibach HI. Fragrance hypersensitivity, Part I. Cosmet Toiletr 106:25–26, 1991.
10. Maibach HI. Fragrance hypersensitivity, Part II. Cosmet Toiletr 106:35–36, 1991.
11. Larsen WG, Maibach HI. Fragrance contact allergy. Semin Dermatol 1:85–90, 1982.
12. Eiermann HJ, Larsen WG, Maibach HI, Taylor JS. Prospective study of cosmetic reactions; 1977–1980. J Am Acad Dermatol 6:909–917, 1982.
13. Wells FV, Lubowe II. Cosmetics and the Skin. New York: Reinhold Publishing, 1964, pp. 370–374.
14. Larsen WG. Perfume dermatitis. J Am Acad Dermatol 12:1–9, 1985.
15. Larsen WG. Perfume dermatitis: A study of 20 patients. Arch Dermatol 113:623–626, 1977.
16. Fisher AA. Patch testing with perfume ingredients. Contact Dermatitis 1:166–168, 1975.
17. Goldner R. Clinical tests. In Jackson EM, Goldner R (eds.). Irritant Contact Dermatitis. New York: Marcel Dekker, 1990, pp. 201–218.
18. Fowler JF. Reading patch tests: Some pitfalls of patch testing. Am J Contact Dermatitis 5:170–172, 1994.
19. Fisher AA. Contact Dermatitis, 3rd ed. Philadelphia: Lea & Febiger, 1986, pp. 686–709.
20. Frosch PJ, Kligman AM. A method for appraising the stinging capacity of topically applied substances. J Soc Cosmet Chem 28:197–209, 1977.
21. Billhimer WL. Phototoxicity and photoallergy. In Waggoner WC (ed.). Clinical Safety and Efficacy Testing of Cosmetics. New York: Marcel Dekker, 1990, pp. 43–74.
22. Elmets CA. Drug-induced photoallergy. Dermatol Clin 4:231–241, 1986.
23. Stephens RJ, Bergstresser PR. Fundamental concepts in photoimmunology and photoallergy. In Jackson EM (ed.). Photobiology of the Skin and Eye. New York: Marcel Dekker, 1986, pp. 41–66.
24. Epstein JH. Phototoxicity and photoallergy in man. J Am Acad Dermatol 8:141–147, 1983.
25. DeLeo VA, Harber LC. Contact photodermatitis. In Fisher AA (ed.). Contact Dermatitis, 3rd ed. Philadelphia: Lea & Febiger, 1986, pp. 454–469.
26. DeLeo VA. Photocontact dermatitis. In DeLeo VA (ed.). Photosensitivity. New York: Igaku-Shoin, 1992, pp. 84–99.

3

Cosmetic Safety Testing

Cosmetic safety testing is an extraordinarily important process designed to ensure the stability and suitability of cosmetic and skin care formulations for human skin (Fig. 3–1). Initially, ingredient selection is of primary importance and should follow the guidelines listed in Table 3–1. Safe formulations must avoid inducing both visible and invisible manifestations of skin disease.[1] This means that objective findings, such as erythema, xerosis, edema, and vesiculation, must be avoided, as must such subjective symptoms as skin tightness, itching, stinging, and burning. Furthermore, the skin must not undergo physiologic changes, such as dehydration, barrier damage, lipid alterations, decreased corneocyte adhesion, protein denaturation, swelling of the stratum corneum, removal or denaturation of water-soluble constituents, enzyme denaturation, or cytokine or mediator release.

Numerous methods have been developed to predict the safety of both individual ingredients and final formulations by assessing the potential activity of such substances to induce irritation or sensitization in humans. Most predictive procedures are done in vitro or on animals, although in some laboratories, tests are performed in humans. For years, predictive tests, properly designed, have been very effective in detecting substances or products likely to be harmful to humans. These tests have been instrumental in enabling the rejection of harmful products, as well as in ensuring appropriate warning labels if the product has weak activity for a particular tissue (e.g., the eyes) (Fig. 3–2). It should be understood that, despite all care in examination of products, such is the diversity of human susceptibility that a few persons will show adverse reactions if sufficient numbers are exposed to the products. Nevertheless, predictive tests for safety in use have ensured that products are harmless to the very great majority. An overall approach to cosmetic safety assessment is presented in Table 3–2.

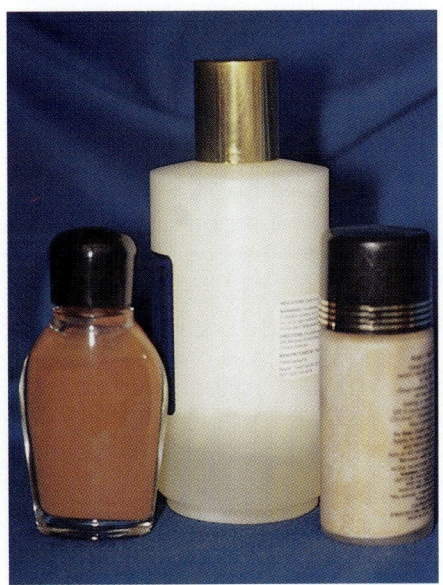

FIGURE 3–1 • These three bottles demonstrate product appearance changes, which are indicative of underlying stability problems. Old cosmetic products, which have degraded in the bottle, are a source of dermatologic difficulty. Problems can be related to breakdown of the emulsifier or preservative.

TABLE 3–1 Ingredient Selection for Safe Skin Products

· · · · · ·

1. Common allergens and irritants must be eliminated from the formulation or, if this is not possible, reduced in concentration.

2. High-quality, pure materials without contaminants should be selected. If it is impossible to eliminate highly allergenic contaminants, a suitable binding agent should be added. For example, nickel contamination can be minimized through the use of a sequestering agent, such as ethylenediamine triacetate.[2]

3. Autoxidation products, which may be responsible for hypersensitivity reactions, should be avoided through the use of suitable antioxidants, such as alpha-tocopherol, butylhydroxyanisole (BHA), or butylhydroxytoluene (BHT).[3,4]

4. Volatile vehicles and substances producing cutaneous stimulation (menthol) should be eliminated or reduced.

5. Solvents that promote skin penetration (propylene glycol, ethanol) should be avoided. If necessary, higher glycols (polyethylene glycols) that do not penetrate the stratum corneum and that may form hydrogen bonds with penetrants should be selected.

6. Surfactants, used either for cleansing purposes or as emulsifiers, should be selected carefully. Anionic surfactants (sodium lauryl sulfate) are strong irritants owing to their ability to penetrate the stratum corneum, bind to skin proteins, induce stratum corneum swelling, and enhance penetration of other substances (antimicrobials).[5] Cationic surfactants are intermediate in their penetration, whereas skin penetration is least with nonionic surfactants.[6] However, nonionic surfactants can change the biosynthetic rate, composition, and content of epidermal phospholipids.[7]

7. Preservatives with low sensitizing potential (parabens) should be selected over those with a higher sensitizing potential (formaldehyde and formaldehyde releasers).[8,9]

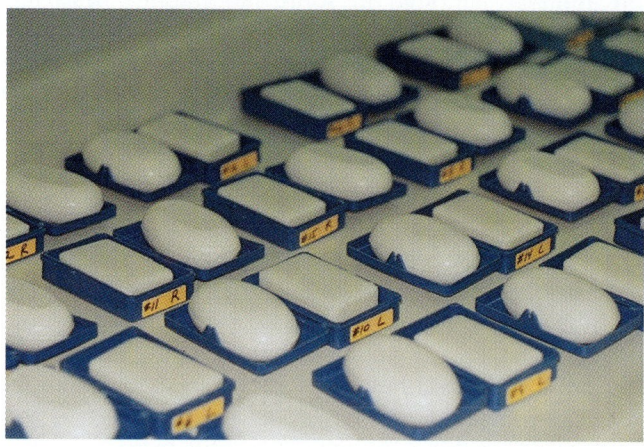

FIGURE 3–2 · Soap must be tested for mildness in large human clinical trials in order to ensure skin compatibility prior to marketing of the final formulation.

TABLE 3–2 Approach for Formulating Safe Skin Products

· · · · · ·

1. Conduct a review of ingredients to minimize irritants and sensitizers.

2. Eliminate unnecessary ingredients.

3. Evaluate the stability of ingredients as formulated.

4. Utilize in vitro methods to predict the final formulations likelihood of causing skin and eye irritation.

5. Utilize in vivo methods to predict the final formulations likelihood of producing skin irritation and sensitization.

6. Utilize sensitive skin panels to confirm results of in vitro and in vivo testing.

7. Conduct pre-market, monitored, large scale testing of consumers.

8. Monitor post-market consumer responses and reports of adverse reactions.

REFERENCES

1. Maes D, Marenus K, Smith WP. Invisible irritation: A new look at product safety. Cosmet Toiletr 105:43–50, 1990.

2. Dooms-Goossens A. Reducing sensitizing potential by pharmaceutical and cosmetic design. J Am Acad Dermatol 10:547–553, 1984.

3. Clark EW, Kitchen GF. Autoxidation and its inhibition in anhydrous lanolin. J Pharm Pharmacol 13:172–183, 1961.

4. Clark EW, Blondeel A, Cronin E, et al. Lanolin of reduced sensitizing potential. Contact Dermatitis 7:80–83, 1981.

5. Rieger M. Human epidermis responses to sodium lauryl sulfate exposure. Cosmet Toiletr 109:65–74, 1994.

6. Bettley FR. The influence of detergents and surfactants on epidermal permeability. Br J Dermatol 77:98–100, 1965.

7. Barry BW. Dermatological Formulations. New York: Marcel Dekker, 1983, pp. 170–172.

8. Fransway AF, Schmitz NA. The problem of preservation in the 1990s: Part II. formaldehyde and formaldehyde-releasing biocides. Am J Contact Dermatitis 2(2):78–88, 1991.

9. Steinberg DC. Cosmetic preservation: Current international trends. Cosmet Toiletr 107:77–82, 1992.

4

Cosmetic Performance Testing

Skin variability frequently complicates the dermatologist's ability to prescribe treatment for a dermatosis, but it also complicates cosmetics and skin care product development.[1] This reality has resulted in the development of a variety of in vitro and in vivo testing protocols designed to assess product performance, and, indirectly, to assess product safety. These methods are used to determine how a finished formulation performs on the skin in terms of physiologic benefits. This testing must also be performed to substantiate marketing claims.

1. In Vitro Techniques

Analysis of cosmetic and skin care product performance should reproducibly and accurately assess small cutaneous changes and preclinical disease, without altering the underlying skin condition.[2] This analytical challenge has led to great interest in the development of noninvasive mechanistic skin assessment. The following section pictorially demonstrates a few of the bioengineering methods of assessing cosmetics and skin care product performance.[3]

a. PROFILOMETRY

Profilometry is a method of assessing changes in skin surface contour, such as wrinkling and scarring.[4] It involves analysis of silicone rubber replicas of the skin surface. These replicas serve as negatives from which are cast plastic positives mirroring the three-dimensional topography of the skin in a selected area (Fig. 4–1). For example, the upper cheek is typically used as the replica site for the assessment of decreased wrinkling following application of a moisturizing treatment cream. These plastic positives are evaluated with the aid of a computerized stylus or laser, producing

a tour tracing of the skin surface. Dramatic two- or three-dimensional topograms can be created for the evaluation of fine lines and wrinkling of the skin (Fig. 4–2). Unfortunately, this method can be inaccurate, as application of silicone rubber to the skin decreases transepidermal water loss and skin wrinkling while flattening the desquamating skin scale.[4]

b. SQUAMETRY

Another technique, known as squametry, is used to assess the number of desquamating corneocytes.[5] Squametry involves analysis of skin squames harvested by pressing a round sticky tape against the skin (D-Square, Cu-Derm, Dallas, Texas). The outermost, loosely adherent skin scale is removed on the tape, which is attached to a black background. The tape provides a specimen that retains the topographic relationships of the skin surface and the pattern of desquamation. Image processing is then used to evaluate the scaliness of the skin (Fig. 4–3).[5] This technique is valuable for documenting claims regarding skin scaliness.

c. ELASTICITY

The skin can be modeled and studied as an elastic material, and its ability to withstand forces of stress and strain can be studied. This is an indirect manner or assessing the moisturization of the skin, as well-moisturized skin is more elastic than dry skin. Reduced elastic properties are seen in aged skin. This technique uses a torsion machine, known as a Twistometer (L'Oreal, Paris, France) (Fig. 4–4). A computer is used to assess the ability of the skin to recover its original state, generating stress-strain curves. This noninvasive technique can substantiate claims of skin

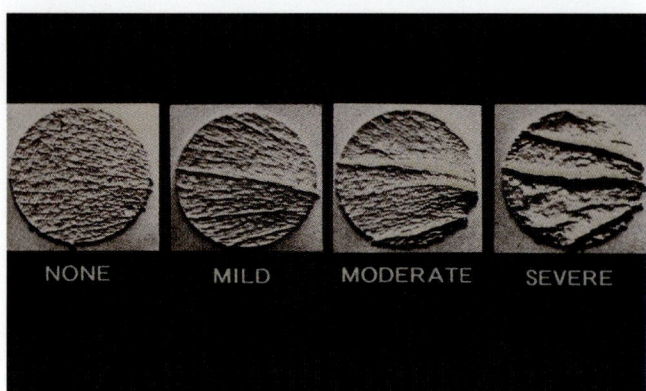

FIGURE 4–1 • These replicas demonstrate progressive photoaging that ranges from mild to moderate to severe. (Photo courtesy of Gary Grove, Ph. D.)

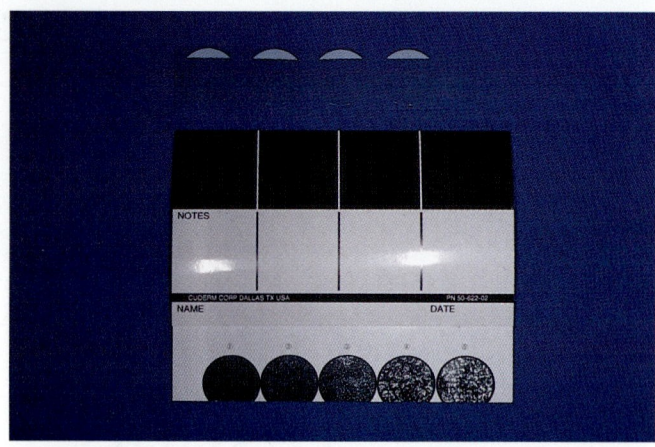

FIGURE 4–3 • The white material on the sticky D-Squame tape represents desquamating corneocytes removed from the skin surface by the adhesive. The more opaque the tape appears on the black background, the greater the amount of retained scale on the skin surface.

moisturization through improved elasticity.[6] Inaccurate data may be obtained, however, because repeated stretching of the skin improves extensibility regardless of product application.

d. IMPEDANCE (CONDUCTANCE)

The skin can be assessed in terms of its mechanical properties, such as elasticity, but it also can be evaluated for its electrical properties, such as impedance or conductance. The impedance of the skin is the total electric resistance of the skin to an alternating current. This noninvasive technique involves the use of a dry electrode, which consists of two concentric brass cylinders separated by a phenolic insulator operating at 3.5M Hz (Skicon, IBS Ltd., Hamamatsu, Japan).[7] The electrode is placed in contact with the skin (Fig. 4–5). Impedance measurements have been found to correlate directly with skin hydration.[8] This technique

can evaluate the efficacy and the duration of effect of moisturizers.[9]

e. EVAPORIMETRY

Evaporimetry is a noninvasive technique assessing cutaneous transepidermal water loss, as opposed to skin water content.[10] This method utilizes a computer attached to a handpiece containing two probes designed to measure changes in water vapor (Evaporimeter, ServoMed, Stockholm, Sweden) (Fig. 4–6). Transepidermal water loss is increased in skin having a damaged stratum corneum barrier. Evaporimetry can be used to assess barrier dysfunction and recovery following application of an ingredient or finished product.[10] It can also measure skin porosity, indirectly predicting the rate of loss of topically applied sub-

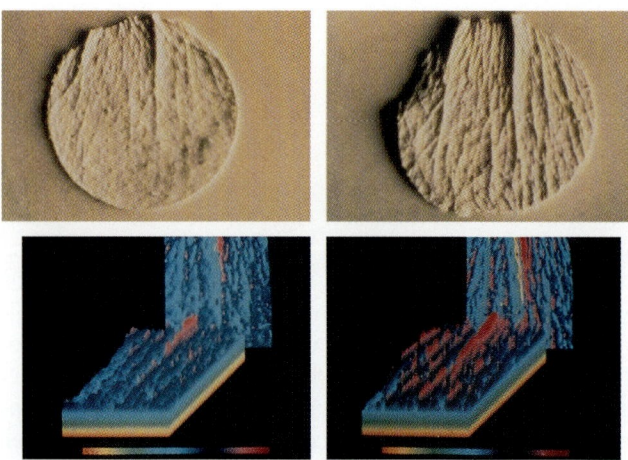

FIGURE 4–2 • Three-dimensional topograms can be created from the replicas via computer imaging techniques. (Photo courtesy of Gary Grove, Ph. D.)

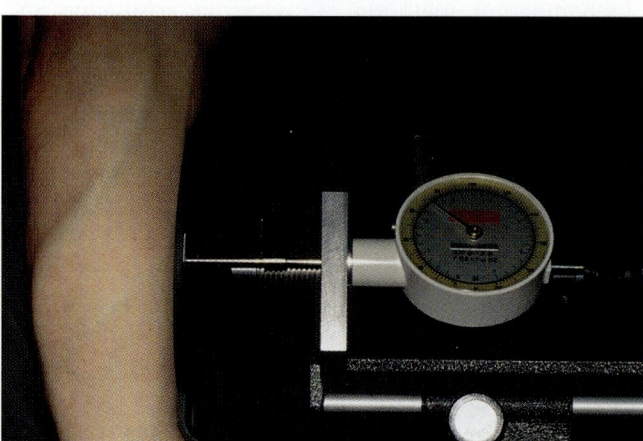

FIGURE 4–4 • This meter measures the amount of force required to twist the skin, an indirect assessment of skin moisturization.

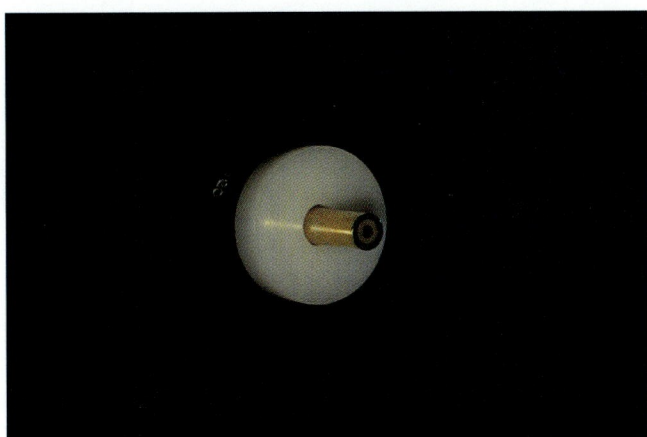

FIGURE 4–5 • Skin impedance is measured using a concentric brass probe. The data obtained indirectly correlates with skin hydration.

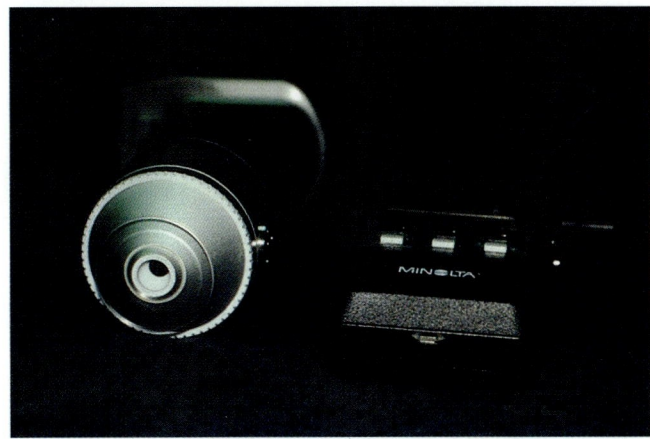

FIGURE 4–7 • This camera measures skin color and can be used to assess pigmentation or erythema.

stances from the skin surface.[11] This technique must be used under careful subject/environmental control, as perspiration can yield incorrect readings of transepidermal water loss.

It is critical to recognize that noninvasive assessment data can be manipulated easily. For example, the application of most moisturizers will result in an immediate and marked reduction in transepidermal water loss. However, this benefit may be lost within 5 minutes if the product is not carefully formulated. Assessments of moisturizer function, then, should be performed at least 6 hours after product application.[12] Furthermore, a product may demonstrate a 25% decrease in transepidermal water loss, but this may not translate into clinical efficacy.

f. COLORIMETRY

An assessment of skin color can be obtained through a technique known as colorimetry (Chromameter,

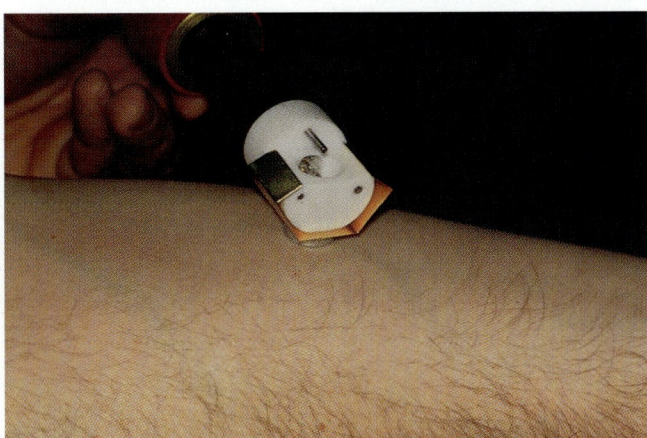

FIGURE 4–6 • This probe measures transepidermal water loss from the skin surface, an indication of the state of the stratum corneum barrier.

Minolta, Osaka, Japan) (Fig. 4–7).[13,14] This is a compact, tri-stimulus, color analyzer that measures reflected object color. It can be used to evaluate color changes in the skin, such as those resulting from sunburn, erythema due to irritation, basic skin color, or the effect of pigmenting or depigmenting agents. This technique is useful when substantiating claims of improved skin color or decreased sallowness.

2. In Vivo Techniques

Even though sophisticated, noninvasive methods of cutaneous evaluation sound appealing, there is no substitute for the opinion of an unbiased dermatologist-observer when evaluating cosmetic and skin care product effectiveness. Computers cannot yet accurately synthesize all the tactile and visual information that can be obtained by human evaluation. Furthermore, slight changes that are apparent with image processing techniques may not significantly alter clinical skin appearance. Thus, noninvasive techniques are another tool for assessing product performance, but should be used in combination with in vivo testing.[15]

This section discusses methods used for clinical assessment of the performance of a cosmetic or skin care product in a human population, utilizing a trained observer. Methods discussed include regression analysis and in vivo image analysis.

a. REGRESSION ANALYSIS

Regression analysis, a method developed by A. M. Kligman,[18] evaluates cosmetic and skin care product efficacy under clinical conditions. Subjects are selected and treated with the test product(s) at a prede-

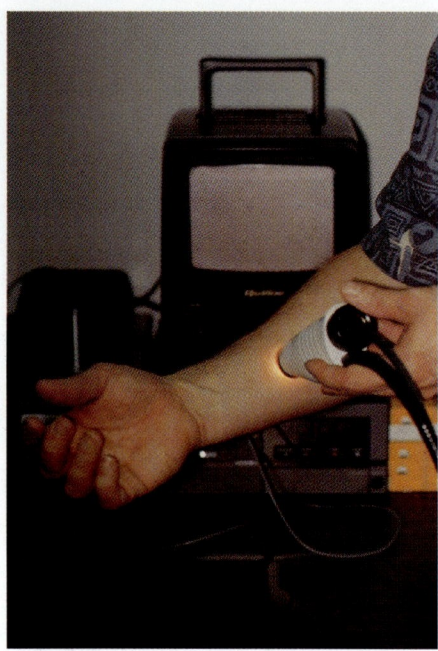

FIGURE 4–8 • Video microscopes allow real-time evaluation of the effect of cosmetics and skin care products on the stratum corneum.

termined test site for 2 weeks. The test site is then evaluated by an objective observer on days 7 and 14. If improvement is noted, product application is discontinued and the test site is evaluated daily for 2 weeks, or until the baseline pathology has reappeared.[16] This method is particularly valuable for efficacy assessment, as product performance may be excellent immediately following application, but true effectiveness can only be assessed with the passage of time.

b. IMAGE ANALYSIS

In vivo image analysis is accomplished by analyzing images produced by a video microscope (Fig. 4–8). This technique is used to evaluate skin surface features.[17] Care must be taken to standardize lighting and imaging angles to ensure accurate data for analysis, as differing exposures can lead to erroneous image processing and faulty data. It should also be remembered that in vivo image analysis is only as good as the video image obtained.

REFERENCES

1. Jackson EM. Hypoallergenic claims. Am J Contact Dermatitis 4(2):108–110, 1993.
2. Green BG. Measuring the chemosensory irritability of the skin. First International Symposium on Cosmetic Efficacy, New York, 1996.
3. Grove GL. Noninvasive methods for assessing moisturizers. In Waggoner WC (ed.). Clinical Safety and Efficacy Testing of Cosmetics. New York: Marcel Dekker, 1990, pp. 121–148.
4. Grove GL, Grove MJ. Objective methods for assessing skin surface topography noninvasively. In Leveque JL (ed.). Cutaneous Investigation in Health and Disease. New York: Marcel Dekker, 1988, pp. 1–32.
5. Grove GL. Dermatological applications of the Magiscan image analysing computer. In Marks R, Payne PA (eds.). Bioengineering and the Skin. Lancaster, England: MTP Press, 1981, pp. 173–182.
6. de Rigal J, Leveque JL. In vivo measurements of the stratum corneum elasticity. Bioeng Skin 1:13–23, 1985.
7. Tagami H. Electrical measurement of the water content of the skin surface. Cosmet Toiletr 97:39–47, 1982.
8. Archer WI, Kohli R, Roberts JMC, Spencer TS. Skin impedance measurement. In Rietschel RL, Spencer TS (eds.). Methods for Cutaneous Investigation. New York: Marcel Dekker, 1990, pp. 121–142.
9. Grove GL. The effect of moisturizers on skin surface hydration as measured in vivo by electrical conductivity. Curr Therap Res 50: 712–719, 1991.
10. Idson B. In vivo measurement of transdermal water loss. J Soc Cosmet Chem 29:573–580, 1976.
11. Rietschel RL, Spencer TS. Correlation between mosquito repellent protection time and insensible water loss from the skin. J Invest Dermatol 65:385–387, 1975.
12. Lazar AP, Lazar P. Dry skin, water, and lubrication. Dermatol Clin 9:45–51, 1991.
13. Babulak SW, Rhein LD, Scala DD, et al. Quantification of erythema in a soap chamber test using the Minolta Chroma (Reflectance) Meter. J Soc Cosmet Chem 37:475–479, 1986.
14. Pierard GE, Nikkels AF. Rating sensitive skin by colorimetry of the skin and of D-squame collections. International Symposium on Irritant Contact Dermatitis, Groningen, Holland, October 1991.
15. Grove GL. Design of studies to measure skin care product performance. Bioeng Skin 3:359–373, 1987.
16. Kligman AM. Regression method for assessing the efficacy of moisturizers. Cosmet Toiletr 93:27–35, 1978.
17. Prall JK, Theiler RF, Bowser PA, Walsh M. The effect of cosmetic products in alleviating a range of skin dryness conditions as determined by clinical and instrumental techniques. Int J Cosmet Sci 8:159–174, 1986.

5

Effects of Cosmetics on the Skin

Cosmetics and skin care products have a variety of effects on the skin. Some of the adverse reactions, such as allergic contact dermatitis, irritancy, contact urticaria, and photoreactions have already been discussed; however, there are other skin reactions of equal concern to the dermatologist. These include comedogenicity, acnegenicity, follicular migration, and sensitive skin.

1. Comedogenicity

Comedogenicity is a major issue in cosmetic and skin care product marketing. Facial foundations frequently bear the label "noncomedogenic," giving the consumer the impression that the product does not cause acne. As most dermatologists know, noncomedogenic simply means that the product does not cause open and closed comedones (Fig. 5–1). A traditional list of comedogenic ingredients found in cosmetics and skin care products in listed in Table 5–1. However, this list is rarely helpful, as it is practically impossible to find formulations that possess none of these ingredients. The list contains some of the most effective emollients (octyl stearate, isocetyl stearate), detergents (sodium lauryl sulfate), occlusive moisturizers (mineral oil, petrolatum, sesame oil, cocoa butter), and emulsifiers found in the cosmetic industry.[1] A product line that avoided all of these substances would exhibit low performance and low cosmetic acceptability.

Unfortunately, the issue of comedogenicity is more complex than a simple ingredient list. Products that do not contain comedogenic substances from this list are not necessarily noncomedogenic. Conversely, products that contain comedogenic substances are not necessarily comedogenic. Comedogenicity can only be evaluated in light of the patient's susceptibility to the formation of comedonal plugs and the concentration of the comedogen in the final formulation.[2,3] However, the formation of comedones following product use is extraordinarily rare compared with the incidence of inflammatory papules and pustules, a condition known as acnegenicity.

2. Acnegenicity

Acnegenicity is a completely separate issue from comedogenicity. Substances that are comedogenic cause open and/or closed comedones (blackheads and whiteheads), whereas substances that are acnegenic cause papules and pustules. Comedogenicity is caused by follicular plugging, whereas acnegenicity is due to follicular irritation.[4] Thus, substances that are comedogenic are not necessarily acnegenic, and the reverse is also true.

Acnegenicity is a complex interaction between the follicular ostia and the cosmetic or skin care product.

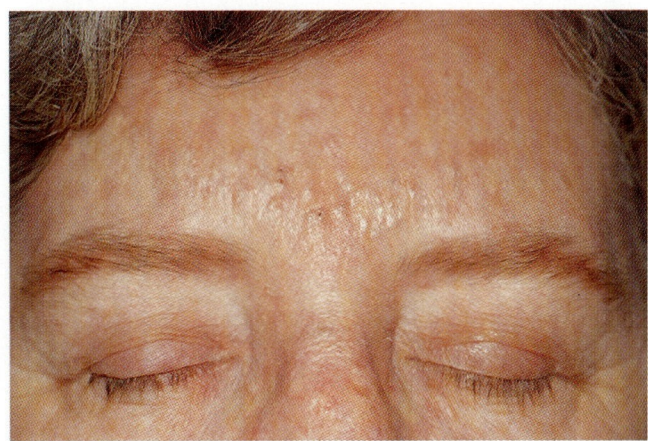

FIGURE 5–1 • The comedones on this patient's forehead may be attributable to the use of vegetable oil as a bedtime moisturizer.

TABLE 5–1 Standard List of Possible Comedogenic Substances

• • • • • •

Butyl stearate	Myristyl ether propionate
Cocoa butter	Myristyl lactate
Corn oil	Myristyl myristate
D&C red dyes	Octyl palmitate
Decyl oleate	Octyl stearate
Isopropyl isostearate	Oleic acid
Isopropyl myristate	Oleyl alcohol
Isostearyl neopentanate	Olive oil
Isopropyl palmitate	Peanut oil
Isocetyl stearate	Propylene glycol stearate
Lanolin, acetylated	Petrolatum
Linseed oil	Safflower oil
Laureth-4	Sesame oil
Mineral oil	Sodium lauryl sulfate
Methyl oleate	Stearic acid

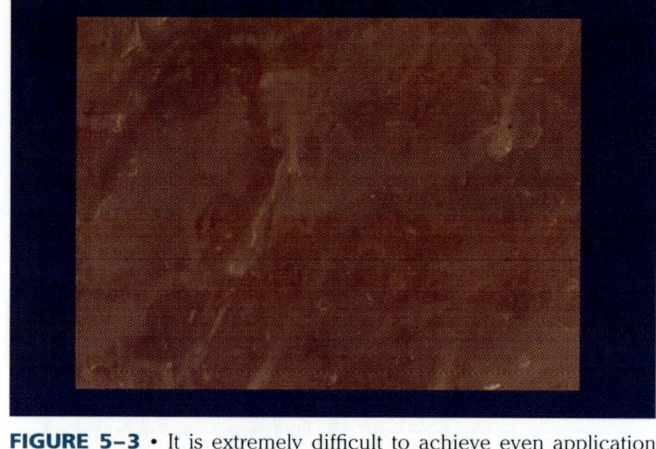

FIGURE 5–3 • It is extremely difficult to achieve even application of sunscreen film for optimal ultraviolet protection.

It is, in actuality, a variant of irritant contact dermatitis, with a more pronounced follicular component (Fig. 5–2). It arises quickly after application of the offending product, whereas formation of comedones may take weeks to develop. Acnegenicity is a more individualized response to topical products and one that has extraordinary variability. It is impossible to develop a list of acnegenic substances. Cosmetics that are acnegenic in one patient are not necessarily acnegenic in another patient. Acnegenicity is, in large part, influenced by the interaction of cosmetics and the skin.

3. Film Formation

The skin is an extremely complex surface full of irregularities created by eccrine ostia, follicular ostia, benign cutaneous tumors, desquamating corneoctyes, etc. The cutaneous effect of many cosmetics and skin

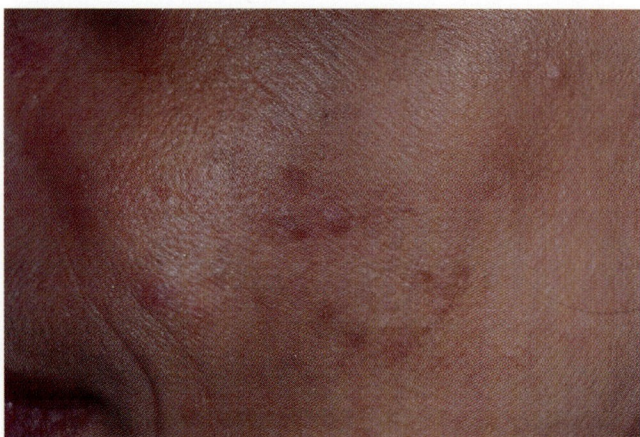

FIGURE 5–2 • An acneiform eruption developed on the cheeks of this patient following the use of a new facial foundation.

care products is determined by how the product interacts with the topography of the skin surface. For example, the performance of a sunscreen is dependent on even, uniform application. Figure 5–3 shows the appearance of a sunscreen film on the skin surface after an attempt to apply the product liberally, with great care taken to spreading the lotion evenly on the skin surface. Notice the areas where the film is thinner, providing less sun protection. This video microscopic image (X400) demonstrates, in part, why sunscreens cannot completely protect the skin against UVB and UVA radiation.

4. Product Movement

Not only is it difficult to achieve an even application of products on the skin surface, but it is even more challenging to prevent migration of the formulation over the skin surface. Figures 5–4 and 5–5 demonstrate video microscopic images (X400) of a facial foundation on the cheek after 4 hours of wear in a patient with combination skin. Notice the large clumps of facial foundation around the follicular ostia and on the hair shafts.

What is the significance of these observations? First, it is important that substances applied to the skin are safe for entry into the body. It is likely that small amounts of facial foundation and other cosmetics are absorbed into the viable epidermis and dermis through the appendageal route. Second, this migration toward the follicular ostia may explain the perifollicular distribution of reactions to cosmetics. The acneiform eruption observed in some patients following the use of certain facial foundations is probably not acne, but rather a follicular irritant contact dermatitis.

The ingredient in facial foundations that is responsible for perifollicular irritant contact dermatitis is diffi-

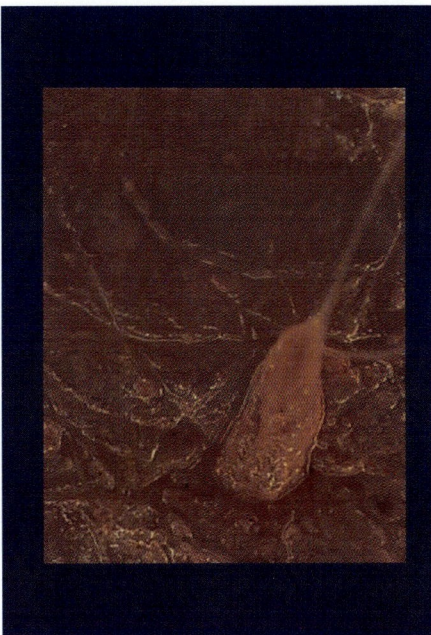

FIGURE 5–4 • Migration of facial foundation toward the follicular ostia occurs over time, increasing the concentration of the cosmetic on the skin in this location.

cult to isolate, and further research is necessary. Yet, it is worthwhile to speculate on the cause. It is possible that one of the potential causes is the emulsifier used to keep the oil-soluble and water-soluble ingredients in a single phase in the formulation. Emulsifiers are basically detergents. It is not unreasonable to think that the emulsifiers are not only emulsifying the facial foundation ingredients, but also the sebum within the follicular ostia and, possibly, the skin proteins around the ostia. Detergents are the common cause of irritant contact dermatitis in both household and occupational settings.

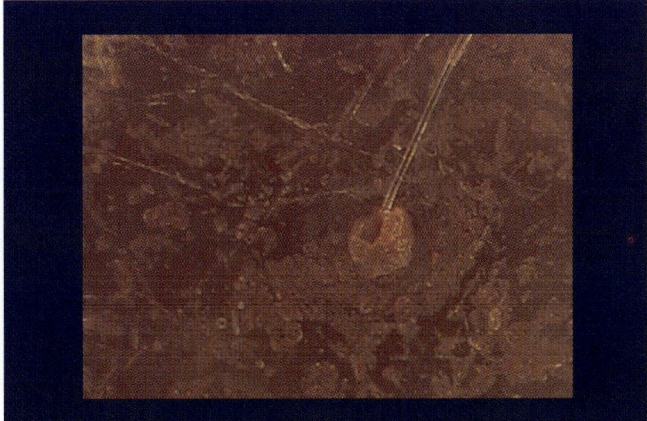

FIGURE 5–5 • The increased concentration of facial foundation around the follicular ostia may account for the irritant phenomena known as acne cosmetica.

5. Sensitive Skin

The patient with sensitive skin presents another challenge for cosmetic and skin care product manufacturers. Skin sensitivity may be clinically manifested by stinging, burning, pruritus, and/or tightness, regardless of the environmental stimulus or underlying medical cause. These symptoms may be noticed immediately following product application, or they may be delayed by minutes, hours, or days. Furthermore, the symptoms may only result following cumulative product application or in combination with products used concomitantly.[5] It is important to note that these symptoms can be present even if there is no visible sign of skin disease.[6] Cosmetic manufacturers have reported that 1% to 10% of facial cosmetic users experience these subjective perceptions, without clinical findings.[7] The most reliable predictor of sensitive skin appears to be a prior history of dermatologic disease, especially eczematous dermatoses related to dry skin.[8]

It is important to understand the physiologic changes that accompany both visible and invisible adverse reactions to cosmetics and skin care products. Sensitive skin may be accompanied by a combination of heightened neurosensory input, increased immune responsiveness, and altered barrier function. Table 5–2 lists some of the physiologic differences that have been noted between various ethnic and age groups in this regard.

Previously, it was thought that women reacted more intensely to irritants than men,[9] presumably because of a relatively higher skin pH, with less buffering capacity in female subjects.[10] However, this thinking was refuted by Bjornberg, who, by evaluating the cutaneous effects of an anionic detergent, cationic detergent, soap, acid, alkali, and other common skin irritants, demonstrated no difference in susceptibility to irritancy between men and women.[11] Lack of gender difference was confirmed by Lammintausta et al., who examined transepidermal water loss (TEWL) and dielectric water content (DEWC) following sodium lauryl sulfate application.[12] Research by Reed et al. further demonstrated that skin type, but neither race nor gender, influenced the epidermal permeability barrier function, as evidenced by tape stripping analysis.[13] Thus, the increased incidence of adverse reactions to cosmetics and skin care products reported in women may be attributable simply to the greater number of products used by this population.

Sometimes, despite rigorous testing and formulation criteria, a dermatologic patient presents who complains of being unable to use a variety of cosmetics and skin care products. To assist in the care of such difficult patients, the author has developed Table 5–3, which lists cosmetic selection criteria. Specific product recommendations are listed in Table 5–4.

TABLE 5–2 Racial and Age-Related Cutaneous Differences

Evaluated Parameter	White Skin[14]	Hispanic Skin[15]	Asian Skin[16]	Black Skin[17]	Aged Skin[18]
SC thickness	7.2 μm			6.5 μm	Epidermis becomes more compact with age
SC layers	17			22	
TEWL following SLS exposure[19]		Higher water loss than in whites following 2% SLS		Higher water loss than in whites following preoccluded skin, 0.5% SLS	Lower water loss in healthy aged skin
TEWL following tape stripping			Higher water loss than in whites	Higher water loss than in whites	
Corticosteroid penetration[20]	Higher level of penetration than in blacks			Lower level of penetration than in whites	
Vessel reactivity	Highest	Same as in white skin		Less	No age-related difference
Stinging susceptibility	Greatest			Reduced	Reduced
Response to irritation	Erythema	Erythema and hyperpigmentation		Hyperpigmentation	Reduced
Sweat glands	Decreased number of apocrine-eccrine glands			Increased number of apocrine-eccrine glands	
Ceramide levels[21]	Intermediate	Intermediate high	Highest	Lowest	Decreased with age

SC, subcutaneous; *TEWL,* transepidermal water loss; *SLS,* sodium lauryl sulfate.

TABLE 5–3 Cosmetic Selection Criteria for Patients with Sensitive Skin

1. When possible, powder cosmetics should be selected over cream or lotion formulations.
2. All cosmetics should be able to be removed easily by water; no waterproof cosmetics should be selected.
3. Old cosmetics should be discarded and fresh products purchased.
4. Eyeliner and mascara should be selected in the color black.
5. Pencil forms of eyeliner and eyebrow cosmetics should be selected.
6. Eye shadows should be selected from the light earth tones, (e.g., tan, peach, light pink, etc.). Deep colors, such as blues, purples, and greens, should be avoided.
7. Select cosmetics without chemical sunscreen agents (e.g., PABA esters, methoxycinnamates)
8. Purchase cosmetic products with no more than 10 ingredients, if possible.
9. Avoid nail polishes.
10. Facial foundations should be of the cream/powder variety or, if of the liquid type, based on silicone derivatives (e.g., cyclomethicone, dimethicone).

TABLE 5–4 Skin and Hair Care Product Recommendations for Patients with Sensitive Skin

1. Bathing soap: Oil of Olay Sensitive Skin Bar (Procter & Gamble)
2. Facial cleanser: Oil of Olay Sensitive Skin Foaming Face Wash (Procter & Gamble)
3. Sunscreen-containing daytime moisturizer: Oil of Olay Complete Daily UV Protectant (Procter & Gamble)
4. Hair shampoo: DHS Clear Dermatological Hair and Scalp Shampoo (Person & Covey)
5. Hair conditioner: DHS Conditioning Rinse (Person & Covey)
6. Facial moisturizer: Cetaphil Moisturizing Cream (Galderma)
7. Body moisturizer: Eucerin Cream and Lotion (Biersdorf)
8. Sunscreen: Sensitive Skin Chemical SPF 17 Free Sunscreen (Neutrogena)

REFERENCES

1. Fulton JE, Pay SR, Fulton JE. Comedogenicity of current therapeutic products, cosmetics, and ingredients in the rabbit ear. J Am Acad Dermatol 10:96–105, 1984.
2. Fulton JE, Bradley S, Aqundez A, Black T. Non-comedogenic cosmetics. Cutis 17:344, 1976.
3. Report of the 1988 American Academy of Dermatology Invitational Symposium on Comedogenicity. J Am Acad Dermatol 20: 272–277, 1989.
4. Mills OH, Berger RS. Defining the susceptibility of acne-prone and sensitive skin populations to extrinsic factors. Dermatol Clin 9:93–98, 1991.
5. Green BG, Bluth BS. Measuring the chemosensory irritability of human skin. J Toxicol Cut Ocul Toxicol 14:230, 1995.
6. Simion FA, Rau AH. Sensitive skin. Cosmet Toiletr 109:43–50, 1994.
7. Amin S, Maibach HI. Cosmetic intolerance syndrome: Pathophysiology and management. Cosmet Dermatolol 9:34–42, 1996.
8. Berardesca E, Maibach HI. Sensitive and ethnic skin. Dermatol Clin 9:89–92, 1991.
9. Beek CH. The sensibility of the skin against soap among patients with eczema. Dermatologica 93:167, 1946.
10. Andersson DS. The acid-base balance of the skin. Br J Dermatol 63:283, 1951.
11. Bjornberg A. Skin reactions to primary irritants in men and women. Acta Dermat Venereol [Stockholm] 55:191–194, 1975.
12. Lammintausta K, Maibach HI, Wilson D. Irritant reactivity in males and females. Contact Dermatitis 17:276–280, 1987.
13. Reed JT, Bhadially R, Elias PM. Skin type, but neither race nor gender, influence epidermal permeability barrier function. Arch Dermatol 131:1134–1138, 1995.
14. Stephens TJ, Oresajo C. Ethnic sensitive skin. Cosmet Toiletr, 109:75–80, 1994.
15. Berardesca E, Maibach HI. Sodium-lauryl-sulphate–induced cutaneous irritation. Contact Dermatitis 19:136–140, 1988.
16. Berardesca E, Maibach H. Racial differences in skin pathophysiology. J Am Acad Dermatol 34:667–672, 1996.
17. Stephens TJ, Oresajo C. Ethnic sensitive skin. Cosmet Toiletr, 109:75–80, 1994.
18. Harvell JD, Maibach HI. Percutaneous absorption and inflammation in aged skin: A review. J Am Acad Dermatol 31:1015–1021, 1994.
19. Berardesca E, Maibach HI. Racial differences in sodium lauryl sulphate–induced cutaneous irritation: Black and white. Contact Dermatitis 18:65–70, 1988.
20. Stoughton RB. Bioassay methods for measuring percutaneous absorption. In: Montagna W, Stoughton RB, Van Scott EJ (eds). Pharmacology of the Skin. New York: Appleton-Century-Crofts, 1969, pp. 542–544.
21. Sugino K, Imosawa G, Maibach HI. Ethnic difference of stratum corneum lipid in relation to stratum corneum function. J Invest Dermatol 100:597, 1993.

6

Cosmetics and Skin Care Product Delivery Systems

Delivery systems provide a mechanism for enhanced exposure of the skin to ingedients designed to produce a specific benefit. They influence the safety and efficacy of products by exposing the skin to active agents, preservatives, fragrances, emulsifiers, and vehicles utilizing unique physical methods. This is a rapidly expanding area within product formulation in both the over-the-counter and prescription skin care market. The delivery systems currently being utilized include liposomes, niosomes, transdermal delivery systems, polyester webs, and microsponges.

1. Liposomes

Liposomes are spherical vesicles, ranging in diameter from 25 to 5000 nm, that are formed from membranes consisting of a bilayer of amphiphilic molecules (Fig. 6–1).[1] The term amphiphilic refers to the fact that the molecules have both polar and nonpolar ends. The polar heads are directed both toward the inside of the vesicle and to its outer surface. The nonpolar, or lipophilic tails, are directed toward the middle of the bilayer. This unique structure thus allows the sustained release of water-soluble chemicals from the liposome structure. Liposomes may be one double layer (unilamellar), two to four double layers (oligolamellar), or multilayered (multilamellar) vesicles.[2]

The primary substances used to form liposomes are phospholipids, such as phosphatidylcholine. Other minor components may include phosphatidylethenolamine, phosphatidylinositol and phosphatidic acid. Vegetable phospholipids are also used, owing to their high concentration of the essential fatty acids, linoleic and linolenic acid. Parameters that influence the function of liposomes in topical preparations are listed in Table 6–1.

Liposomes can also be incorporated into cosmetics, bath products, moisturizers, and sunscreens. Empty liposomes have possibilities as bath oils, emollients, and wound healing aids owing to their rich concentrations of phospholipids. Loaded liposomes can be devised to release their contents at specific temperatures or at specific pH levels, a concept known as "triggering." These liposomes can be loaded with sunscreens to enhance distribution within the stratum corneum, or with moisturizers to reduce transepidermal water loss. The liposome concentration in such formulations is usually 1% to 10%.

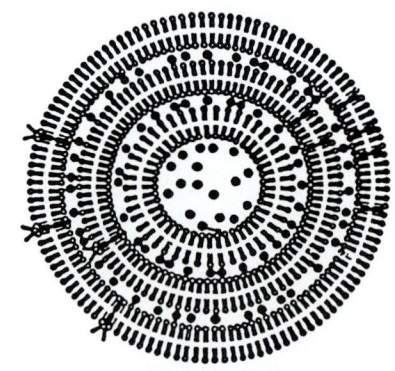

- • **hydrophilic active or drug molecule**
- — **lipophilic active or drug molecule**
- ⟩O— **amphiphilic active or drug molecule, the hydrophobic part is immobilized in the lipophilic domain of the bilayer**

FIGURE 6–1 • The structure of a liposome or a niosome is illustrated. Notice that the structure can deliver both water-soluble and oil-soluble substances, depending on how the bilayer membranes are loaded during the manufacturing process.

TABLE 6-1 Properties Influencing Liposomes and Niosomes

• • • • • •

Chemical composition
Vesicle size
Shape
Surface charge
Lamellarity
Homogeneity
Active agent location
   Inside the vesicles
   In the membrane
   On the outer surface of the vesicle
Chemical nature of the active agent
   Hydrophilic
   Amphiphilic
   Lipophilic

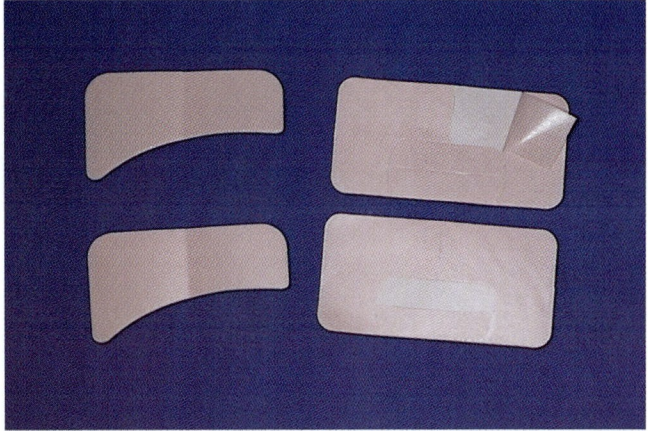

FIGURE 6-2 • Transdermal delivery patches are marketed to deliver vitamins, such as vitamin C, to the skin in a time-released fashion. However, the efficacy of such products has not been demonstrated in clinical trials.

2. Niosomes

Niosomes represent a specialized form of liposomes composed of nonionic surfactants. Their main components are ethoxylated fatty alcohols and synthetic polyglycerol ethers (polyoxyethylene alkylester, polyoxyethylene alkylether). They share the same properties as the liposomes listed in Table 6-1. Although their formulation is different, their chemical structure and impact on the skin is identical to those of liposomes (see Fig. 6-1).

3. Transdermal Delivery

Transdermal delivery differs from liposomes or niosomes in that, rather than targeting specific skin sites, a physical barrier is applied to the skin to encourage penetration. Transdermal delivery systems utilize a barrier that prevents transepidermal water loss and increases hydration of the stratum corneum to facilitate penetration. A reservoir with the active agent is present beneath the plastic barrier, which continuously releases into the stratum corneum. Transdermal delivery systems are commonly utilized to deliver nitroglycerin or estrogen to the body, but have been adapted to the over-the-counter market for the delivery of vitamins to the skin. Figure 6-2 demonstrates a patch that, when worn all night, is designed to deliver vitamin C and protein to the skin. Enhanced moisturization of the skin under such a patch occurs until it is removed. It is unknown whether transdermal vitamin delivery is efficacious; oral administration is certainly more direct.

4. Polyester Webs

Polyester webs are similar to transdermal delivery systems in that both are used to provide a constant infusion of an active agent into the skin. Polyester webs, however, are invisible to the human eye. They create a thin film over the skin surface that can constantly release a desired active agent onto the stratum corneum. This technique is especially effective at maintaining long-term skin moisturization.

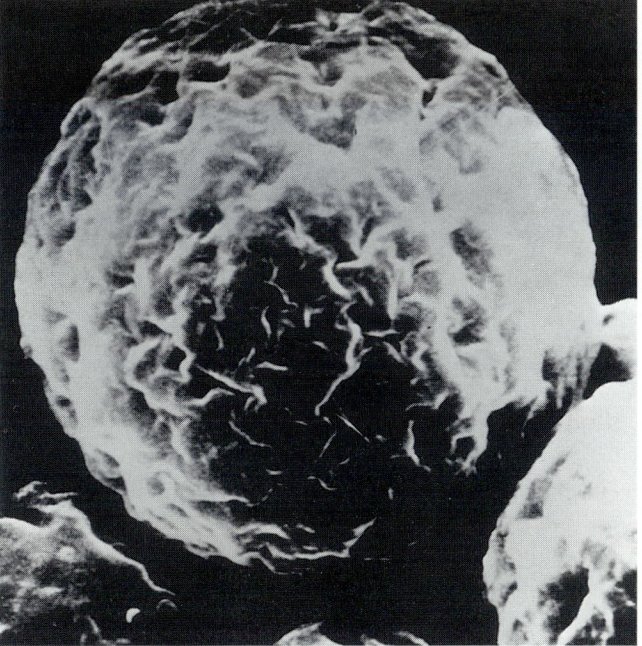

FIGURE 6-3 • Microsponges are loaded with substances for time-released application to the stratum corneum (X5000).

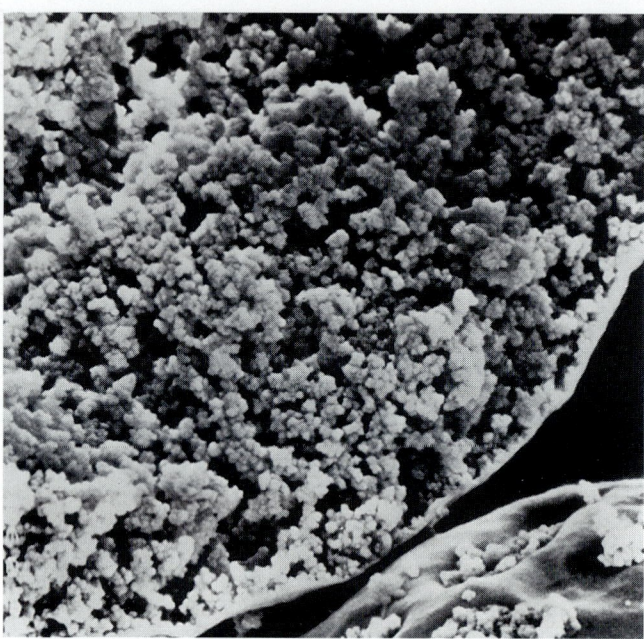

FIGURE 6–4 • The interior of a microsponge contains macropores for storage and eventual delivery of active agents (X6000).

5. Microsponges

Another method of maintaining long-term delivery of an active agent is through the use of microsponges. These microscopic sponges are loaded with an active agent that is continually released onto the stratum corneum (Figs. 6–3 and 6–4). The benefit of this delivery system is its ability to sustain low-level release of active agents that may be slightly irritating. One widely marketed use of this technology is the delivery of topical tretinoin (Retin-A Micro, Ortho Pharmaceuticals). The only problem with the use of microsponges is that they dissolve with continued rubbing into the skin, prematurely releasing all of the active agent.

REFERENCES

1. Junginger HE, Hofland HEJ, Bouwstra JA. Liposomes and niosomes: Interactions with human skin. Cosmet Toiletr 106:45–50, 1991.
2. Hayward JA. Potential of liposomes in cosmetic science. Cosmet Toiletr 105:47–54, 1990.

Colored Cosmetics

7

Facial Foundations

Facial foundations are designed to add color, cover blemishes, and blend uneven facial color. However, they can also provide the therapeutic benefits of sun protection, oil control, and moisturization. They represent the class of cosmetics about which patients most frequently question their dermatologist. This section pictorially demonstrates the formulation, cutaneous appearance, and application of facial foundations.

1. Formulation

There are four basic facial foundation formulations: oil-based, water-based, oil-free, and water-free forms. Oil-based foundations are water-in-oil emulsions containing pigments suspended in oil, such as mineral oil or lanolin alcohol (Fig. 7–1). The water evaporates from the foundation following application, leaving the pigment in oil on the face, providing excellent moisturization for patients with eczema.

Water-based facial foundations are oil-in-water emulsions containing a small amount of oil in which the pigment is emulsified with a relatively large quantity of water. These are the most popular foundations and are appropriate for normal/combination skin (Fig. 7–2).

Oil-free facial foundations contain no animal, vegetable, or mineral oils, and are based on silicones, such as dimethicone or cyclomethicone. Most new facial foundations entering the marketplace are of this

type, as the silicones exhibit tremendous versatility (Fig. 7–3). The silicones are noncomedogenic, nonacnegenic, and hypoallergenic.

Oil-control foundations are a subset of facial foundations, containing ingredients, such as talc, kaolin, starch, or polymers, to absorb facial sebum (Fig. 7–4). Oil-control foundations are not necessarily oil-free, however.[1]

Water-free or anhydrous foundations are waterproof. These foundations provide superior sun protection, making them useful in patients with photosensi-

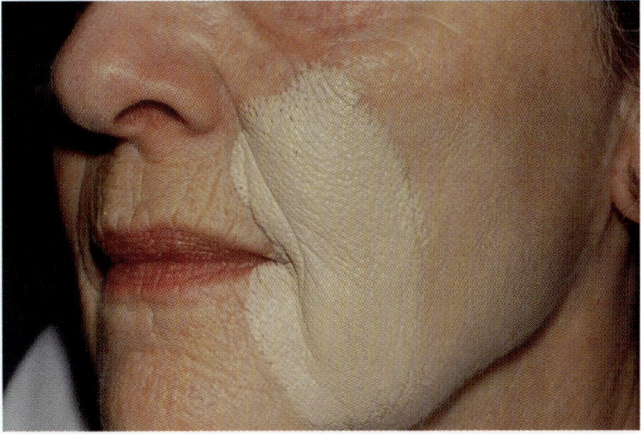

FIGURE 7–1 • Oil-based facial foundations leave a moist shine on the skin surface and can decrease transepidermal water loss. However, the shiny finish can accentuate skin surface irregularities, such as the prominent follicular ostia demonstrated here.

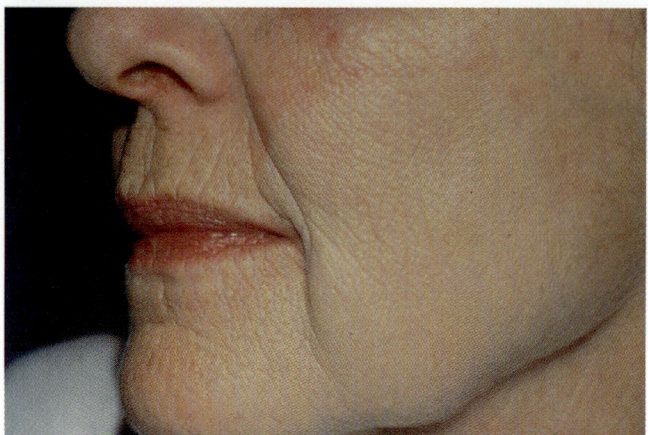

FIGURE 7–2 • Water-based facial foundations provide less moisturization than oil-based varieties, but their matte finish does not accentuate surface irregularities. Mature patients with dry skin may wish to use a moisturizer under their facial foundation to achieve a better cosmetic appearance.

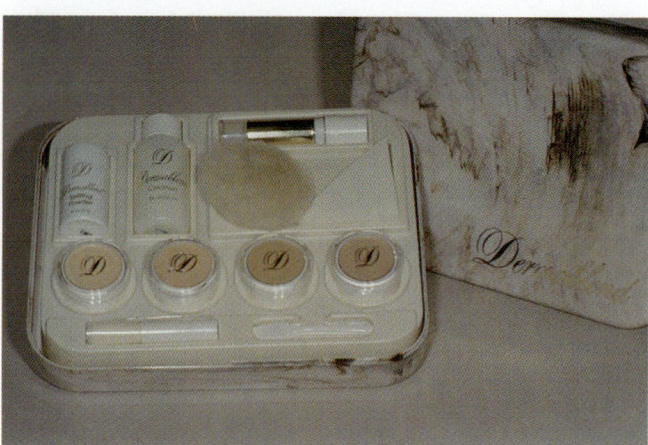

FIGURE 7–5 • Anhydrous facial foundations are used for surgical camouflaging and theatrical purposes.

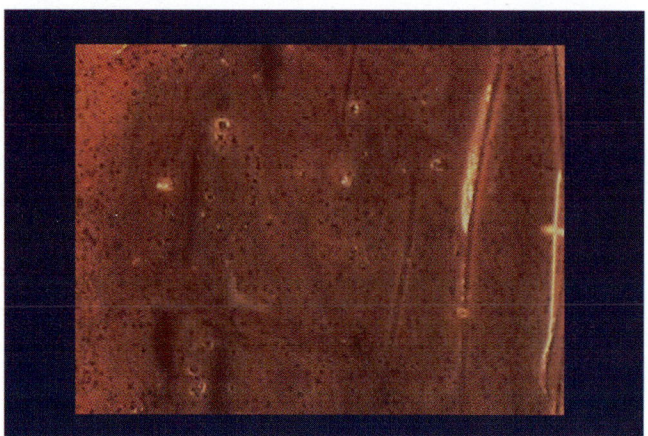

FIGURE 7–3 • This video microscopic image (X400) demonstrates the appearance of a silicone-based facial foundation on the skin.

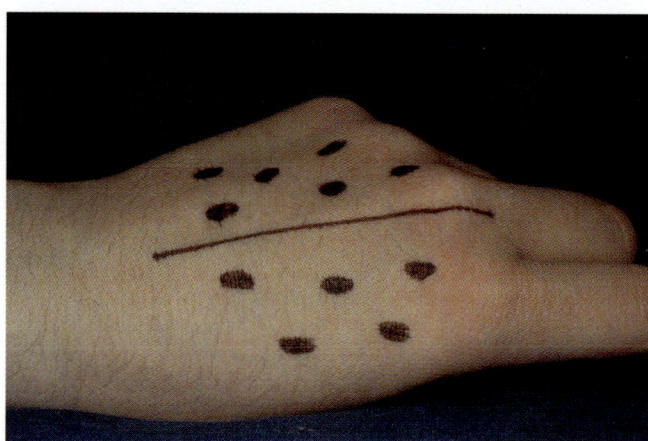

FIGURE 7–6 • This model demonstrates the coverage of various facial foundations. Coverage can be assessed as the ability of the cosmetic to hide the black dots placed on the dorsum of the hand.

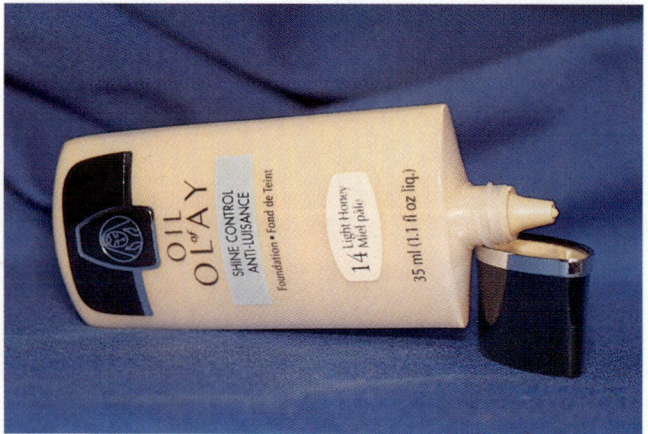

FIGURE 7–4 • Oil-control or shine-control facial foundations incorporate an oil-absorbing polymer to prevent the development of facial shine.

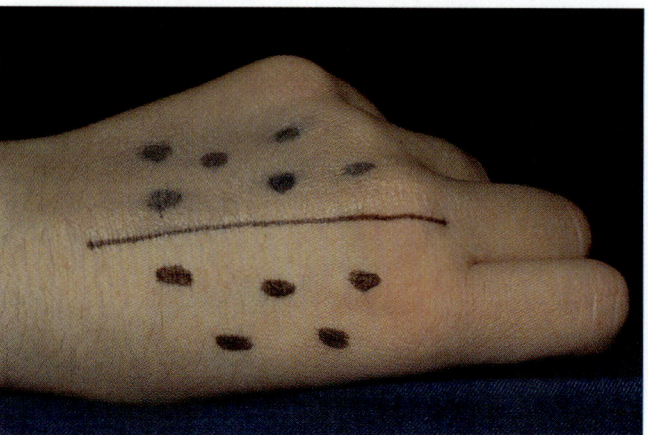

FIGURE 7–7 • A sheer-coverage facial foundation has been applied to the upper hand, which has basically pigmented the skin.

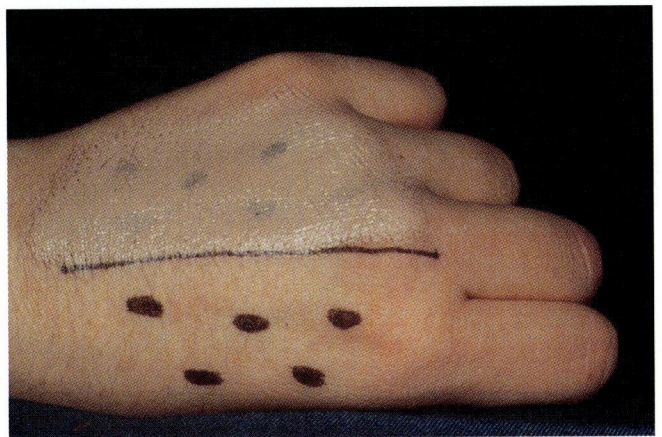

FIGURE 7–8 • A moderate-coverage facial foundation has been applied to the upper hand, providing some camouflage of the black dots.

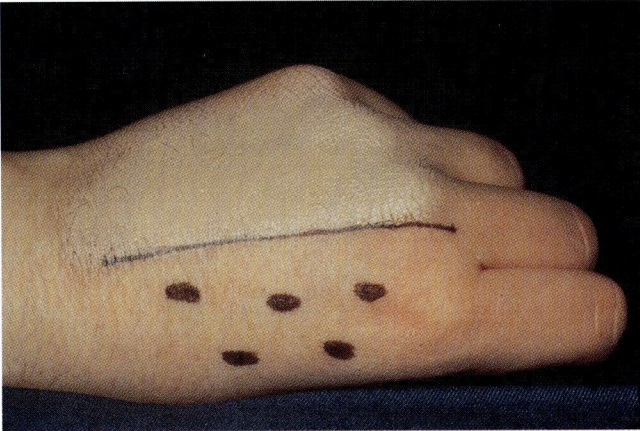

FIGURE 7–9 • A high-coverage facial foundation completely obscures the black dots on the upper hand.

tive dermatoses and in patients requiring postsurgical camouflaging (Fig. 7–5).

2. Coverage

Coverage, which refers to the ability of a facial foundation to conceal or cover the underlying skin, is proportional to the amount of titanium dioxide, zinc oxide, talc, kaolin, and/or precipitated chalk in the formulation (Fig. 7–6). Sheer coverage foundations with minimal titanium dioxide are almost transparent and have a sun protection factor (SPF) of approximately 2 (Fig. 7–7). Moderate coverage foundations

are translucent and have an approximate SPF of 4 to 5 (Fig. 7–8), whereas anhydrous, high-coverage foundations with large amounts of titanium dioxide are opaque, acting as a total physical sunblock (Fig. 7–9). Additional sun protection can be provided by incorporating chemical sunscreens, such as oxybenzone and octyl methoxycinnamate, to achieve an SPF of 15.

3. Types

Facial foundations are available in a variety of forms: liquid, mousse, water-containing cream, soufflé, anhy-

TABLE 7–1 **Types of Facial Foundations**

Type	Coverage	Wearability	Skin Type	Main Ingredients
Liquid	Sheer to moderate	Moderate	Any	Water, oil, TiO_2
Mousse	Shear	Short	Oily to normal	Aerosolized liquid formulation
Water-containing cream	Moderate	Moderate to long	Dry to normal	Water, oil, wax, TiO_2
Soufflé	Moderate	Moderate	Dry to normal	Whipped cream formulation
Anhydrous cream	Full	Long	Dry	Mineral and vegetable oils, synthetic esters, wax, TiO_2
Stick	Full	Long	Dry	Mineral oil, wax, TiO_2
Cake	Full	Moderate to long	Oily to normal	Talc, kaolin, chalk, zinc oxide, TiO_2
Shake lotion	Sheer	Short	Oily	Talc, water, solvent

Coverage key: sheer = semitransparent; moderate = translucent; heavy = semiopaque; full = opaque.
Wearability key: short = 3 hours; moderate = 4 hours; long = 8 hours.

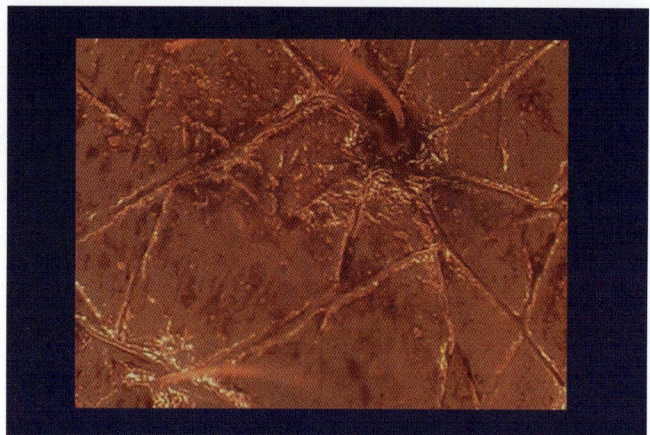

FIGURE 7–10 • Shake lotion facial foundations place a thin layer of pigment on the skin surface, as seen in this video microscopic image (X400). Notice that the facial foundation is migrating to the follicular ostia and collecting in the skin folds in this elderly patient after only 2 hours of wearing the cosmetic.

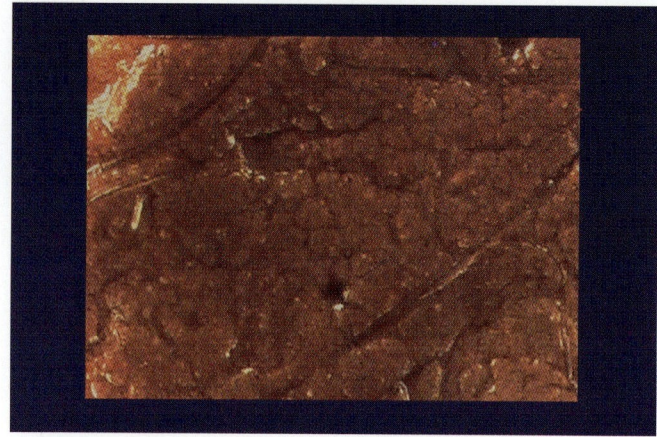

FIGURE 7–12 • Cream/powder facial foundations provide the most complete coverage of the skin surface, as seen in this video microscopic image (X400).

drous cream, stick, cake, and shake lotion (Table 7–1).[2] Shake lotions contain pigmented talc suspended in water and solvents that evaporate, leaving a thin layer of powder on the face (Fig. 7–10). Liquid formulations are most popular because they are the easiest to apply, provide sheer to moderate coverage, and create a natural appearance (Fig. 7–11). Cream/powder foundations, which are wiped from a compact with a sponge, can be used to achieve increased coverage of underlying cutaneous defects (Fig. 7–12). However, all facial foundations tend to migrate over the face as perspiration and oil combine with the cosmetic (Figs. 7–13A–C).

4. Finishes

Facial foundations are manufactured in a variety of finishes: matte, semimatte, moist semimatte, and shiny (Table 7–2). The finish is the surface appearance and characteristics of the cosmetic (see Figs. 7–1, 7–2).

5. Application

Proper application of facial foundation is key to achieving the appearance of natural, unblemished skin. The foundation should be selected to match the natural skin, as closely as possible, at the jawline, as this is where blending into the neck must occur (Fig. 7–14). Proper color selection can only be made under natural sunlight, as the fluorescent lights found in most stores distort color perception. Usually, a darker color than desired is selected under these conditions. Patients should be advised to apply a sample of the cosmetic in the store and walk outside to examine the color match with a compact mirror.

In general, facial foundation should be applied with the fingertips. A dab of foundation should be placed on the forehead, nose, cheeks, and chin and then blended with a light circular motion until it is evenly spread over all the facial skin, including the lips. Products applied under the facial foundation should not alter the appearance of the cosmetic (Fig. 7–15). Finally, a puff or sponge should be used, stroking in a downward direction, to remove any streaks and to flatten vellus facial hair (Fig. 7–16). Special care should be taken to rub the foundation into the hair-

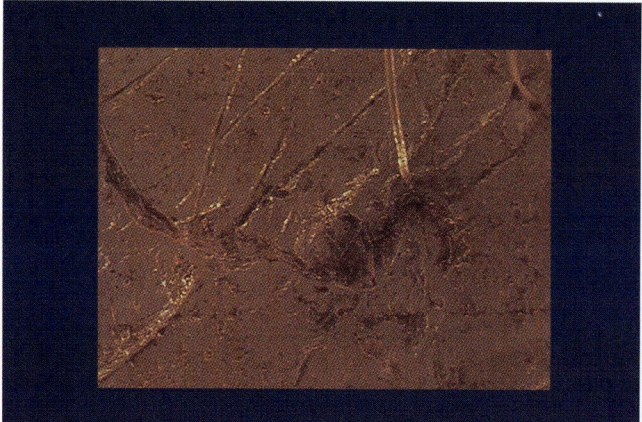

FIGURE 7–11 • Liquid facial foundations also migrate over the skin surface, as seen in this video microscopic image (X400) taken 2 hours after cosmetic application.

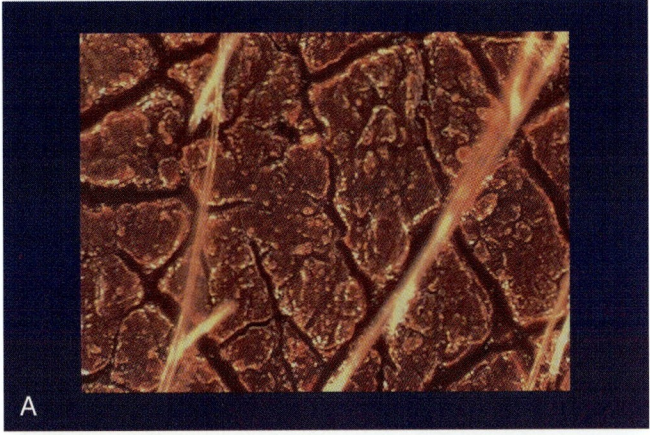

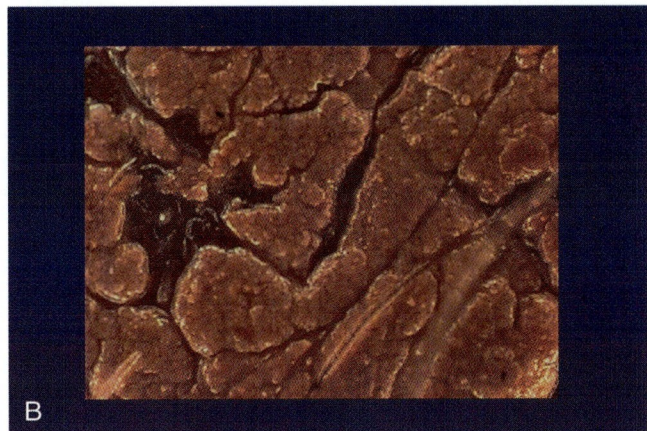

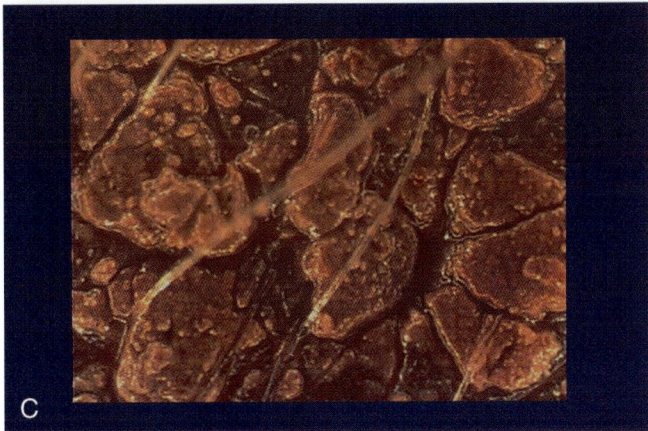

FIGURE 7–13 • These sequential video microscopic images (X400) show the changes in the appearance of a cream/powder facial foundation on the skin surface at 30 minutes (A), 2 hours (B), and 4 hours (C) following application. Notice how the sebum and perspiration lift the cosmetic from the skin surface.

TABLE 7–2   **Facial Foundation Finishes**

	Appearance	Formulation	Skin Type	Moisturizing Ability	
Matte	Flat, no shine	Generally oil-free	Oily	↑	Least
Semimatte	Minimal shine	Oil-free or water-based	Oily to normal		
Moist semimatte	Dewy shine	Generally water-based	Normal to dry		
Shiny	Obvious shine	Generally oil-based	Dry	↓	Most

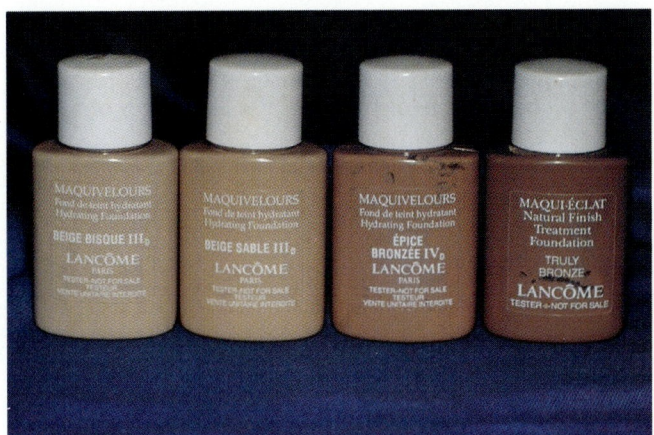

FIGURE 7–14 • Facial foundations are available in a variety of colors to match all skin tones.

line, over the tragus, and beneath the chin. Foundation should also be blended around the eyes and may even be applied to the entire upper eyelid, if desired. The foundation should be allowed to set or dry until it can no longer be removed with light touch. If additional coverage is desired, a second layer of foundation can be applied.

6. Selection

The facial foundations the author recommends are arranged in table form according to skin type: oily (Table 7–3), normal/combination (Table 7–4), and dry (Table 7–5).

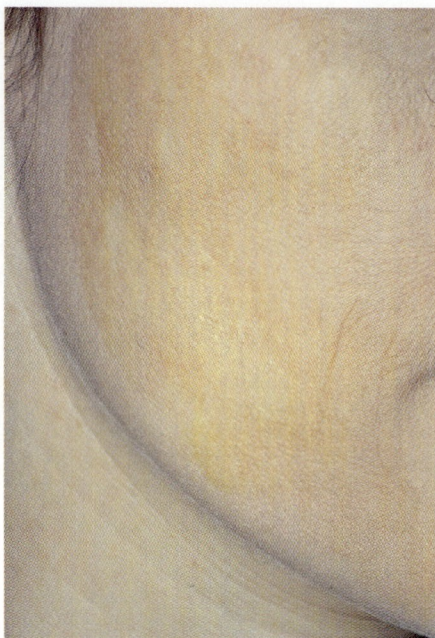

FIGURE 7–15 • Gel sunscreens and acne treatments may alter the color of the overlying facial foundation. Select products that have been tested for their cosmetic compatibility.

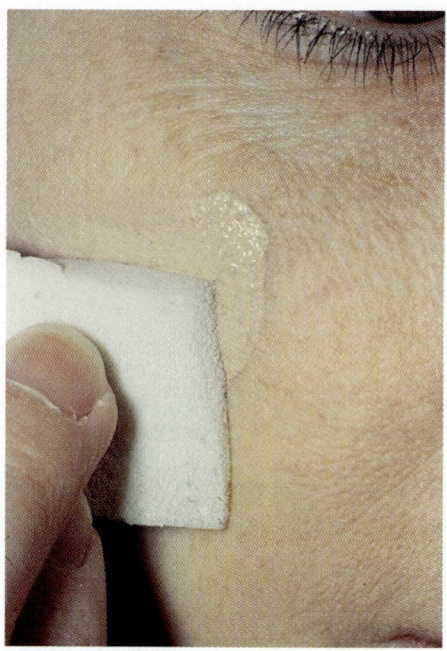

FIGURE 7–16 • A makeup sponge can be stroked in a downward direction to smooth the vellus hairs on the face. Latex-containing makeup sponges can be a cause of allergic contact dermatitis, however.

TABLE 7–3 **Facial Foundations for Patients with Oily Skin**

• • • • • •

1. Oil of Olay Shine Control (Procter & Gamble)
2. Maquicontrole (Lancôme)
3. Stay True (Clinique)
4. Mattique (L'Oreal)
5. Oil Control Makeup (Almay)
6. Demimatte (Estée Lauder)
7. Oil-free Foundation (Mary Kay)
8. Shake-It Regular Normalizer (Erno Lazlo)
9. Teint Pur (Chanel)
10. Shine Free (Maybelline)

TABLE 7–5 **Facial Foundations for Patients with Dry Skin**

• • • • • •

1. Oil of Olay All Day Moisture (Procter & Gamble)
2. Moisture Renew Makeup (Almay)
3. Moisture Whip Makeup (Maybelline)
4. Moisture Wear Cream (Cover Girl)
5. Polished Performance (Estée Lauder)
6. Teint Lumiere Creme (Chanel)
7. Day Radiance Cream Foundation (Mary Kay)
8. Healthy Skin Cream/Powder Foundation (Neutrogena)
9. Country Mist (Estée Lauder)
10. Touch and Glow (Revlon)

TABLE 7–4 **Facial Foundations for Patients with Normal/Combination Skin**

• • • • • •

1. Visuelle (L'Oreal)
2. Sheer Essentials (Maybelline)
3. Moisture Balance Makeup (Almay)
4. Balanced Makeup (Clinique)
5. Day Radiance Liquid Foundation (Mary Kay)
6. Fresh Air Makeup (Estée Lauder)
7. Maquimat Ultra Naturel (Lancôme)
8. Healthy Skin Liquid Makeup (Neutrogena)
9. Colorstay Makeup (Revlon)
10. Clean Makeup (Cover Girl)

REFERENCES

1. Fulton JE, Bradley S, Aqundez A, Black T. Non-comedogenic cosmetics. Cutis 17:344–351, 1976.
2. Fiedler JG. Foundation makeup. In Balsam MS, Sagarin E. (eds.). Cosmetics, Science and Technology, Vol. 1, 2nd ed. New York: Wiley-Interscience, 1972, pp. 317–334.

8

Facial Cosmetics

Facial colored cosmetics attempt to deemphasize facial defects and to accentuate attractive facial features. Effective use of facial colored cosmetics can reshape a poorly proportioned face or minimize facial scarring. The basic facial cosmetics that are pictorially presented in this section are powder, blush, bronzing gel, bronzing powder, concealer, self-tanning cream, and tinted moisturizer (Table 8-1).

1. Powder

Facial powders provide coverage of complexion imperfections, oil control, a matte finish, and tactile smoothness to the skin. They are removed from a compact with a puff (Fig. 8-1) or are dusted loosely from a container with a brush (Fig. 8-2). Patients with dry complexions may wish to avoid facial powder, as it can further dry the skin; however, the oil-absorbing qualities of facial powder are valuable for the patient with an oily complexion (Fig. 8-3).

2. Blush

Facial blush is pinkish powder designed to enhance rosy cheeks (Fig. 8-4). For a natural appearance, cheek color should be applied beginning at a point directly beneath the pupil on the fleshy part of the cheek, sweeping upward beyond the lateral eye (Fig. 8-5).[1,2] Blush containing rough-edged, light-reflective particles can contribute to perifollicular irritation and an acneiform eruption on the upper cheeks. This problem can be avoided by selecting matte finish blush products over the frosted formulations (Figs. 8-6 and 8-7).

Bronzing powders, also known as highlighter powders, are more intensely pigmented than facial blushes. They are available in deep burgundy, bronze, or brown and are used to color and contour the face and body. For example, a bronze facial highlighter can be applied to the central forehead, nasal tip, and central chin to create the appearance of a tan.

3. Bronzing Gel

Facial bronzing gels are products used to add facial color, without coverage. The brownish gel is rubbed into the skin to stain the surface and simulate a tan (Fig. 8-8). The cosmetic must be applied quickly and evenly to yield a satisfactory result. Inadvertent staining of the fingertips and clothing is a common problem.

TABLE 8-1 Facial Colored Cosmetics

Facial Colored Cosmetic	Intended Use	Formulation
Powder	Covering facial imperfections, imparting skin smoothness, and absorbing oil	Talc, zinc stearate, kaolin, titanium dioxide, pigment, pearl
Blush	Adding color to cheeks	Talc, zinc stearate, titanium dioxide, pigment, pearl
Bronzing gel	Adding transparent color to face	Water, alcohol, neutral aqueous gel, light esters, color
Concealer	Covering facial color imperfections	Mineral oil, wax, titanium dioxide, pigment
Self-tanning Cream	Creating the illusion of a tan	Dihydroxyacetone, mineral oil, glycerin
Tinted moisturizer	Adding color to the face without coverage	Water, silicone, glycerin, pigment

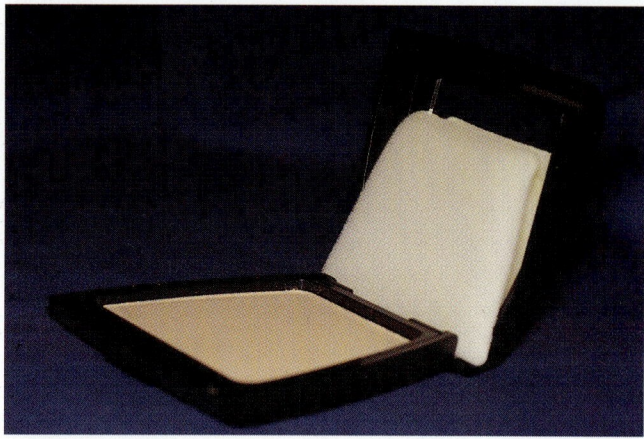

FIGURE 8–1 • Compact powder can be used to remove an oily shine from the nose, improve the color match of a facial foundation, create a matte finish, or increase coverage of the underlying skin.

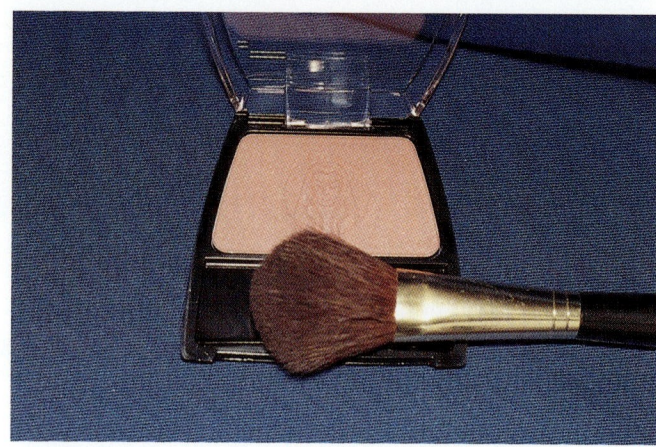

FIGURE 8–4 • Blush can be used to accentuate the appearance of rosy cheeks, especially in mature individuals with a sallow complexion.

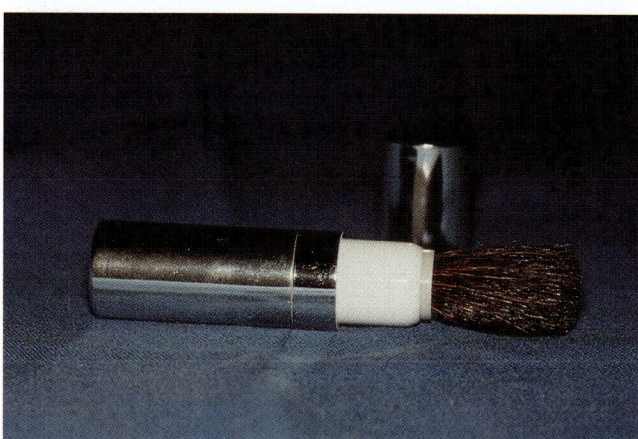

FIGURE 8–2 • A loose brush can be used to dust powder over the entire face, following application of a facial foundation, to increase the wear of the cosmetics.

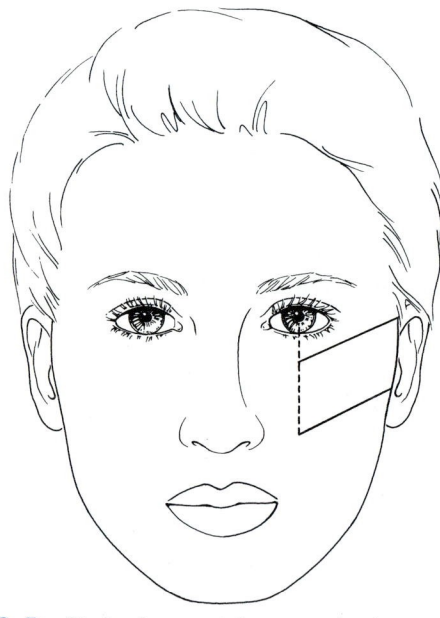

FIGURE 8–5 • Blush placement for an optimal cosmetic appearance.

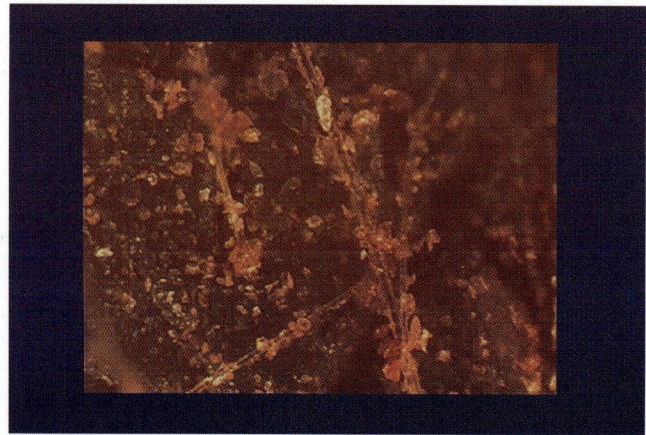

FIGURE 8–3 • The powder can be visualized along the vellus hair shafts and on the skin surface using a video microscope ($\times 400$). The light-reflective properties of the added pearl can also be appreciated.

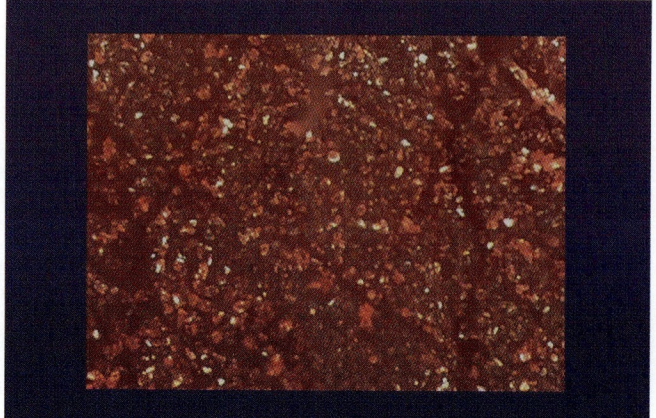

FIGURE 8–6 • Blush with numerous light reflective particles has a distinct appearance when viewed with a video microscope ($\times 400$).

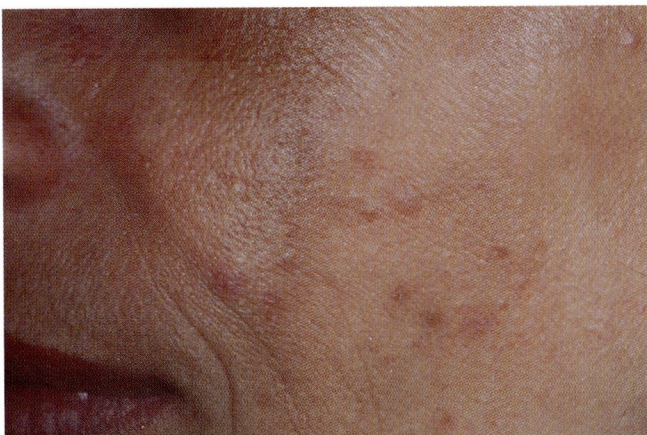

FIGURE 8–7 • Follicular irritation can result from the rough-edged, light-reflective particles in blushes and bronzing powders that lodge within the follicular ostia. The eruption can be confused with acne, but is generally limited to the cheeks where the blush is applied.

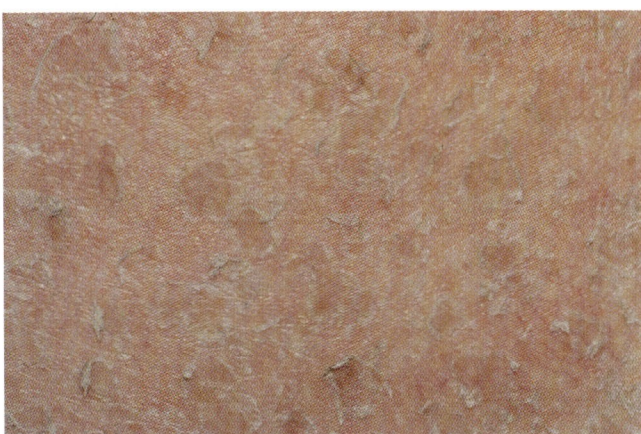

FIGURE 8–10 • Skin scale is high in protein and thus will stain a deeper color than the surrounding skin when a self-tanning cream is applied. To achieve even application with a self-tanning cream, it is best to exfoliate any desquamating corneocytes prior to application.

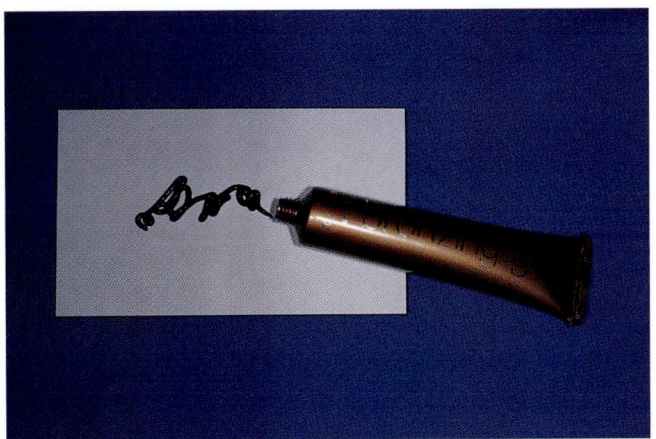

FIGURE 8–8 • Bronzing gels provide sheer color to the face and can be used by both men and women to simulate a tan. The stain produced is water-resistant.

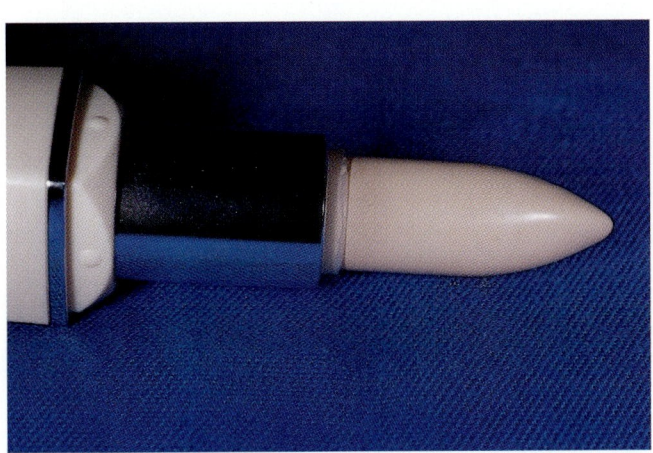

FIGURE 8–9 • Concealer sticks are useful in camouflaging under-eye shadows.

4. Concealer

Facial concealer sticks are intended for use under a facial foundation to cover imperfections. For example, under-eye concealers are matched to the skin color and applied to camouflage the darkness of under-eye circles (Fig. 8–9).[3] Concealers can also be used to hide the red papules and pustules of acne while delivering comedolytic agents, such as sulfur, salicylic acid, or resorcinol.

5. Self-tanning Cream

Self-tanning creams produce a golden skin color overnight, without sun exposure. The active ingredient is 3% to 5% dihydroxyacetone, which is incorporated into a glycerin and mineral oil base to form a white cream that turns the stratum corneum golden.[4] Chemically, the dihydroxyacetone acts as a sugar, interacting with amino acids in the stratum corneum to produce melanoidins.[5–8] The color is not permanent and is lost as the stratum corneum desquamates; thus, continued use is necessary. The major disadvantages of the product are that it stains all contacted skin surfaces, including the palms of the hands, if it is not quickly removed, and it produces deeper staining of the follicular ostia, seborrheic keratosis, actinic keratosis, porokeratosis, and icthyotic skin (Fig. 8–10).

6. Tinted Moisturizer

Some moisturizers contain brown pigment, providing a sheer tanned appearance in addition to moisturiza-

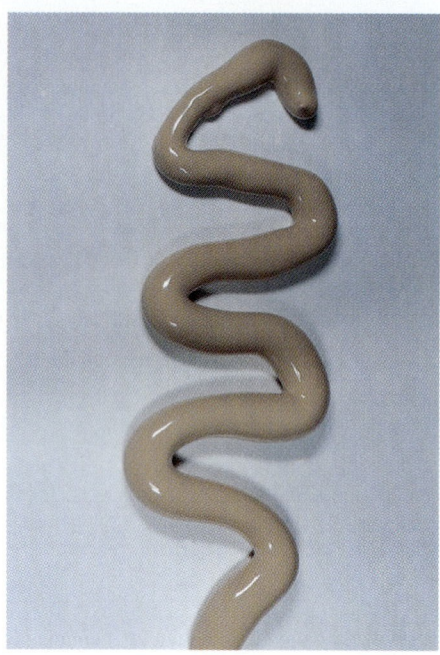

FIGURE 8–11 • Tinted moisturizers are an excellent method of improving facial color in mature individuals with excessive facial wrinkles, as facial foundations tend to migrate rapidly into the furrows, accentuating them.

tion. Technically, a tinted moisturizer is a moisturizing facial foundation without coverage (Fig. 8–11). These products are recommended for facial coloring in mature patients with numerous wrinkles and benign lesions.

REFERENCES

1. Begoun P. Blue Eyeshadow Should Be Illegal. Seattle, WA: Beginning Press, 1986, pp. 62–64.
2. Soldo BL, Drahos M. The Inside-Out Beauty Book. Old Tappan, NJ: Fleming H. Revell Company, 1978, pp. 78–79.
3. Wesley-Hosford Z. Face Value. Toronto: Bantam Books, 1986, pp. 148–150.
4. Levy SB. Dihydroxyacetone-containing sunless or self-tanning lotions. J Am Acad Dermatol 27:989–993, 1992.
5. Maibach HI, Kligman AM. Dihydroxyacetone: A suntan-simulating agent. Arch Dermatol 35:161–164, 1960.
6. Goldman L, Barkoff J, Blaney D, et al. The skin coloring agent dihydroxyacetone. GP 12:96–98, 1960.
7. Wittgenstein E, Berry HK. Reactions of dihydroxyacetone (DHA) with human skin callus and amino compounds. J Invest Dermatol 36:283–286, 1961.
8. Wittgenstein E, Berry HK. Staining of skin with dihydroxyacetone. Science 132:894–895, 1960.

9

Eyelid Cosmetics

The eyes, more than any other body part, reveal inner thoughts and emotion and, therefore, are the focus of cosmetic decoration. Basic eyelid cosmetics are listed in Table 9–1.

1. Eye Shadow

Eye shadows are available as pressed powders that are applied to the eyelid with a sponge-tipped applicator or brush (Fig. 9–1). Color variety is extensive, but no coal tar derivatives can be used in the eye area (Fig. 9–2). Fashion and eye color dictate the preferred eye shadow color (Table 9–2). Eye shadow surface texture can range from dull to a pearled shine to an iridescent finish. Titanium dioxide is used in matte-finish eye shadows to improve coverage, and bismuth oxychloride, mica, and/or fish scale essence

are the standard materials used to produce a pearly shine (Fig. 9–3). A metallic finish is provided by copper, brass, aluminum, gold, or silver powders.

In the author's experience, powdered eye shadow preparations with a matte finish and a light tan or cream color are the preferred choices for patients with eyelid dermatitis. Ideally, the cosmetic should be applied with a soft brush applicator (Fig. 9–4). Powdered eye shadows are also recommended to achieve an optimal cosmetic result in mature patients with redundant upper eyelid skin (Fig. 9–5). Contact lens wearers should avoid the use of pearlescent or iridescent eye shadows, as the reflective material particles can cause corneal abrasions if trapped beneath a contact lens.

The eyelid skin is the thinnest skin on the body and so is frequently affected by irritant contact dermatitis (Fig. 9–6), as well as allergic contact dermatitis

TABLE 9–1 Eyelid Cosmetics

Form	Application Technique	Wearability	Main Ingredients
Pressed powder	Brush	Long	Talc, pigment in oily base (mineral oil, beeswax, or lanolin) with surface finish additives (titanium dioxide, bismuth oxychloride, mica, fish scale essence, ground metal particles)
Anhydrous cream	Finger	Waterproof, short	Pigment in petrolatum, cocoa butter, or lanolin
Automatic emulsion	Wand	Waterproof, moderate	Petroleum distillate, cyclomethicone, beeswax, pigment
Stick	Pencil type	Waterproof, short	Petrolatum, mineral oil, wax, pigment
Pencil	Pencil type	Waterproof, moderate	Petrolatum, wax, pigment
Unpigmented setting cream	Finger	Long	Beeswax, talc, cyclomethicone

Wearability key: short = 3 hours; moderate = 4 hours; long = 8 hours.

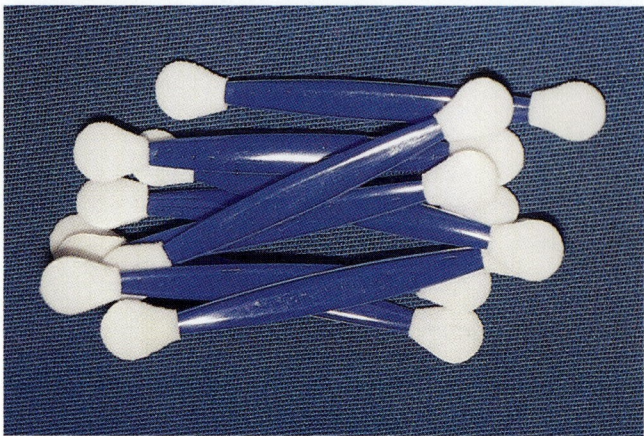

FIGURE 9-1 • Sponge-tipped applicators can irritate the eyelid as a result of their rough surface. A soft, sable brush applicator is preferred for patients with recurrent eyelid dermatitis.

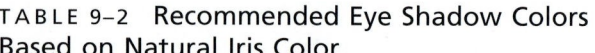

TABLE 9-2 **Recommended Eye Shadow Colors Based on Natural Iris Color**

Eye Color	Shadow Color	Effect
Blue	Brown	Intensifies blue
	Beige	Intensifies gray
	Pink	Provides contrast
	Plum	Provides contrast
Green or hazel	Charcoal	Intensifies green
	Brown	Intensifies gold
	Pink	Intensifies green
Brown	Light gray	Provides contrast
	Pink	Provides contrast
	Plum	Provides contrast

(Fig. 9-7).[1,2] The North American Contact Dermatitis Group has determined that 12% of cosmetic reactions occur on the eyelid, but only 4% of these reactions have been linked to eye makeup use.[3] Eye cosmetic ingredients associated with allergic contact dermatitis are listed in Table 9-3.[4,5]

For patients in whom eyelid dermatitis is thought to be attributable to the use of an eyeshadow, use testing is recommended. The patient is instructed to apply the cosmetic at the lateral corner of the eye for 5

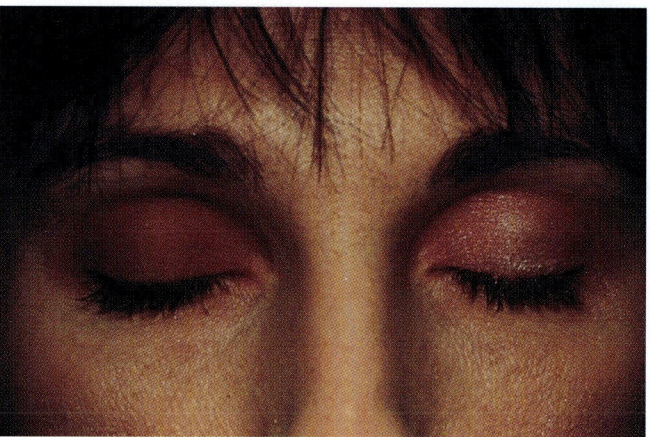

FIGURE 9-3 • The dull surface of a matte-finish eye shadow can be appreciated on the left eyelid, whereas reflective particles in the eye shadow applied to the right eyelid produce a frosted shine.

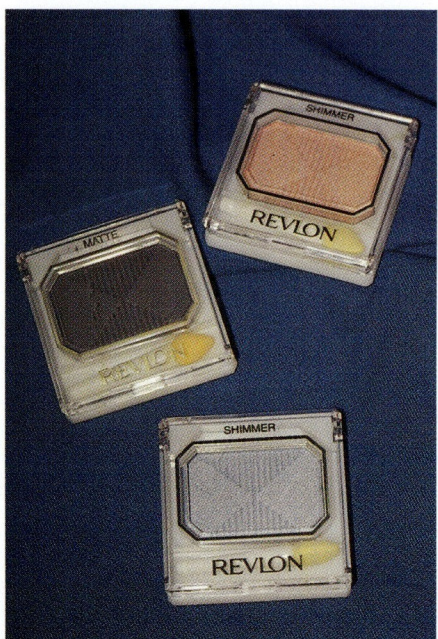

FIGURE 9-2 • Tremendous variety is available in eye shadow color. More deeply pigmented colors generally have an increased chance of inducing irritation in patients with sensitive skin.

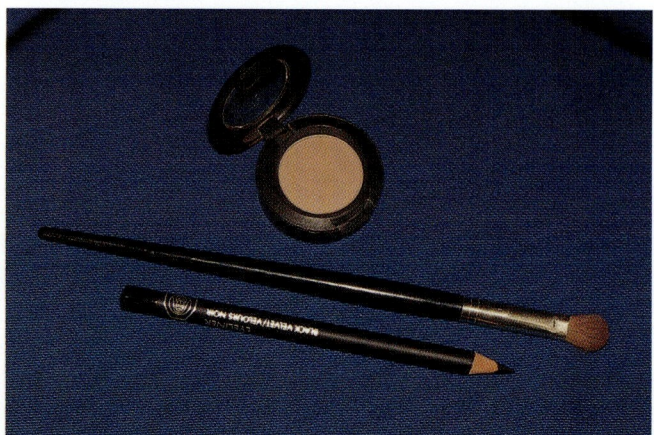

FIGURE 9-4 • Eyelid cosmetics recommended for patients with recurrent eyelid dermatitis: a light tan to pink eye shadow, a brush applicator, and a black eyeliner pencil.

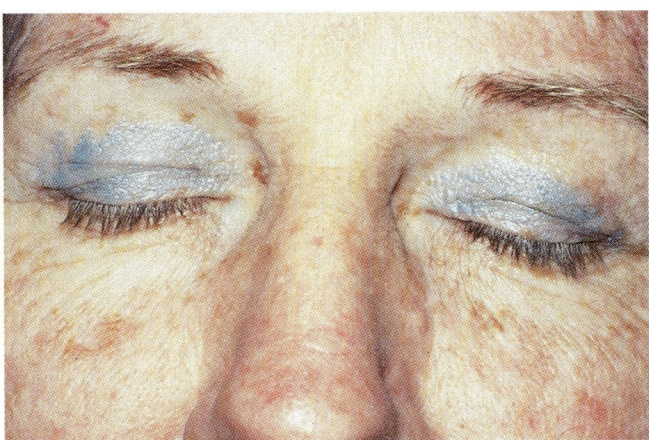

FIGURE 9–5 • Creamy, frosted, deeply pigmented eye shadows accentuate the redundant folds of the upper eyelids in a mature patient.

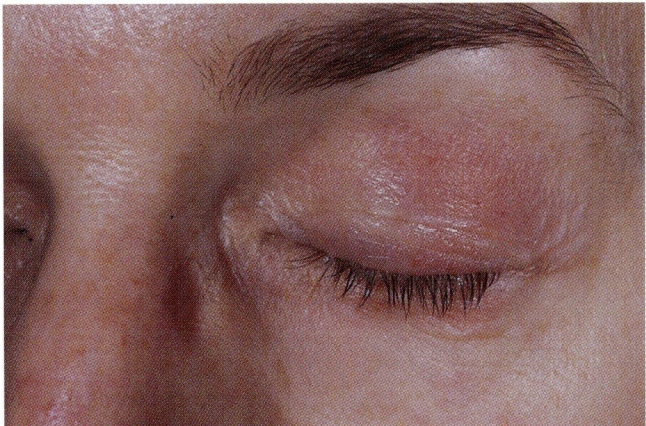

FIGURE 9–7 • Allergic contact dermatitis secondary to a preservative in a cream, automatic-emulsion eye shadow.

consecutive nights, after which the cutaneous reaction is evaluated.

2. Eye Shadow Setting Cream

Eye shadow setting creams are unpigmented and are designed to provide an adherent base over which pigmented eye shadow can be applied. They increase the wearability of eye shadows and are most useful in oily complected patients or those with redundant eyelid skin who experience migration of eye shadow into eyelid creases.

3. Eyelid Cosmetic Remover

Eyelid cosmetic remover is one of the most common causes of eyelid dermatitis, as it not only removes the

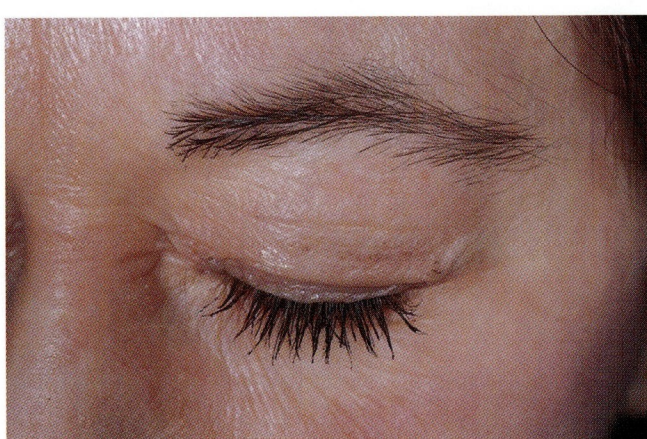

FIGURE 9–6 • Irritant contact dermatitis induced by the mica present in a frosted-finish eye shadow. The particles can be seen on the upper eyelid, even after thorough washing.

cosmetic, but also damages the eyelid cutaneous barrier (Fig. 9–8). In general, patients who experience difficulty with eyelid dermatitis should avoid waterproof eyelid cosmetics and use a lipid-free cleanser for product removal (Cetaphil [Galderma]).

4. Eye Cosmetic Camouflage Techniques

Eye cosmetics can be used to correct the appearance of eye defects arising from surgery, congenital anoma-

TABLE 9-3 Ingredients Causing Eyelid Allergic Contact Dermatitis

• • • • • •

Preservatives[8]
Parabens
Phenyl mercuric acetate
Imidazolidinyl urea
Quaternium-15
Potassium sorbate

Antioxidants
Butylated hydroxyanisole[9]
Butylated hydroxytoluene[10]
di-tert-Butyl-hydroquinone[10]

Resins
Colophony[11]

Pearlescent Additives
Bismuth oxychloride[12]

Emollients
Lanolin[13]
Propylene glycol[14]

Fragrances[15]

Pigment Contaminants
Nickel[16]

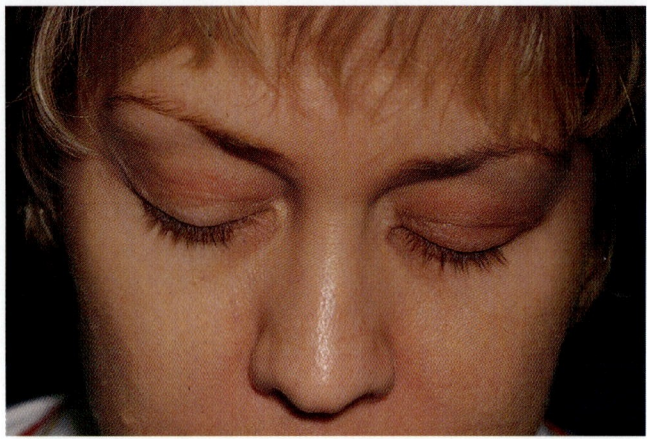

FIGURE 9–8 • Eyelid cosmetic removers can cause pruritic, erythematous eyelids owing to barrier damage from excess intercellular lipid removal.

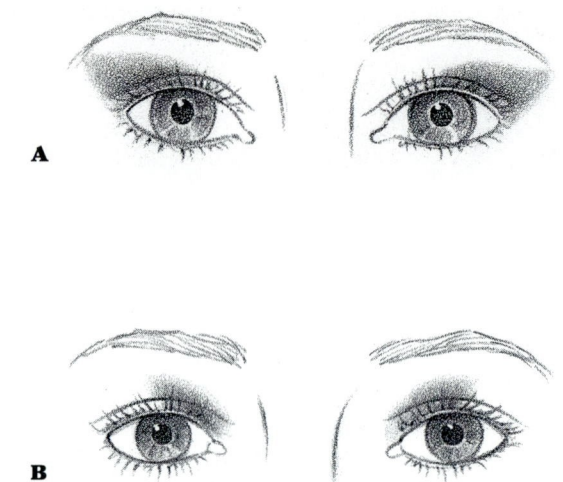

FIGURE 9–10 • Artistic eye shadow application in patients with hypoteloric eyes (*A*) and hyperteloric eyes (*B*).

lies, or dermatoheliosis. Camouflaging is achieved by careful color selection and application techniques.

An attractive appearance can only be achieved if the dimension and location of the eyes fit proportionally on the face. Ideally, the eyes should be positioned on the face so that the inner canthal distance is equal to the width of one eye (Fig. 9–9). If the eyes are closer together, the patient appears hypoteloric; if the eyes are further apart, the patient appears hyperteloric. Hypoteloric eyes can be optically corrected by sweeping deeply colored eye shadow up and out from the center to the outer corners of the lid (Fig. 9–10*A*). Hyperteloric eyes are deemphasized by placing deeply

colored eye shadow from the inner canthus to the central eyelid (Fig. 9–10*B*).[6]

Deeply colored eye shadows can also be used effectively to correct the size of the eyes. The eyes can be made to appear larger if deeply colored eye shadow is placed along the lateral orbital ridge and eyebrow, with a small amount placed beneath the lateral lower lash line (Fig. 9–11*A*). A light-colored eye shadow should be placed medially beneath the eyebrow. Large eyes in a female patient with exophthalmos secondary to hyperthyroidism can be made to appear smaller by applying a dark eye shadow only in the crease and on the lateral eyelid (Fig. 9–11*B*). A light eye shadow is then placed on the medial eyelid.[7]

Probably the most common cosmetic eye problem seen in female patients is blepharochalasis, commonly

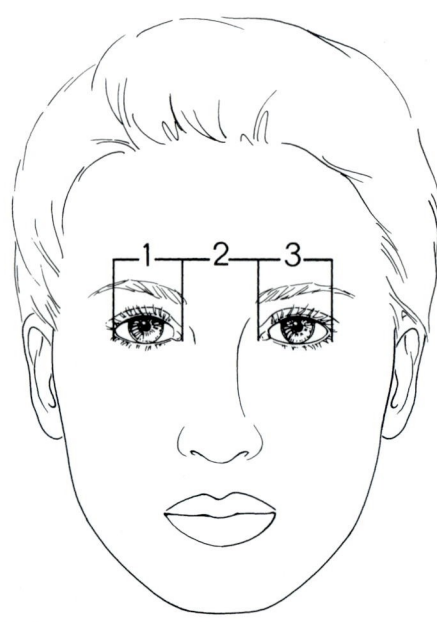

FIGURE 9–9 • Proper placement of the eyes on a well-proportioned face (see text).

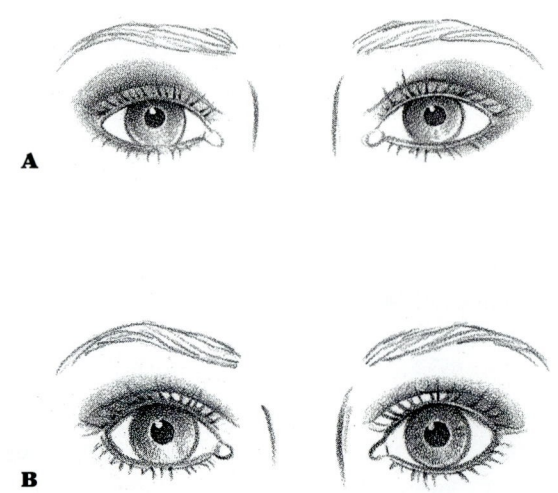

FIGURE 9–11 • Camouflage technique for small eyes (*A*) and large eyes (*B*).

should be used on the drooping eyelid to apply a line in the crease and above the lash line (Fig. 9–12B).

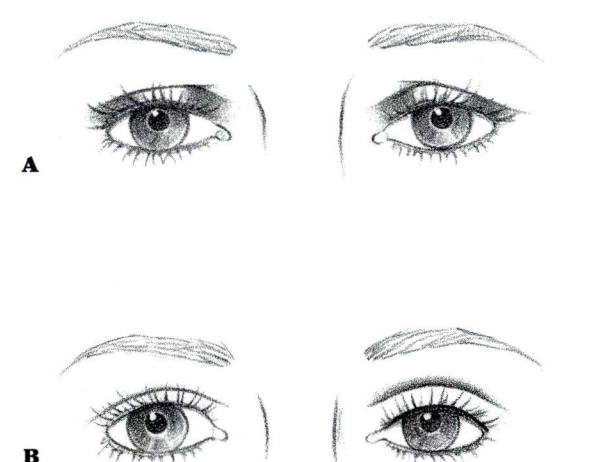

FIGURE 9–12 • Cosmetic correction for blepharochalasis (A) and a unilateral, drooping, upper eyelid (B) (see text).

known as drooping or hooded eyelids. A drooping eyelid can be corrected cosmetically by covering the entire eyelid from the lash line to the crease with a light, matte-finish eye shadow (Fig. 9–12A). A complementary matte-finish eye shadow two to three shades darker should then be applied on the medial and lateral eyelids, leaving the area above the iris a lighter color. Sometimes, unilateral ptosis develops following Bell's palsy or surgery. Normally, the upper eyelid should touch the superior border of the iris and the lower eyelid should touch the inferior border of the iris. More dramatic eye makeup should be applied to the drooping eyelid. A brown eye shadow crayon

REFERENCES

1. Fisher AA. Cosmetic dermatitis of the eyelids. Cutis 34:216–221, 1984.
2. Valsecchi R, Imberti G, Martino D, Cainelli T. Eyelid dermatitis: An evaluation of 150 patients. Contact Dermatitis 27:143–147, 1992.
3. Adams RM, Maibach HI. A five-year study of cosmetic reactions. J Am Acad Dermatol 13:1062–1069, 1985.
4. deGroot AC, Weyland JW, Nater JP. Face cosmetics. In Unwanted Effects of Cosmetics and Drugs Used in Dermatology. Amsterdam: Elsevier, 1994, pp. 513.
5. Pascher F. Adverse reactions to eye area cosmetics and their management. J Soc Cosmet Chem 33:249–258, 1982.
6. Greene A, Pomerance M. The Successful Face. New York: Summit Books, 1985, pp. 67–73.
7. Arpel A. 851 Fast Beauty Fixes and Facts. New York: GP Putnam's Sons, 1985, pp. 97–100.
8. Marks JG, DeLeo VA. Preservatives and vehicles. In Contact and Occupational Dermatology. St. Louis: CV Mosby, 1992, pp. 107–133.
9. White IR, Lovell CR, Cronin E. Antioxidants in cosmetics. Contact Dermatitis 11: 265–267, 1984.
10. Calnan CD. Ditertiary butylhydroquinone in eye shadow. Contact Dermatitis Newslett 14: 402, 1973.
11. Fisher AA. Allergic contact dermatitis due to rosin (colophony) in eyeshadow and mascara. Cutis 42:505–508, 1988.
12. Eiermann HJ, Larsen W, Maibach HI, Taylor JS. Prospective study of cosmetic reactions: 1977–1980. J Am Acad Dermatol 6: 909–917, 1982.
13. Schorr WF. Lip gloss and gloss-type cosmetics. Contact Dermatitis Newslett 14:408, 1973.
14. Hannuksela M, Pirila V, Salo OP. Skin reactions to propylene glycol. Contact Dermatitis 1:112–116, 1975.
15. Larsen WG. Cosmetic dermatitis due to a perfume. Contact Dermatitis 1:142–145, 1975.
16. Goh CL, Ng SK, Kwok SF. Allergic contact dermatitis from nickel in eyeshadow. Contact Dermatitis 20:380–381, 1989.

10

Eyelash Cosmetics

The physiologic role of eyelashes is to protect the eyeball from foreign objects; however, long eyelashes are considered desirable in women. This has led to the development of cosmetics designed to darken, lengthen, and curl the eyelashes. Presently available eyelash cosmetics include mascaras, eyeliners, and artificial eyelashes (Table 10–1).

1. Mascara

Mascara is designed to create luxuriant eyelashes, attracting attention to the expressive nature of the eyes. Mascaras are available in two modern formulations: cake and liquid. Cake mascara, demonstrated in Figure 10–1, is a pressed pigmented powder, much like

eye shadow. The cake is stroked with a water-moistened brush and applied to the eyelashes. Black cake mascara is an excellent choice for patients who have had difficulty wearing some of the newer mascara formulations.

Liquid mascara, the most popular formulation, is stroked on the eyelashes from a tube into which a round brush is inserted through a small aperture to remove a metered amount of product (Fig. 10–2).[1] The liquid mascaras can be further divided into water-based, solvent-based, and water/solvent hybrid formulations.

Water-based mascaras, in which water is the first ingredient listed, are classified as oil-in-water emulsions. These formulations allow the water to evaporate readily, creating a fast-drying product that thickens

TABLE 10–1 Eyelash Cosmetics

Eyelash Cosmetic	Main Ingredients	Function	Adverse Reactions
Cake mascara	Soap and pigments	To darken and thicken eyelashes	Irritation secondary to soaps
Cream mascara	Vanishing base and pigment	To darken and thicken eyelashes	Irritant contact dermatitis
Water-based liquid mascara	Waxes, pigments, and resins	To darken and thicken eyelashes	Irritant and allergic contact dermatitis
Solvent-based liquid mascara	Petroleum distillates, pigments, and waxes	To darken and thicken eyelashes	Irritant and allergic contact dermatitis
Water/solvent mascara	Water-in-oil or oil-in-water emulsion	To darken and thicken eyelashes	Irritant and allergic contact dermatitis
Cake eyeliner	Talc, pigment, and binders	To define the eyelash line	Minimal
Liquid eyeliner	Latex or other polymers and pigment	To define the eyelash line	Irritant contact dermatitis
Pencil eyeliner	Waxes and pigment	To define the eyelash line	Minimal
Artificial eyelashes	Human or synthetic hair fibers	To thicken eyelashes	Irritant contact dermatitis to lashes; allergic contact dermatitis to glue

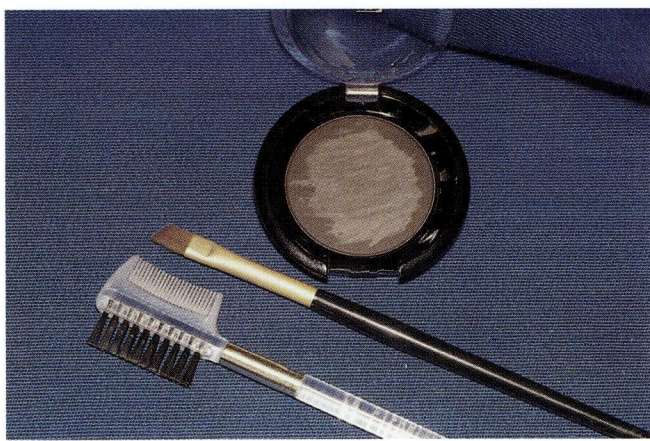

FIGURE 10–1 • A black, compressed, powdered cake can be stroked with the brush shown in the bottom of the picture and applied to the eyelashes as a mascara substitute in patients with eye cosmetic sensitivities.

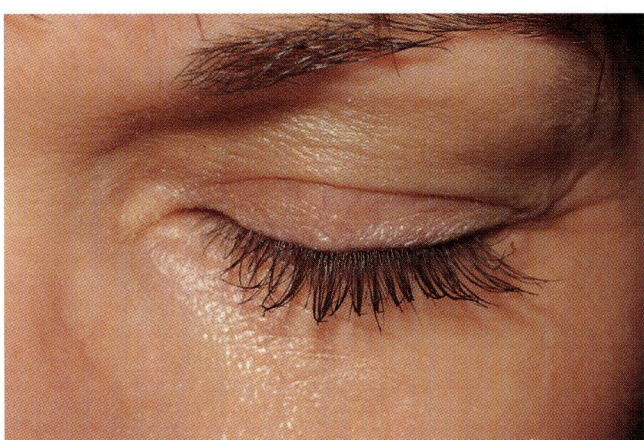

FIGURE 10–3 • Mascara produces a dramatic lengthening of the eyelashes.

and darkens the lashes. The product is water-soluble, allowing for easy removal, but unfortunately, it smudges with perspiration and tearing. Some water-based mascaras are labeled "water-resistant" if they contain an increased amount of wax or a polymer to improve adherence of pigment to the lashes. Water-based mascaras are easily contaminated with bacteria, which readily grow in water, and must include preservatives, usually parabens. Water-based mascaras are generally the least sensitizing of the mascara types and are recommended for patients with eye cosmetic problems.

Solvent-based mascaras are formulated with petroleum distillates to which pigments and waxes are added, thus making them waterproof (Fig. 10–3). As a result, the product performs well with perspiration and tearing, but special removal products are required. Preservatives are still added, but microbial contamina-

tion is not a great problem as the petroleum-based solvent is antibacterial. Individuals with recurrent bacterial infections secondary to colonization should select solvent-based mascaras and discard used mascara tubes after 3 months.[2]

Some mascaras combine both solvent-based and water-based systems to form either a water-in-oil or oil-in-water emulsion. The idea is to create an optimal product that thickens with a short drying time, like the water-based mascaras, but that provides waterproof lash separation, like a solvent-based mascara. The water in the formulation requires incorporation of a good preservative.

2. Eyeliner

Eyeliner defines the margins of the eye. It is placed immediately outside the lower and, possibly, along the upper lash line (Fig. 10–4). Eyeliner is available in

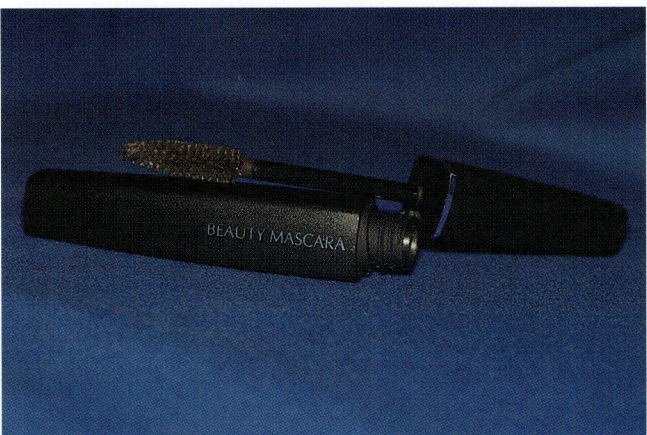

FIGURE 10–2 • The modern mascara tube applies a metered amount of cosmetic to the wand. The product can become contaminated, however, as the wand is reinserted into the tube. Mascaras should be discarded every 3 months.

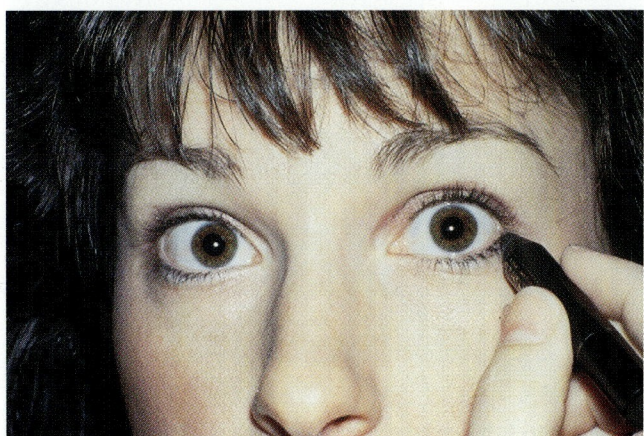

FIGURE 10–4 • Eyeliner can be applied to dramatize and frame the upper and lower eyelids.

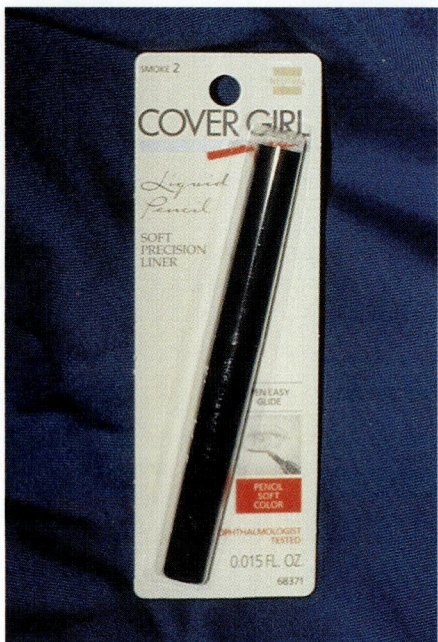

FIGURE 10–5 • In patients with eyelid dermatitis, the pencil-type eyeliner shown in Figure 10–4 is preferred over the automatic eyeliner pen shown here.

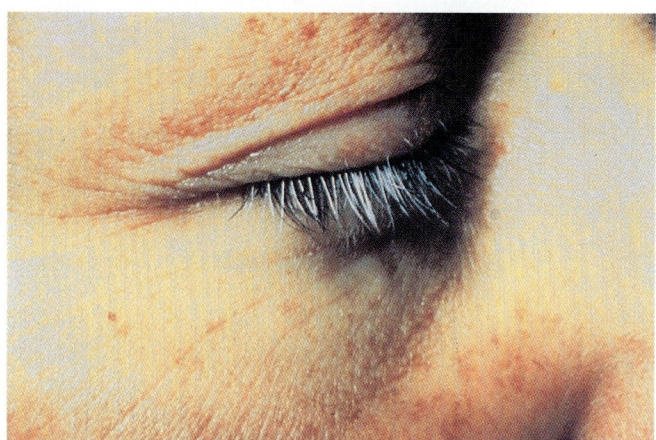

FIGURE 10–7 • Whitening of the eyelashes caused by eyelid vitiligo, which can be camouflaged by eyelash dyeing.

cake, liquid, and pencil forms. Cake eyeliner is used as a compressed powder that is stroked with a moistened brush to create a paste (see Fig. 10–1). It is the eyeliner of choice in patients with eyelid cosmetic problems.

Latex-based liquid eyeliners are packaged as marking pens or in the same form as mascaras, with a cylindrical tube and a unitufted applicator brush (Fig. 10–5). These eyeliners are a common source of both allergic and irritant contact dermatitis, but provide long lasting wear.

Pencil-type eyeliners are the most popular form due to their ease of application. New cosmetic is exposed

by sharpening the pencil, which also decreases the chances of contamination (see Fig. 10–4).

3. Eyelash Dyes

Eyelash dyes, identical to scalp hair dyes, are available to darken the color of the eyelashes; however, their use is not approved owing to the associated risk of blindness. Nevertheless, eyelash dyeing kits (Fig. 10–6) may be found in salons and are used to restore color to graying eyelashes (Fig. 10–7).

4. Artificial Eyelashes

Artificial eyelashes can be fashioned from synthetic or human hair and glued to the natural eyelashes with a clear or pigmented, methacrylate-based glue. The lashes are available as singlets (Fig. 10–8), demi-

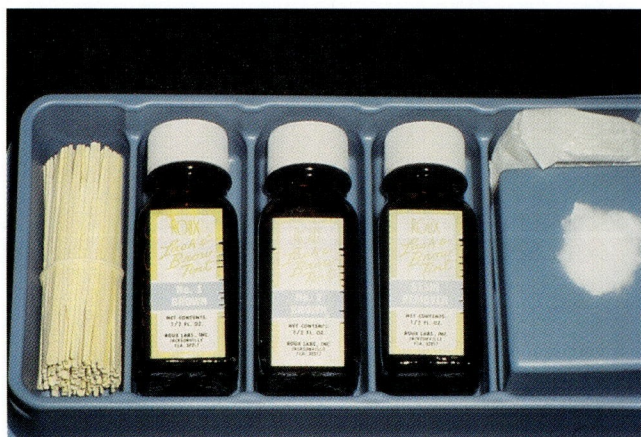

FIGURE 10–6 • Eyelash dyeing kits may be found in commercial salons. These kits are not approved by the FDA.

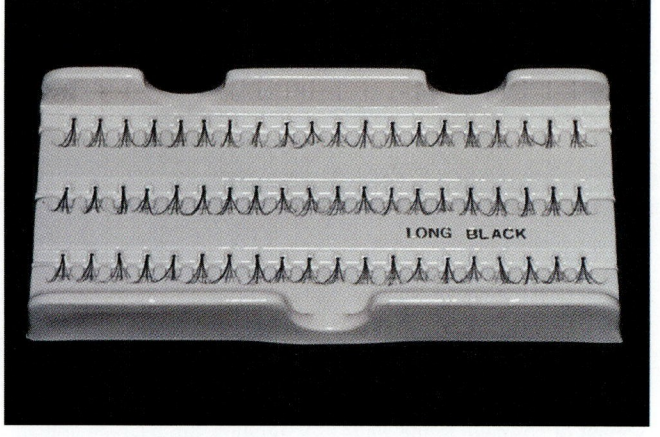

FIGURE 10–8 • Artificial eyelash singlets.

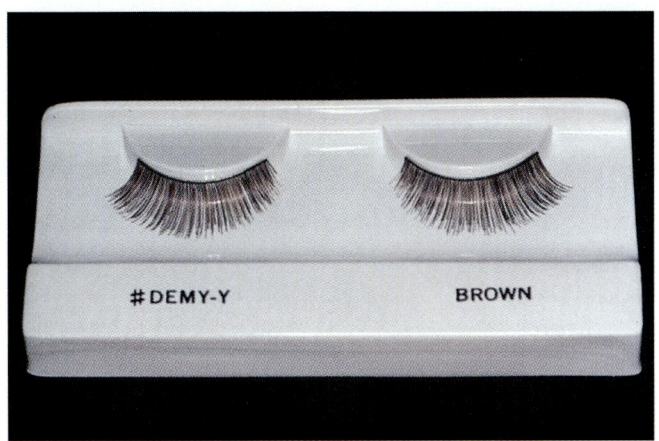

FIGURE 10–9 • A complete set of artificial eyelashes.

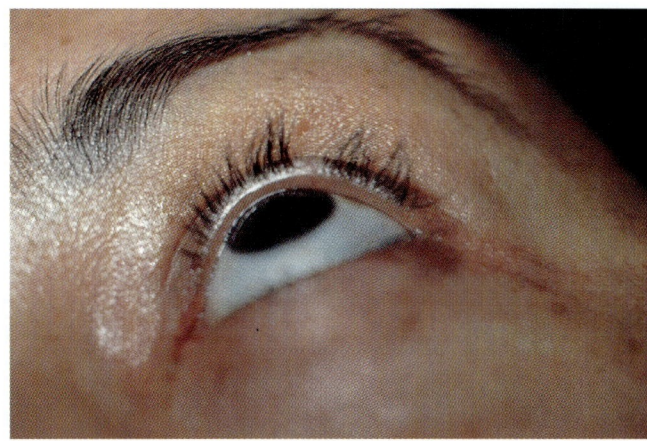

FIGURE 10–12 • Focal eyelash loss due to surgical scarring.

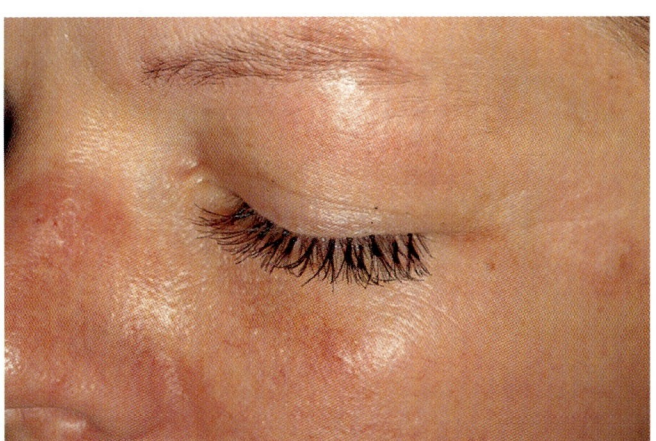

FIGURE 10–10 • The appearance of eyelash singlets in a patient with thinning eyelashes.

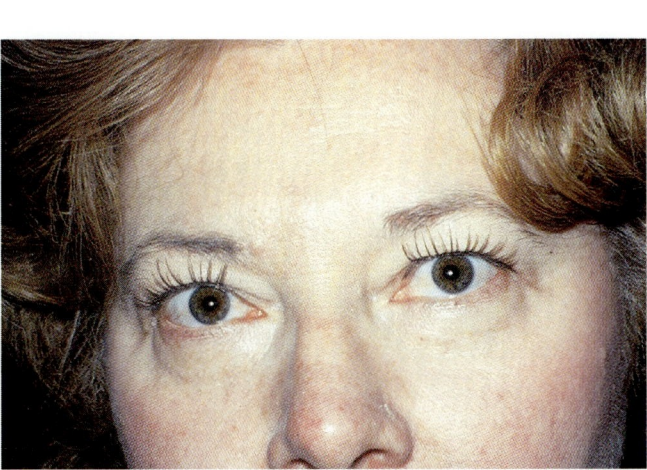

FIGURE 10–11 • The appearance of demilashes in a patient with almost complete absence of the eyelashes.

lashes, or complete eyelashes (Fig. 10–9). If lash singlets are used, several artificial lashes are glued to the patient's existing natural eyelashes (Fig. 10–10). Demilashes, which are sparse artificial lashes, and complete lashes, which are dense artificial lashes, are glued immediately above the existing lash line (Fig. 10–11). The eyelashes are removed with a solvent that is specially designed to remove the adhesive. Artificial eyelashes can easily be trimmed and customized with scissors.

5. Eyelash Camouflaging Cosmetics

Eyelashes function cosmetically as a frame for the eye. Unfortunately, they may thin due to age, alopecia areata, or eyelid scarring secondary to surgery or infections (Fig. 10–12). Eyeliner can be used to place dots where the eyelashes would normally appear (Fig. 10–13A). In female patients in whom all the eyelashes are missing, a brown or black liquid or pencil eyeliner should be used to rim the entire eye, except for one-quarter inch around the inner canthus on the upper and lower eyelids (Fig. 10–13B). Eyeliner can also be used to contour the eyes. For example, small eyes can be enlarged by lining the entire upper lash line and the lateral half of the lower lash line (Fig 10–13C). Hypoteloric eyes can be widened by lining the lateral half of both the upper and lower lash lines (Fig. 10–13D).

The apparent length of the eyelashes can also be increased by curling the lashes so that they are angled more acutely to the eyelid. Eyelash curlers may contain latex rubber and cause allergic contact dermatitis (Fig. 10–14).

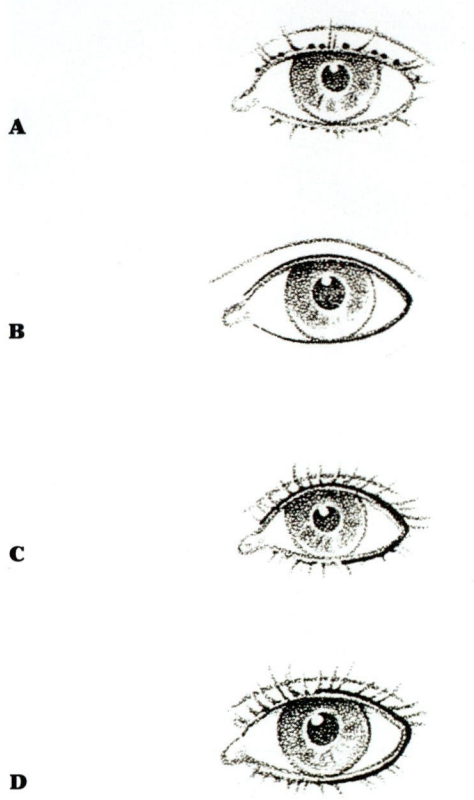

A

B

C

D

FIGURE 10–13 • Cosmetic camouflaging techniques for the eyelashes (see text).

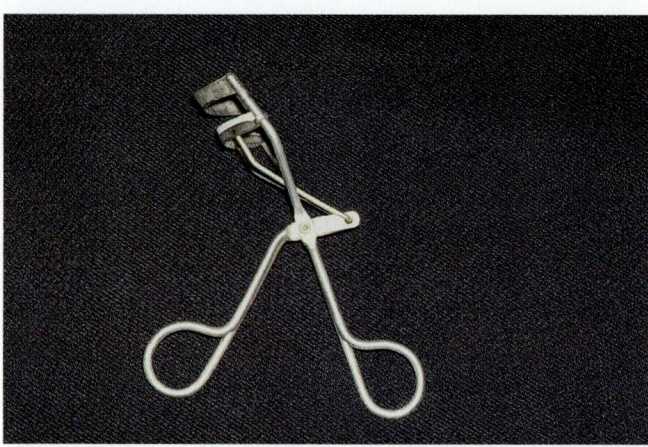

FIGURE 10–14 • Eyelash curlers can be used by mature individuals with shorter eyelashes to increase their apparent length.

REFERENCES

1. Lanzet M. Modern formulations of coloring agents: Facial and eye. In Frost P, Horwitz SN (eds.). Principles of Cosmetics for the Dermatologist. St. Louis: CV Mosby, 1982.
2. Ahem DG, Wilson LA, Julian AJ, et al. Microbial growth in eye cosmetics: Contamination during use. Dev Ind Microbiol 15:211–216, 1974.

11

Eyebrow Cosmetics

The eyebrows frame the eyes and, therefore, are the object of cosmetic adornment. Currently popular eyebrow cosmetics include pencils, sealers, dyes, and artificial eyebrows (Table 11–1).

1. Eyebrow Pencil

Eyebrow pencils are used to darken light or gray eyebrows, fill in sparse or absent eyebrow hairs, and reconstruct malformed or misshapen eyebrows (Fig. 11–1). They are stroked over the skin in the eyebrow region to color both the skin and eyebrow hairs (Fig. 11–2).[1]

2. Eyebrow Sealer

Eyebrow sealers are intended as a grooming agent for unruly eyebrows and a glossening agent to add shine to eyebrow hairs. A brush is used to stroke the product over the eyebrow hairs and groom the eyebrows (Fig. 11–3).

3. Eyebrow Dye

Eyebrow hair can be dyed in the same manner as scalp hair. This service is offered by many professional salons; however, hair dye packaging specifically states that the dyestuff is not to be used in the eye area and contains the following warning:

> "Caution—This product contains ingredients which may cause skin irritation on certain individuals, and a preliminary test according to accompanying directions should first be made. This product must not be used for dyeing the eyelashes or eyebrows; to do so may cause blindness."

The same dyes used for eyelashes (see Fig. 10–6) are also used for eyebrows.

4. Corrective Eyebrow Cosmetics

Corrective eyebrow cosmetics are designed to create the illusion of proper eyebrow placement on the face. Before cosmetic reconstruction can begin, it is important to identify the proper location of the eyebrow on the face, as demonstrated in Figure 11–4. Any hair removal to improve eyebrow appearance should be from the inferior aspect of the eyebrow. Hairs should never be removed from the superior border, as this will disturb the natural eyebrow contour.

TABLE 11–1 Eyebrow Cosmetics

Eyebrow Cosmetic	Main Ingredients	Function	Adverse Reactions
Eyebrow pencil	Pigment, wax, petrolatum, lanolin	To darken and thicken eyebrows	Minimal
Eyebrow sealer	Synthetic polymer	Used as an eyebrow hair grooming agent	Minimal
Eyebrow dye	Metallic dyes, stains, or permanent dyes	To darken eyebrow hairs	May be illegal and may cause blindness, contact dermatitis

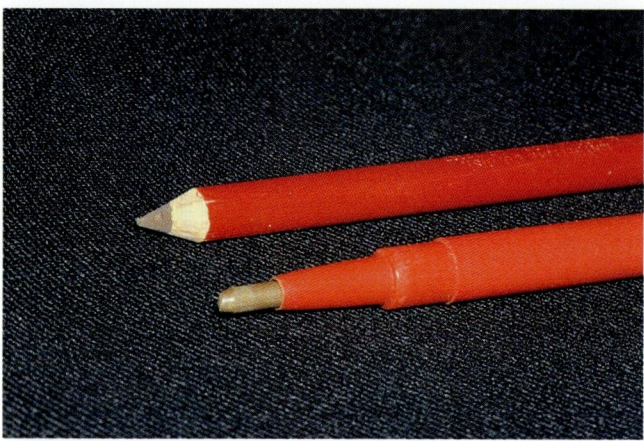

FIGURE 11–1 • Eyebrow pencils are pigmented wax sticks used to draw eyebrow hairs on the skin surface.

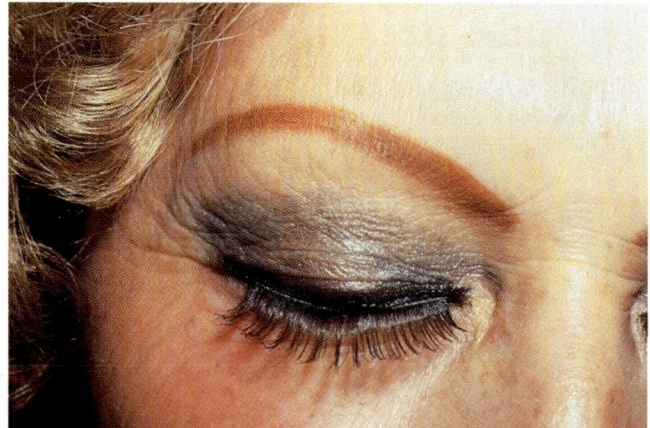

FIGURE 11–2 • This patient with leprosy has used an eyebrow pencil to reconstruct the appearance of eyebrows and is also wearing artificial eyelashes.

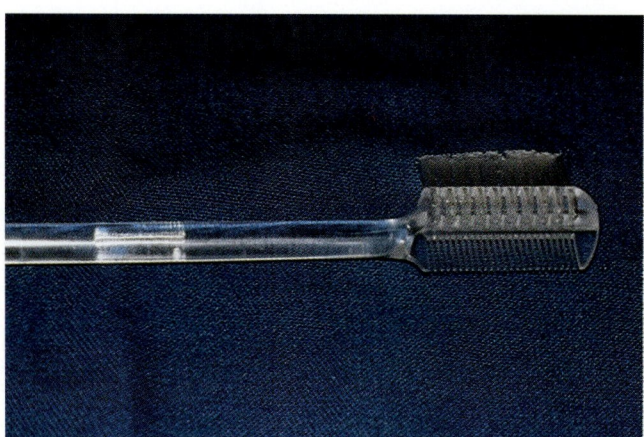

FIGURE 11–3 • An eyebrow brush may be useful in grooming the eyebrows, which can then be held in place by a fixative, such as an eyebrow sealer or a small amount of hair styling gel.

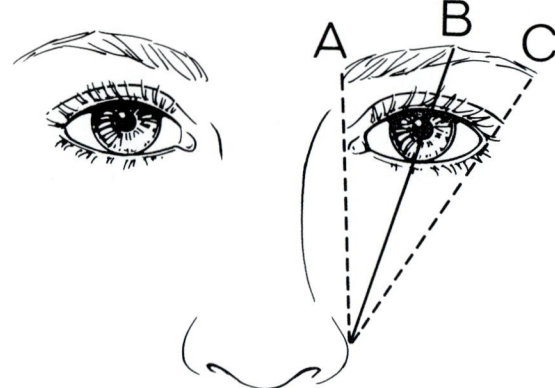

FIGURE 11–4 • The eyebrows must be reconstructed in the proper position on the face. The medial aspect of the eyebrow should begin at a point defined by a straight line drawn from the lateral nose upward. The eyebrow should maximally arch at a point defined by a line drawn from the lateral nose through the pupil. The eyebrow should end at a point defined by a line drawn from the lateral nose through the lateral aspect of the eyeball.

Improper placement of the eyebrows can alter facial expression and the appearance of the eyes (Fig. 11–5). Eyebrows that are placed too far apart give the impression of surprise and can make the patient appear hyperteloric (Fig. 11–5*B*), whereas eyebrows that are too close together give an angry, intense look and impart hypotelorism (Fig. 11–5*C*).

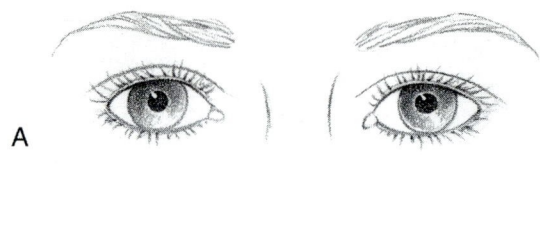

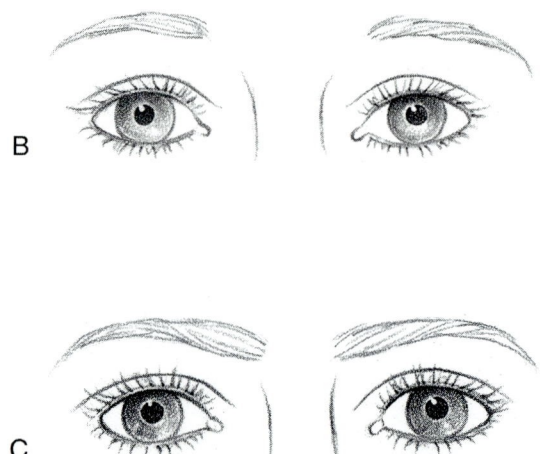

FIGURE 11–5 • Proper spacing of the eyebrows (*A*) is illustrated. Eyebrows that are too far apart (*B*) or too closely spaced (*C*) create an unattractive facial expression (see text).

The illusion of normal eyebrow placement may be achieved with an eyebrow pencil, which can be used to draw absent hairs. A more natural appearance is created if the pencil is used in short strokes, rather than one straight line.[2] The eyebrow pencil will wear longer if the skin is first covered with a facial foundation.

REFERENCES

1. Klarmann EG. Cosmetic Chemistry for the Dermatologist. Springfield, Il: Charles C Thomas, 1962, pp. 53–54.
2. Allsworth J. Skin Camouflage. Cheltenham, England: Stanley Thornes Ltd, 1985, pp. 41–42.

12

Lip Cosmetics

Lip cosmetics are valuable, not only for accentuating the lips, but also for providing lip lubrication and sun protection. There are several types of lip cosmetics, including lipsticks, lip crayons, lip creams, lip liners, and lip sealers, as pictorially demonstrated (Table 12–1).

1. Lipstick

Lipstick is an extruded rod of color dispersed in a blend of oils, waxes, and fats and packaged in a roll-up tube. It is applied by stroking the pigmented rod across the lips (Fig. 12–1). The product must be artistically applied to color the entire vermilion border, yet create a smooth, even, pleasant lip outline. The out-line of the lips can be drawn in any fashion desired, making lipstick a useful camouflage cosmetic in patients with a lip deformity.

Lip cosmetics can be formulated to impart color to the lips for 8 hours or more. Obviously, the lipstick film will not stay on the lips this long, but the lips can be stained to impart long-lasting color. The most common stain employed is acid eosin, a tetrabromo derivative of fluorescein, unfortunately it is also a source of allergic contact dermatitis (Fig. 12–2).

Opaque lipsticks can be created by adding high concentrations of titanium dioxide to the formulation. These lipsticks provide excellent sun protection and can be used to camouflage underlying lip pigmentation defects (Fig. 12–3).

TABLE 12–1 Lip Cosmetics

Lipsticks	Appearance	Coverage	Wearability	Main Ingredients
Lipsticks				
Pigmented	Matte	Full	Moderate	Wax, oil, pigment
Frosted	Pearlescent	Full	Moderate	Wax, oil, pigment
Transparent	Shiny	Very sheer	Short	High percentage of oil, soluble dyes
Indelible	Matte	Moderate	Very long	Wax, oil, bromo acid dyes
Lip crayons	Pearlescent or matte	Full	Moderate	Wax, less oil than in lipsticks, pigment
Lip liners	Matte	Not applicable	Long	Wax, pigment
Lip creams and gloss pots	Shiny	Sheer	Very short	Petrolatum, oil, pigment
Lip sealants	Matte	Not applicable	Long	Water, glycerin, wax, oil, dimethicone
Lip balm	Matte	None	Long	Wax, mineral oil, chemical sunscreen

Reprinted from Draelos ZD. Cosmetics in Dermatology, 2nd ed. New York: Churchill Livingstone, 1996, with permission.

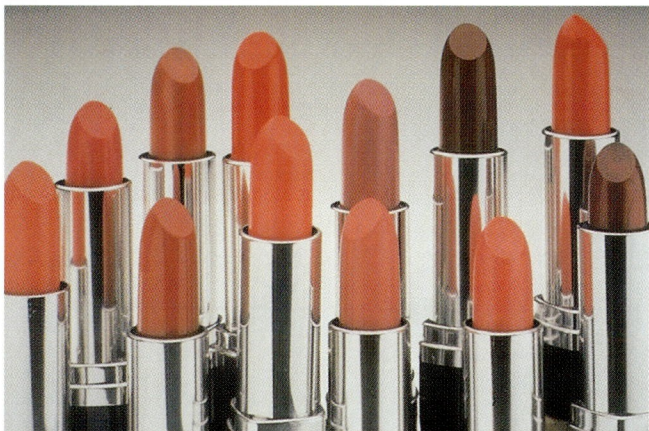

FIGURE 12–1 • Lipsticks are available in a tremendous variety of colors to suit every mood.

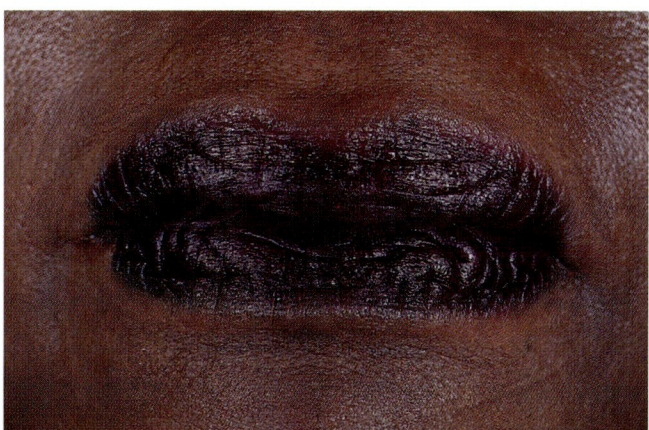

FIGURE 12–2 • A case of allergic contact dermatitis caused by a long-wearing lipstick containing eosin.

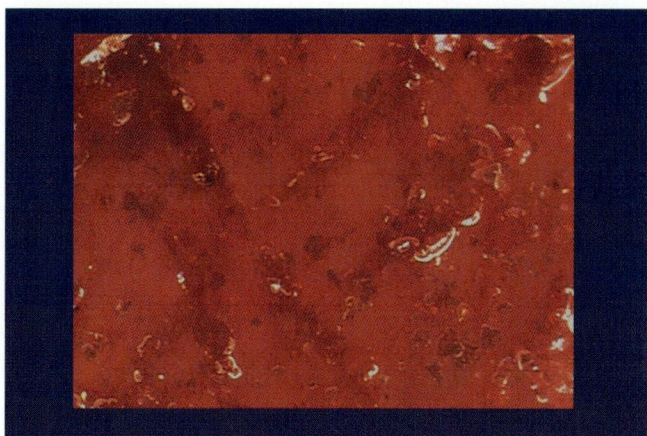

FIGURE 12–3 • As shown by video microscope (X400), lipstick leaves an even opaque film over the lips, providing excellent sun protection.

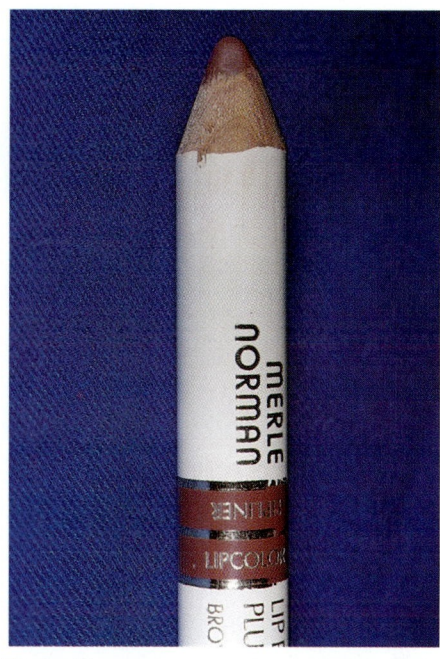

FIGURE 12–4 • Lip crayons contain waxes encased in a wood tube, which is then sharpened to expose new cosmetic, thereby decreasing the chances of contamination.

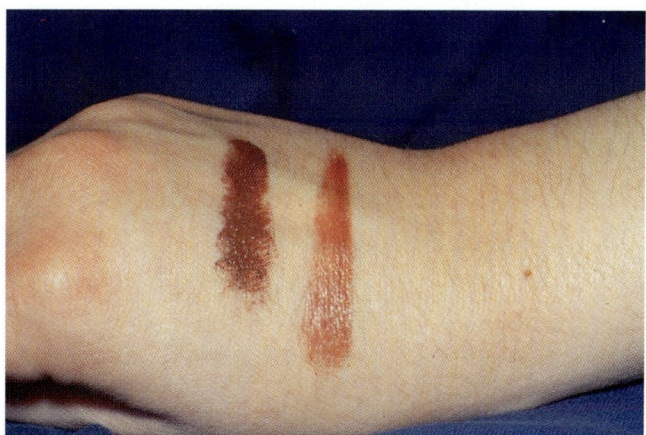

FIGURE 12–5 • Lip creams create opaque color when applied to the skin.

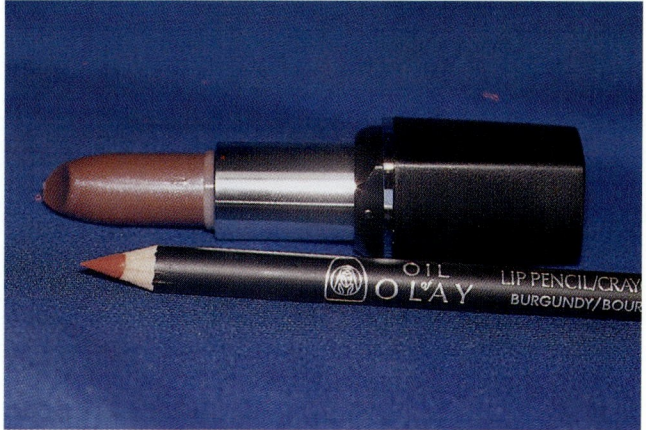

FIGURE 12–6 • Lip liners prevent lipstick from migrating into the furrows on the upper and lower lips.

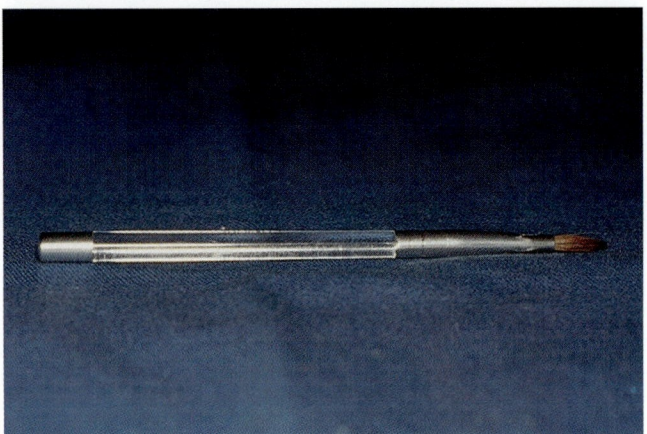

FIGURE 12–7 • A lip brush is a valuable tool when performing lip camouflage.

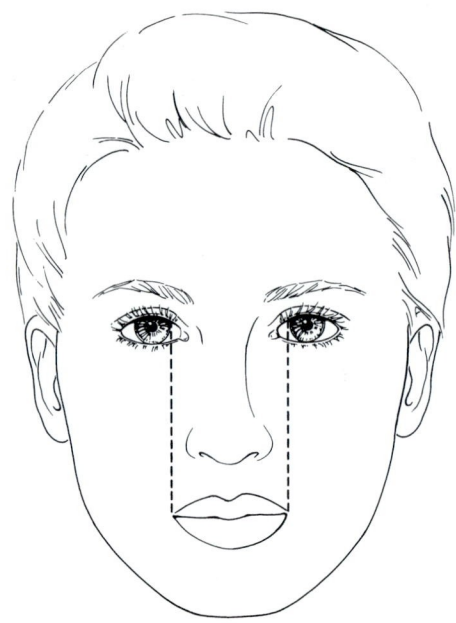

FIGURE 12–8 • The ideal position of the lips on the face.

2. Lip Crayons

Lip crayons are formed by encasing the extruded rod in wood. Sharpening with a pencil-type sharpener is required to expose the product. Lip crayons allow precise application of lip color and are useful for camouflaging purposes (Fig. 12–4).

3. Lip Cream and Lip Gloss

Lip creams and glosses differ from lipsticks and lip crayons in that they are packaged in a small jar and rolled on or applied with the finger. The cream formu-

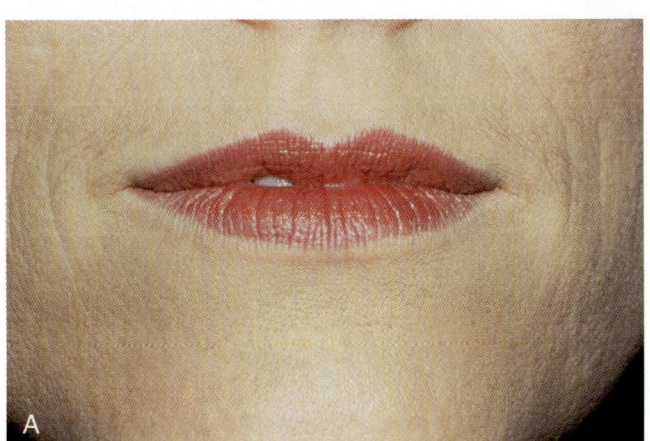

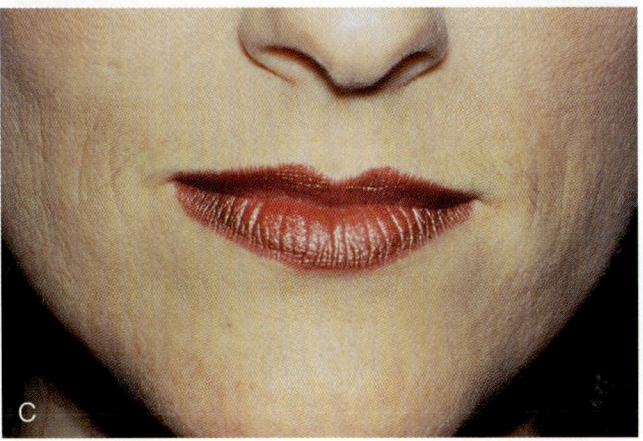

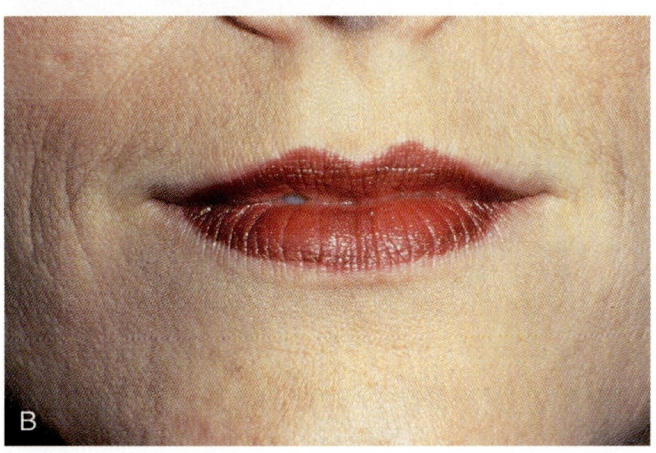

FIGURE 12–9 • The lips lined at the vermilion border (A). Notice that lining the lips inside the vermilion border shrinks the size of the lips (B), whereas lining them outside the vermilion border enlarges the apparent size of the lips (C).

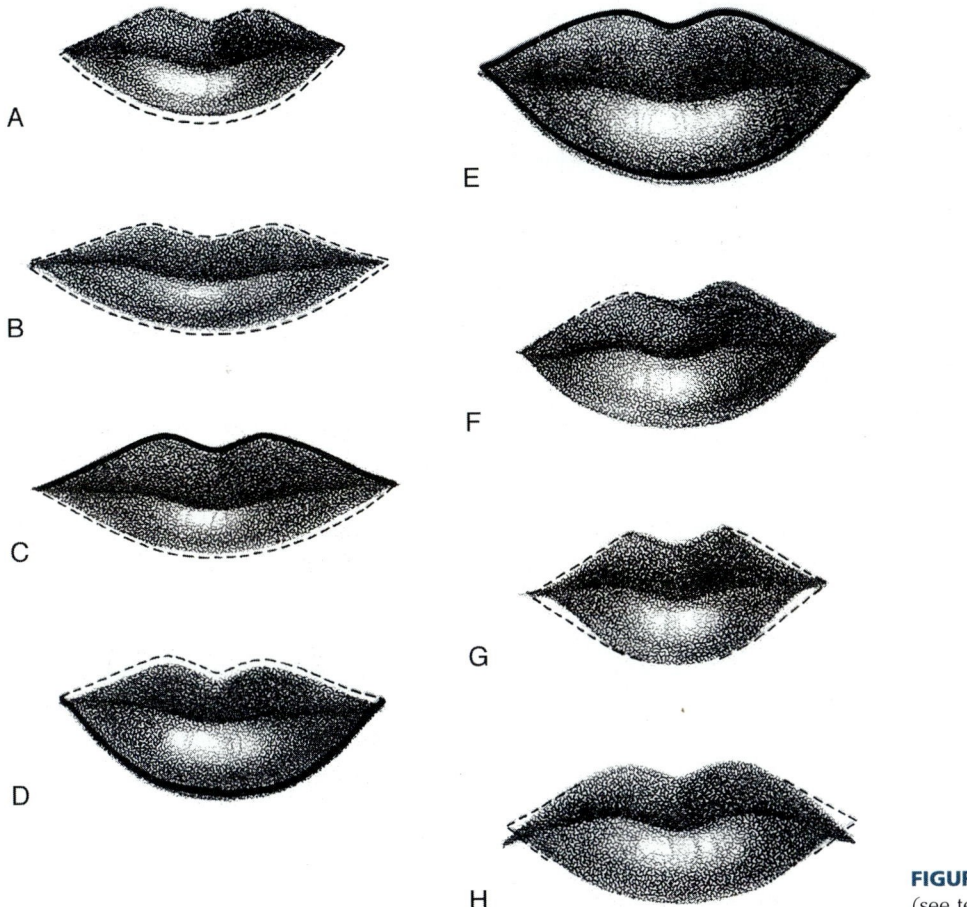

FIGURE 12–10 • Methods of lip camouflage (see text).

lation is obtained by lowering the wax content, increasing the oil content, and using waxes with a lower melting point. Lip cream is usually an opaque lip cosmetic, whereas gloss pots provide transparent color to the lips (Fig. 12–5).

4. Lip Liner

Lip liners are thin extruded rods encased in wood or placed in an automatic pencil-type holder. Their formulation is similar to that of lipsticks except that stiffer waxes with higher melting points are used, with minimal oil. This creates an extremely hard rod that applies a thick layer of pigment to the lips. Lip liners are used to define the outer edge of the lips and are valuable in reconstructing a normal lip contour (Fig. 12–6). The thick wax layer applied around the lips also prevents creamier lip products from bleeding. A lip liner that is one to two shades darker than the lipstick is usually selected.

5. Lip Sealant

Lip sealants prevent movement of lipstick into the fine lines around the lips. This is especially important in mature women. The cream is applied to the lips like lipstick or with the finger and allowed to dry before a pigmented lip cosmetic is applied.

6. Lip-contouring Cosmetics

Abnormal lip shape secondary to congenital causes or surgery can be masked by effective application of lip cosmetics utilizing a lipstick brush (Fig. 12–7). A well-proportioned mouth in a closed, relaxed state is ideally positioned between the medial aspect of the irises (Fig. 12–8).[1] Lips that do not extend this distance are perceived as either small or large (Fig. 12–9). Small lips can be enlarged by using a lip liner to draw the lip boundary on the outer edge of the vermilion border and then filling in with a deeply pigmented, matte-finish lipstick (Fig. 12–10A). Uniformly thin lips (Fig. 12–10B), a thin lower lip, possibly due to lip advancement surgery (Fig. 12–10C), or a thin upper lip (Fig. 12–10D) can be thickened by also lining outside the vermilion border where required, and by selecting a lighter, frosted-finish lipstick. Conversely, thick lips, possibly due to a congenital hemangioma, may be lined inside the vermilion border (Fig. 12–10E). Also demonstrated is the lip lining technique (see the dashed line) for crooked (Fig. 12–10F), bow (Fig. 12–10G), and down-turned lips (Fig. 12–10H).

REFERENCE

1. Powell N, Humphreys B. Proportions of the Aesthetic Face. New York: Thieme-Stratton, 1984, pp. 32–34.

13

Micropigmentation

Dermatologic micropigmentation refers to the art of implanting small amounts of color into the skin for cosmetic adornment, camouflaging, or reconstructive purposes. In other words, micropigmentation is medical tatooing utilizing the same basic techniques, equipment, and pigments as the nonmedical tatoo artist.

A number of companies manufacture equipment and pigments specifically for micropigmentation, although some tatoo artists use a more traditional tatoo machine and traditional tatoo pigments (Fig. 13–1). Companies that manufacture micropigmentation products for the medical community are Permark; Dermouflage Clinics, Inc.; Natural Eyes (Alcon); Lasting Impressions I; and Accents. The pigments used to obtain the various colors are standardized and listed in Table 13–1. They can be mixed in 70% isopropyl alcohol or ethyl alcohol and glycerin. Pigments must be combined and blended to match the color of the structure to be reconstructed or enhanced. For example, placing pigment in vitiliginous skin requires matching the

existing skin color created by endogenous pigment sources (Table 13–2). Color mixing is certainly part of the art of micropigmentation.

Micropigmentation may be used for a variety of reasons. It can be used to enhance normal facial structures in the form of permanent color for the lips (Fig. 13–2), eyebrows, and eyelids (Fig. 13–3). Surgical deformities may also be corrected through the use of color applied to simulate eyelashes, eyebrows, or the breast areola. Dermal pigmentation can be performed to restore color to burn contractures, surgical scars, or skin affect by vitiligo.

The histologic reaction produced by the introduction of inert pigment into the skin is an acute inflammatory response initiated by the mechanical disruption of the skin secondary to the micropigmentation needle. This reaction continues for 1 to 2 weeks and is followed by aggregation of lymphocytes and macrophages around the pigment granules. Some of the granules are phagocytized by the macrophages and moved toward vascular and lymphatic structures. Mild

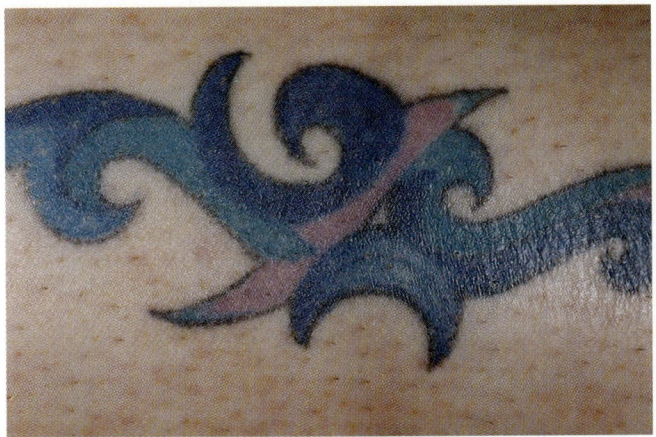

FIGURE 13–1 • Traditional tatoo pigments are blended for use in micropigmentation.

TABLE 13–1 Micropigmentation Color Composition

White	Yellow
Titanium dioxide	Cadium sulfate
Zinc oxide	Iron oxide
Barium sulfate	Red
Black	Mercuric sulfide (cinnabar)
Carbon	Cadmium selenide
Iron Oxide	Alizarin
Brown	Violet
Iron oxide (ochre)	Manganese oxide
Blue	Green
Cobaltous aluminate	Chromic oxide
	Chromium sesquioxide

Adapted from Zwerling CS, Walker AC, Goldstein NF. Micropigmentation. Hands on Productions, 1993.

TABLE 13–2 **Endogenous Skin Pigments**

· · · · · ·

Skin Color	Endogenous Pigment
Brown, black	Melanoproteins
Yellow, red	Pheomelanins
Yellow	Indoles
Red	Dopachromes
Red, blue	Hemoglobins, vasculature
Yellow	Carotenes

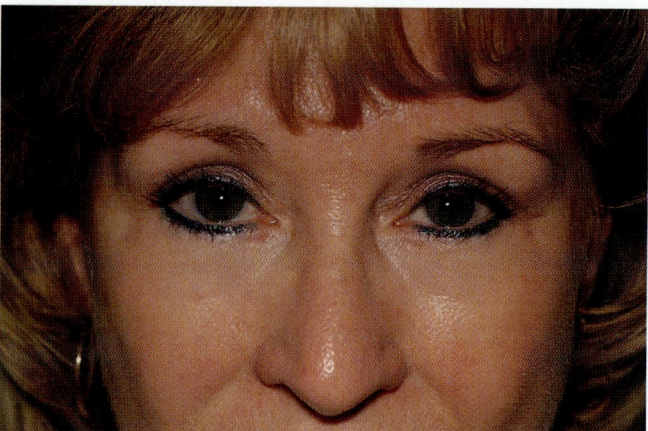

FIGURE 13–3 • Blue and green pigments can be blended to produce permanent eyeliner on the upper and lower lids in fashionable colors.

fibrosis persists indefinitely in the papillary dermis. Untoward histologic reactions may include the formation of giant epithelioid cells, granulomatous inflammation, and a foreign body–type reaction.

For all practical purposes, micropigmentation is permanent, and both the practitioner and patient should keep this fact in mind at all times. It is better to apply too little pigment than too much; likewise, it is better to apply subtle color rather than bold color, and understatement is preferred to overstatement (Fig. 13–4). In most cases, extensive pigment placement should be performed in stages, over a period of weeks to months, to allow the patient to evaluate each phase of micropigmentation.

Expected side effects include pigment migration and loss. The pigment granules for micropigmentation are intentionally sized at 6 μm or larger, as tissue macrophages have a limited ability to phagocytize and move particles of this size. Nevertheless, some migration does occur. Pigment migration occurs as granules are moved along the ducts of sebaceous glands, a phenomenon most pronounced in eyelid micropigmentation, which creates a "halo" around the eyelashes. Pigment placement too deep on the eyelids can allow the granules to migrate along connective tissue planes.

Infection and scarring can occur if the micropigmentation practitioner is careless. Micropigmentation needles and pigments should be sterilized prior to use to prevent the spread of both bacterial and viral disease.

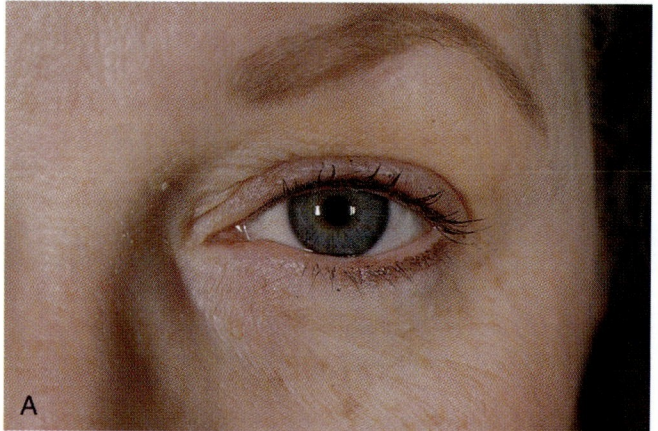

A

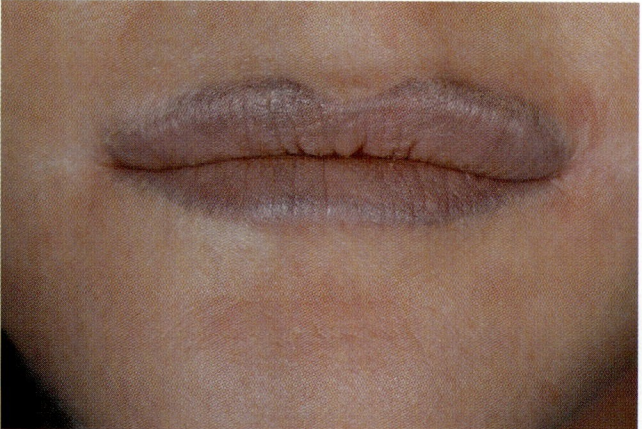

FIGURE 13–2 • Micropigmentation can be performed outside the vermilion border of the lips to create permanent lip liner and enlarge the appearance of the lips.

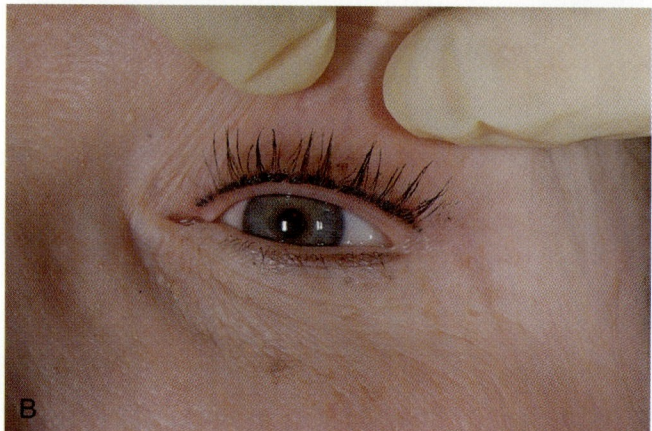

B

FIGURE 13–4 • Subtle eyeliner placement (*A*) is accomplished by placing the pigment beneath the eyelashes on the edge of the tarsal plate (*B*).

14

Postsurgical Cosmetics

The postsurgical patient emerges with a new self-image, regardless of whether the surgery was therapeutic or cosmetic.[1] Often, the patient may view therapeutic surgery as deforming and may experience a period of depression during which he/she withdraws from social situations with family and friends. Even when an elective cosmetic procedure is performed, there is a brief time when uncertainty about the positive outcome of the surgery may cause emotional problems for the patient. The dermatologist should anticipate these difficulties and provide recommendations for the use of postsurgical cosmetics.

1. Immediate Postoperative Period

Skin in the postsurgical patient no longer functions as a barrier to the external environment. Therefore, all applied substances have much greater access to the dermal vasculature. This increases the probability of experiencing adverse reactions to topical products, including irritation (stinging, burning, itching, tingling), sensitization, and urticaria. Products must be carefully selected to meet the strictest standards of hypoallergenicity in the postsurgical patient. Unusual erythema or vesicle formation in and around the postsurgical site should clue the clinician to look for cutaneous adverse reactions to a topically applied cosmetic, skin care product, or medicament (Fig. 14–1).

Immediately following surgery, cosmetics should not be applied to wounds that are healing by either primary or secondary intention. This generally is not a problem, as cosmetics will not adhere to skin until serous drainage from the wound has stopped. Premature application of cosmetics can create problems related to foreign bodies or milia due to the particulate matter in the formulations (Fig. 14–2). Therefore, facial foundations and all other cosmetics should be avoided until reepithelialization has occurred or the sutures have been removed.

2. Cleansers

Cleansers in the postoperative period should be nonirritating so as to minimize damage to newly formed epithelium. In the immediate postoperative period, lukewarm water may be the only cleanser required (Fig. 14–3). As serum crusting begins, however, a synthetic detergent soap (Oil of Olay Sensitive Skin Foaming Fash Wash [Procter & Gamble]) can provide gentle cleansing without damaging the healing cutaneous barrier. If infection is suspected, an antibacterial soap containing triclosan (Dial Liquid [Dial Corporation]) may speed resolution.

3. Moisturizers

Moisturizers are an important part of skin care in the postsurgical patient, as the barrier to transepidermal water loss is absent. Loss of the barrier allows in-

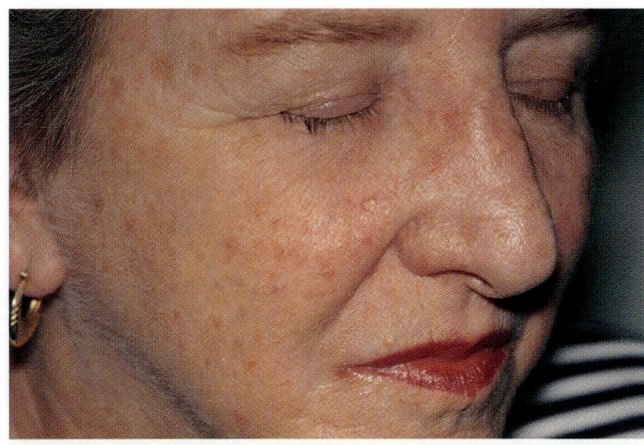

FIGURE 14–1 • This patient developed an irritant contact dermatitis secondary to using her alpha-hydroxy acid facial moisturizer too soon following a trichloroacetic (TCA) face peel.

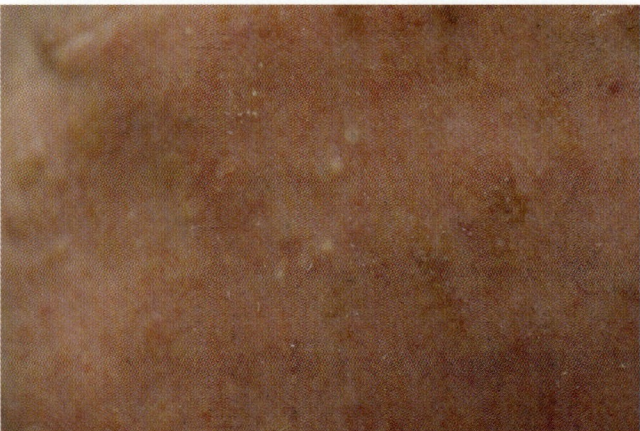

FIGURE 14–2 • Milia, frequent sequelae of dermabrasion, may be more numerous if facial foundation is applied before initial reepithelialization is complete.

creased water evaporation from the skin, producing tightness, stinging, and pruritus. Furthermore, desiccation impedes wound healing, which proceeds most rapidly in a moist environment (Fig. 14–4).

In the immediate postoperative period, pure white petroleum jelly may be the best moisturizer. It is an excellent occlusive agent, temporarily providing a barrier to transepidermal water loss. It is used as a negative control for dermatologic patch testing; thus, its irritation and sensitization potentials are low.

Once reepithelialization has begun, oil-in-water formulations that are more cosmetically pleasing may be substituted (Cetaphil cream [Galderma]). Creams should be selected over lotions, as they have greater moisturizing ability and are less likely to contain irritating vehicles. Products should be chosen for their paucity of ingredients. Therefore, creams with fragrances, herbal or biological additives, and specialty

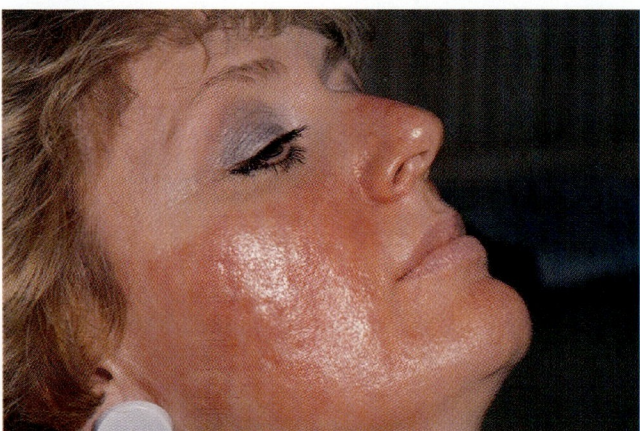

FIGURE 14–3 • Mild cleansing is important following dermabrasion.

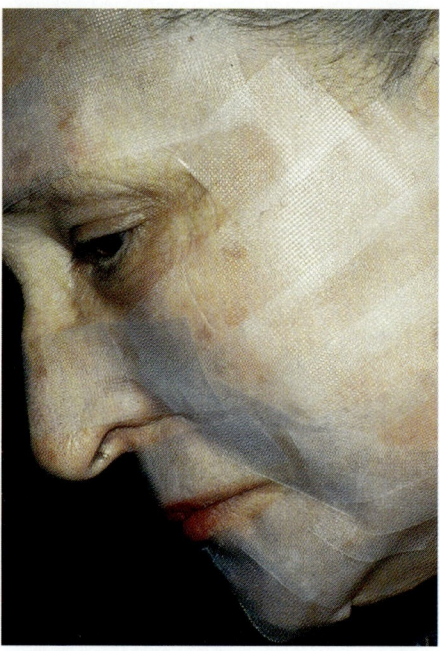

FIGURE 14–4 • White petroleum jelly provides excellent control of transepidermal water loss immediately following a taped TCA peel.

ingredients should be avoided until complete healing has occurred.

4. Sunscreens

Sun exposure of the surgical site should be avoided immediately following surgery, as the skin cannot protect against photodamage. Once reepithelialization has occurred, sun exposure should be minimized to prevent postinflammatory hyperpigmentation and the recurrence of melasma, both of which are ultraviolet (UVA) light–induced phenomena (Fig. 14–5). Daily application of a sunscreen, containing moisturizer with a broad-spectrum particulate sun block (such as microfine zinc oxide), is recommended over the reepithelialized site (Oil of Olay Daily Complete UV Protectant [Procter & Gamble]).

5. Facial Foundations

Facial foundations are designed to add color, cover blemishes, and blend uneven facial color. Postsurgical patients have all of these needs, and facial foundations are an excellent method of camouflaging postsurgical erythema (Fig. 14–6). Facial foundations appropriate for blending erythema do not require the high coverage necessary for surgical camouflaging. Table 14–1 lists product recommendations.

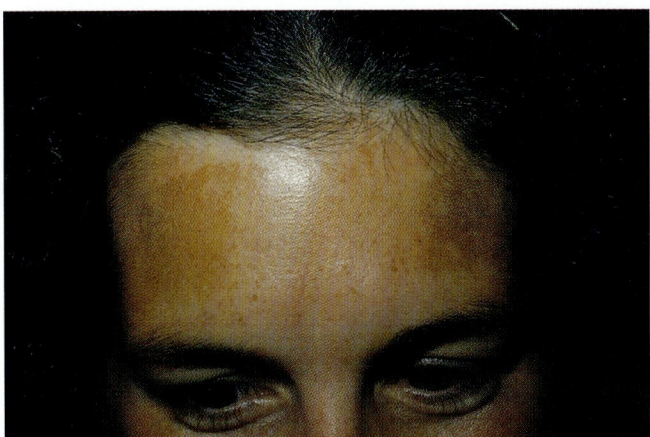

FIGURE 14–5 • Broad-spectrum UVB/UVA protection, in the form of a sunscreen containing moisturizer, is especially important following face peels to prevent the recurrence of melasma.

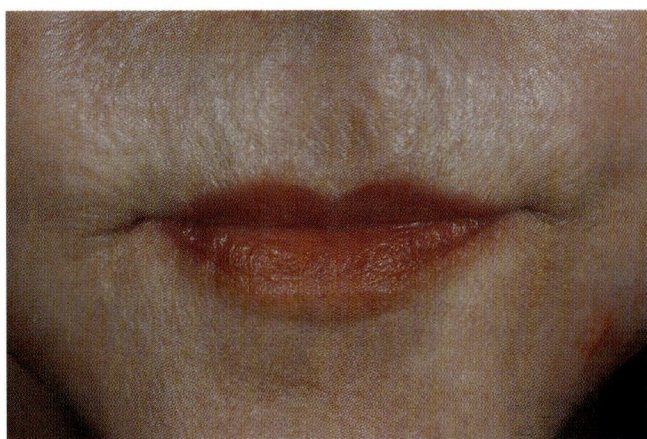

FIGURE 14–6 • The permanent, long-term hypopigmentation seen following laser resurfacing, especially around the mouth, can be camouflaged with use of a high-coverage facial foundation.

6. Postsurgical Cover Creams

Cover creams are also facial foundations, except that they are designed to provide opaque cover, thus completely obscuring the underlying skin. They are formulated as creams, sticks, and compressed powders. Cream and stick formulations may be waterproof, whereas the compressed powders are not. Table 14–2 lists recommendations for postsurgical cover creams.[2] Additional discussion and photographs relating to the use of postsurgical cover creams may be found in Chapter 15.

7. Color Correctors

Color correctors are liquid or cream facial foundations in specialty colors designed to aid in the blending of unwanted skin tones.[3] They contain pigment complementary to the color of the defect because the combination of complementary colors yields brown. Table 14–3 lists appropriate color correctors based on the color of the underlying skin deformity. This topic is more fully discussed in Chapter 15.

8. Camouflage Techniques for Dermatologic Procedures

Surgical dermatologic procedures may require short-term camouflaging until complete healing occurs. Table 14–4 details recommendations for camouflaging abnormalities created by a variety of common dermatologic procedures.

Some dermatologic surgical procedures, such as Moh's surgery or flaps or grafts, destroy appendageal

TABLE 14–1   Recommended Facial Foundations for Postsurgical Patients

Foundation Name	Formulation	Color Selection	Purchase Site
Waterproof Creme Makeup (Max Factor)	Cream	Medium	Mass merchandiser
Workout Makeup (Clinique)	Cream	Fair to medium	Cosmetic counter
Soft Finish Compact Makeup (Estée Lauder)	Cream/powder	Fair to medium	Cosmetic counter
Flawless Finish (Elizabeth Arden)	Cream/powder	Medium to dark	Cosmetic counter
Dual Finish Creme/Powder Makeup (Lancome)	Cream/powder	Fair to dark	Cosmetic counter
Perfect Finish Cream Makeup (Fashion Fair Cosmetics)	Cream	Dark	Cosmetic counter

TABLE 14–2 Recommended Postsurgical Cover Creams

Trade Name	Company Address	Trade Name	Company Address
Corrective Concepts	Pattee Products European Crossroads 2829 West Northwest Highway Dallas, Texas 75220	Dermablend	Dermablend Corrective Cosmetics PO Box 3008 Lakewood, New Jersey 08701
Coverette	Ben Nye Company, Inc. 5935 Bowcroft Street Los Angeles, California 90016	Dermaceal	Joe Blasco Cosmetics 1708 Hillhurst Avenue Hollywood, California 90027
Covermark	Lydia O'Leary 1 Anderson Avenue Moonachie, New Jersey 07074	Dermacolor	Kryolan Corporation 132 Ninth Street San Francisco, California 94103
Cover Tone	Fashion Fair Cosmetics 820 South Michigan Avenue Chicago, Illinois 60605	Natural Cover	LS Cosmetics PO Box 32203 Baltimore, Maryland 21208
Cream Makiage	Il-Makiage PO Box 1064 Long Island City, New York 11101	Veil	Atelier Esthetique 386 Park Avenue South Suite 209 New York, New York 10016

TABLE 14–3 Color Corrector Selection for Postsurgical Dyspigmentation

Color of Dyspigmentation	Surgical Situation	Color Corrector Selection
Red	Healing cutaneous wound	Green
Blue	Postsurgical bruising	Peach
Tan	Postinflammatory hyperpigmentation	White
Yellow/gold	Hemosiderin deposition	Purple
White	Pigment cell loss	Brown

TABLE 14–4 Postsurgical Camouflaging for Dermatologic Procedures

Procedure	Postsurgical Deformity	Camouflage Technique
Cryosurgery	Crust and erythema	Two applications of patient's usual facial foundation
Electrosurgery	Crust and erythema with some remaining telangiectasia	Green color correcter covered by two applications of patient's usual facial foundation
Incisional surgery	Erythematous linear scar	Surgical cover cream selected from Table 14–2
Chemical peel	Generalized erythema	Postsurgical facial foundation selected from Table 14–1
Dermabrasion	Generalized erythema	Green color correcter covered by a postsurgical facial foundation selected from Table 14–1
Liposuction, lipotransfer	Bruising and incisional erythema	Peach color correcter covered by a postsurgical facial foundation selected from Table 14–1
Laser surgery	Erythema	Green color corrector covered by postsurgical facial foundation selected from Table 14–1

structures, creating skin of a different texture once healing has occurred. For example, scarred skin may be devoid of hair. If the male beard is missing in a key area on the side of the face, cover creams alone will not be able to reproduce the color or texture of beard stipple. Beard stipple can easily be added by dipping a coarse sponge into black theatrical powder and then pressing the sponge into the surgical foundation.

Patients who will be left with long-term contour abnormalities may wish to seek the services of a paramedical camouflage artist who can assist them in cosmetic selection, color blending, and cosmetic application.[4]

REFERENCES

1. Cash TF, Cash DW. Women's use of cosmetics. Int J Cosmet Sci 1982;4:1.
2. Allsworth J. Skin Camouflage. Great Britain: Stanley Throes, Ltd., 1985, pp. 19–33.
3. Draelos ZK. Cosmetic camouflaging techniques. Cutis 52:362–364, 1993.
4. Rayner V. Clinical Cosmetology. Albany, NY: Milady Publishing Company, 1993, pp. 116–122.

15

Camouflage Cosmetics

A knowledge of camouflage cosmetics is important to the surgical dermatologist, who performs both cosmetic and medically necessary procedures. Camouflage cosmetics attempt to recreate a natural, attractive appearance. They do not, however, duplicate the appearance of a freshly washed, unadorned face. Camouflage cosmetics are designed to minimize facial defects while accentuating attractive features of the face.

Two types of facial defects require camouflaging: contour defects and pigmentation defects. Defects of contour are defined as areas where scarred skin is hypertrophic or atrophic and may or may not have an abnormal texture or decreased appendageal structures. Pigmentation defects are abnormalities solely in the color of the skin, with no texture abnormalities.

1. Contour Defect Camouflaging

Contour defect camouflaging is predicated on the fact that dark colors make surfaces recede, whereas light colors make surfaces appear to project (Fig. 15–1).[1] Thus, lighter colors will minimize depressed areas of scarring, whereas darker colors will minimize protuberant areas of a scar. Figure 15–2 demonstrates this technique on a patient who has sustained a depressed scar following an injury to the cheek. The scar itself is lightened to compensate for decreased light reflection.

2. Pigmentation Defect Camouflaging

Pigmentation defects can be camouflaged by applying an opaque cosmetic that allows none of the abnormal underlying skin tones to be appreciated (see Table 14–2). The most popular camouflage facial foundations are creamy products that are scooped from a jar or tin with a spatula and applied to the hand for warming. Figure 15–3 demonstrates the application of a typical camouflage makeup in a young woman who developed hypopigmentation following a burn injury to the chest during childhood.

Camouflage of pigmentation defects can also be achieved by applying foundations of complementary colors, based on the artist's color wheel. For example, permanent erythema can be camouflaged by applying a green foundation, which is the complementary color to red (Fig. 15–4). The blending of the red skin with the green foundation yields a brown tone, which can readily be covered by a more conventional facial foundation. Yellow skin tones can be blended with a complementary purple foundation, and bluish bruising can be blended with a complementary peach-colored foundation (Fig. 15–5). Table 15–1 listed pigmentation defects associated with various dermatologic conditions.[2]

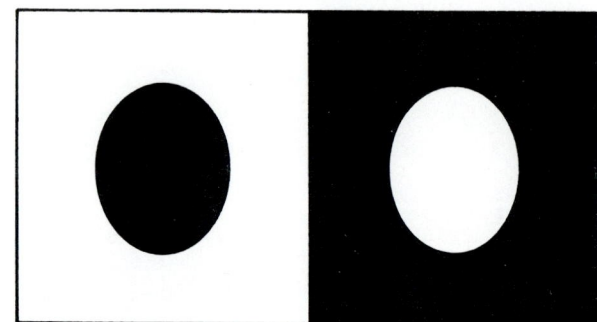

FIGURE 15–1 • Lightly colored areas tend to project, whereas darkly colored areas tend to recede. This is the basic principle underlying cosmetic camouflaging of contour defects.

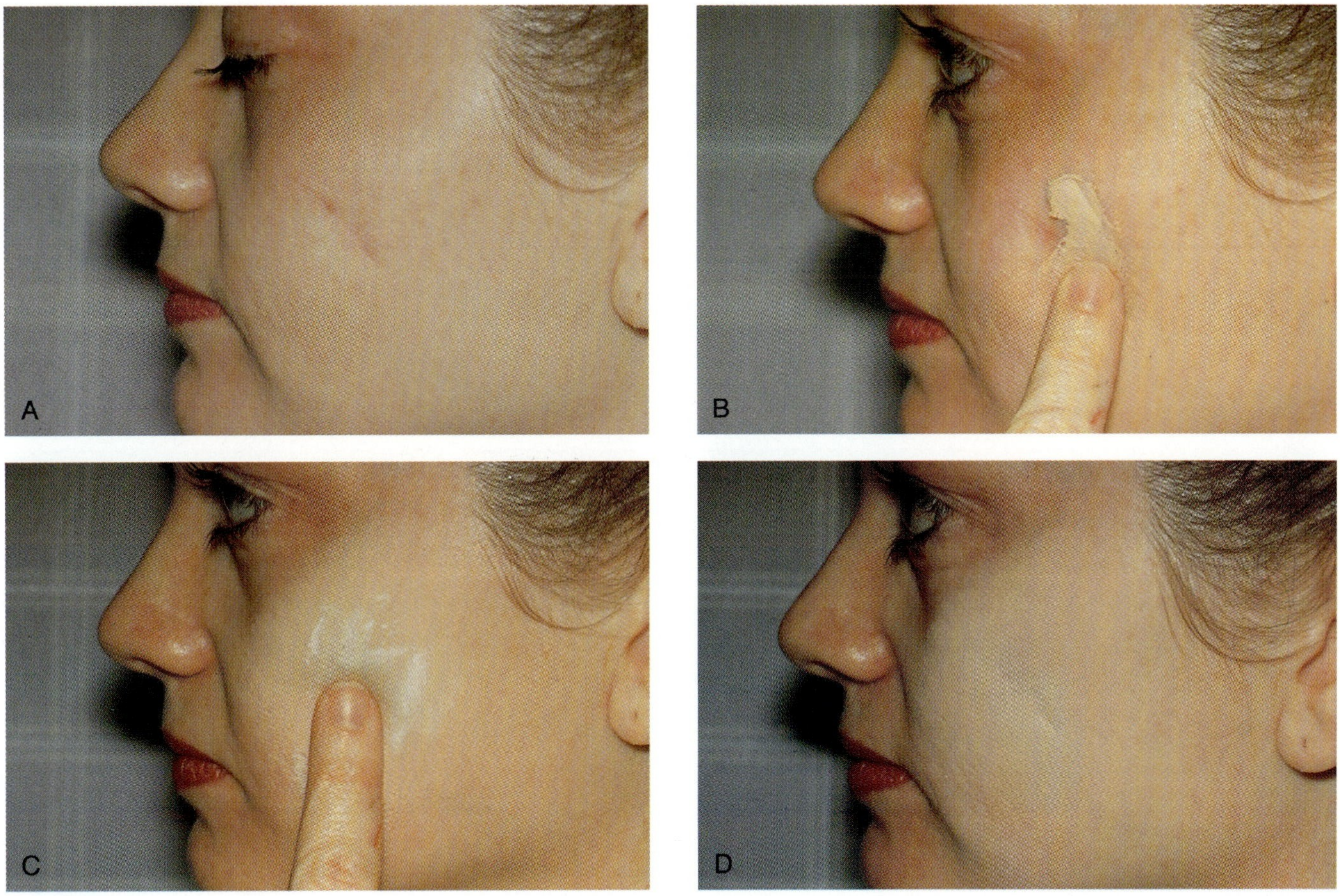

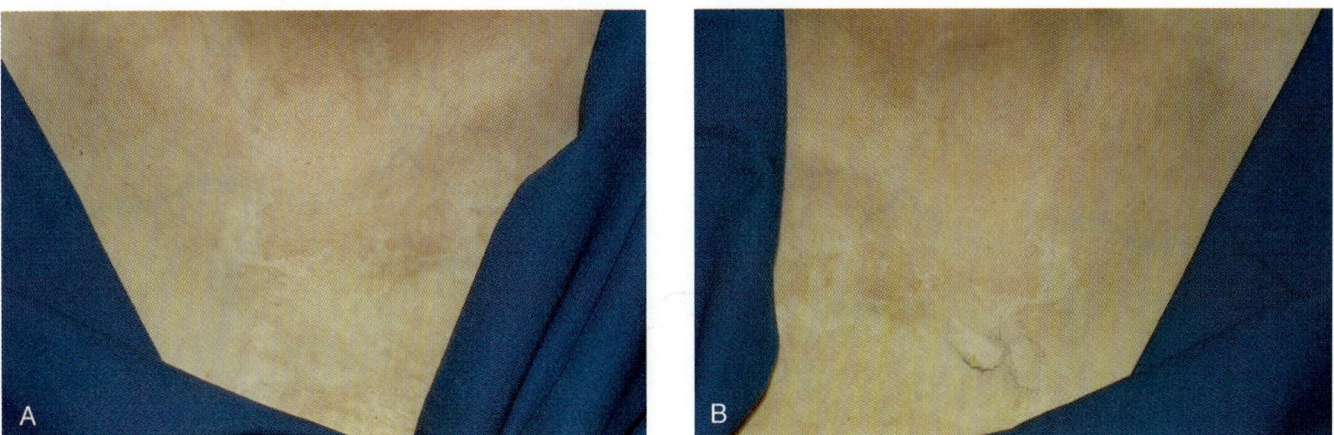

FIGURE 15–2 • A depressed defect is present on the face of a patient following surgery for an injury. *A,* The appearance of the scar without any cosmetics. *B,* Stock foundation colors have been blended to achieve a skin color match. No more than three foundation colors should be mixed. The final foundation color is then dabbed, not rubbed, over the scarred area. *C,* The cosmetic must be set with an unpigmented, finely-ground, talc-based powder to prevent smudging, improve wearability, provide waterproof characteristics, and impart a matte finish. *D,* The scar appears darker than the surrounding skin, even though the same color foundation has been applied, owing to the presence of shadows. Thus, a lighter, powdered rouge is applied over the scar.

FIGURE 15–3 • A hypopigmented scar on the chest, secondary to a burn suffered during childhood, requires camouflaging. *A,* Mottled hypopigmentation is present around the burn scar. *B,* The camouflage cosmetic is warmed on the skin to increase application ease.

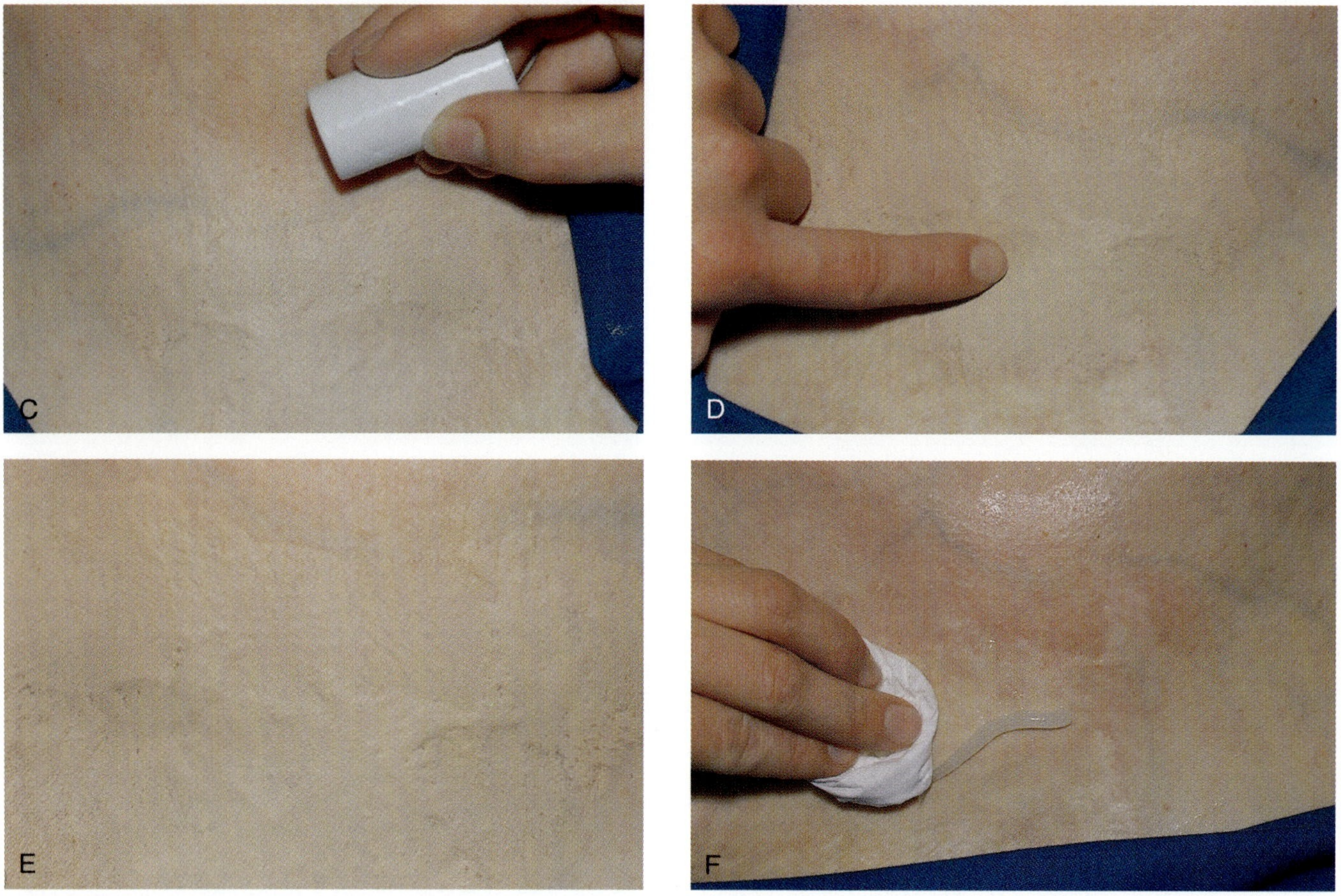

FIGURE 15–3 Continued • *C,* The cosmetic is then gently dabbed with the fingertips until the entire scarred area is covered. *D,* Setting powder is used to impart waterproof characteristics to the cosmetic. *E,* A close look at the final appearance of the camouflaged site. *F,* Removal of camouflaging cosmetics requires more than washing with soap and water owing to the waterproof nature of the product. Most companies provide an oily cleanser for cosmetic removal, and then recommend soap-and-water cleansing of the skin. The cosmetic should only be worn when needed and should be removed at bedtime.

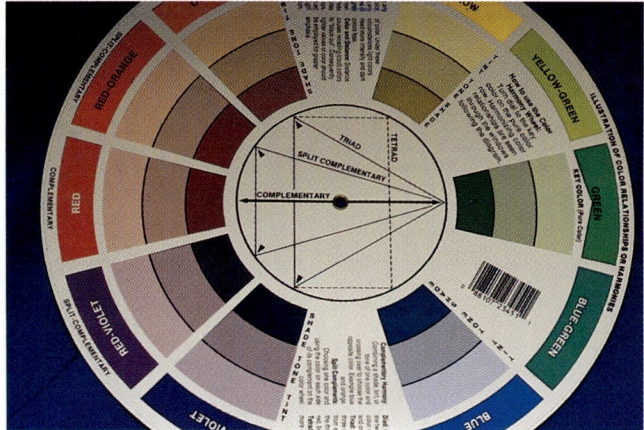

FIGURE 15–4 • The artist's color wheel shows that green and red are complementary colors. Thus, green foundation is applied underneath a traditional brown foundation to camouflage erythema.

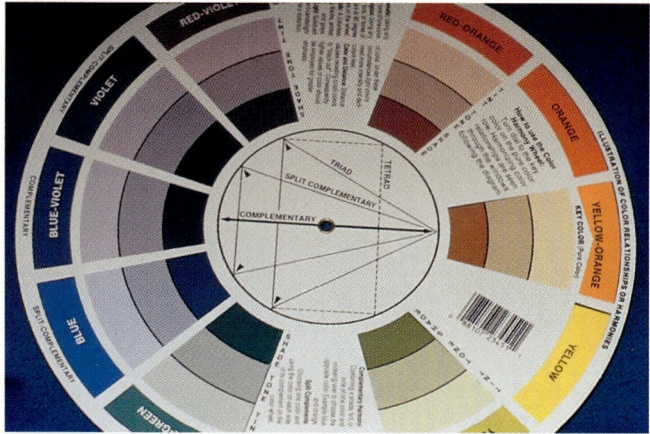

FIGURE 15–5 • Blue-violet is the complementary color to yellow-orange. Thus, peach-colored foundation is applied under a traditional brown foundation to camouflage bluish structures, such as veins.

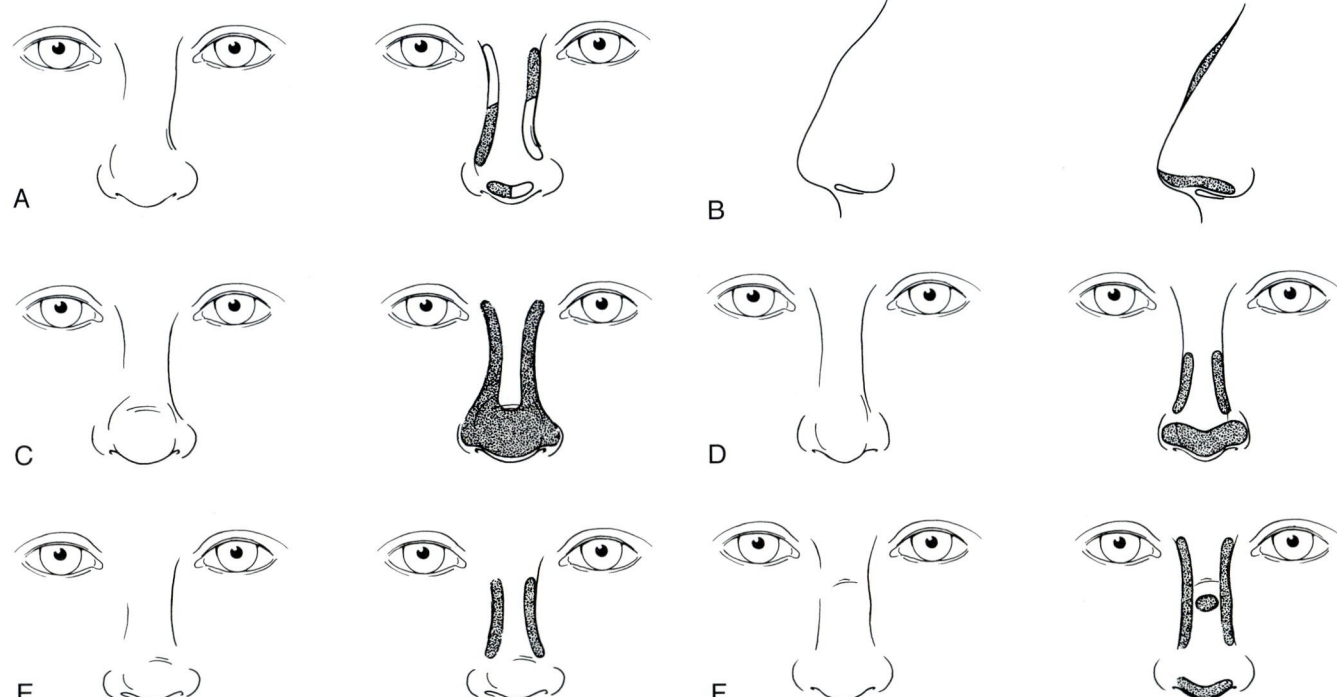

FIGURE 15–6 • Facial contouring principles are demonstrated on the nose. The outlined hatched areas require darker shading. *A*, This patient's broken nose has healed crookedly with a deviation to the left. The prominent upper left side of the nose is darkened, along with the lower right side and right tip. The opposite sides are lightened. *B*, A hooked nose or aquiline nose can be minimized by darkening the hook, along with the lateral nasal tips. *C*, A bulbous nose can be improved by shading the entire bulb on the tip and the lateral margins to the nasal root. *D*, Shading to minimize a long nose. *E*, Shading to elongate a short nose. *F*, Camouflaging for a hypertrophic scar on the nose.

TABLE 15–1 Facial Pigmentation Defects

Facial Color	Disease Process	Foundation Color
Red	Psoriasis, lupus, rosacea	Green undercover foundation
Yellow	Solar elastosis, chemotherapy, dialysis	Purple undercover foundation
Brown hyperpigmentation	Chloasma, lentignes, nevi	White undercover foundation
Hypopigmentation and depigmentation	Postinflammatory changes, congenital conditions, vitiligo	Brown undercover foundation

3. Facial Contouring

Facial contouring, utilizing the principles of highlighting and shading, is most successful in optimizing the shape of the face, the size of the forehead and chin, or the contour of the nose. Figure 15–6 illustrates shading techniques. Areas to be darkened are cross-hatched, whereas areas to be lightened are outlined.[3]

REFERENCES

1. Buchman H. Stage Makeup. New York: Watson-Guptill Publications, 1992, pp. 15–18.
2. Draelos ZK. Cosmetic camouflaging techniques. Cutis 52:362–364, 1993.
3. Newman A, Ebenstein RS. Adrian Arpel's 851 Fast Beauty Fixes and Facts. New York: G. P. Putnam's Sons, 1985, p. 47.

16

Cosmetics for Adolescents

Cosmetic lines and personal care products (Fig. 16–1) are now available that specifically cater to the fashion whims of adolescent girls. These are heavily perfumed, boldly colored products with little camouflage value. Nail polishes are available in the entire color spectrum from red to green to yellow to blue (Fig. 16–2). Lip glosses, designed to add shine to the lips, are both flavored and fragranced for impact (Fig. 16–3). Unfortunately, lip gloss can either cause or intensify perioral dermatitis or vermilion border comedones.

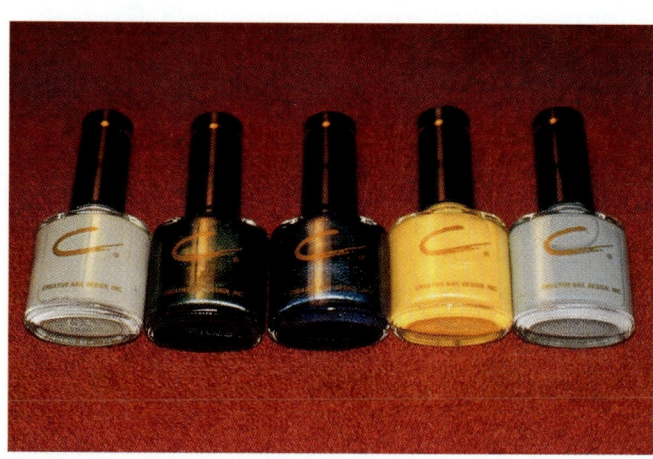

FIGURE 16–2 • Boldly colored nail polishes are popular among adolescents.

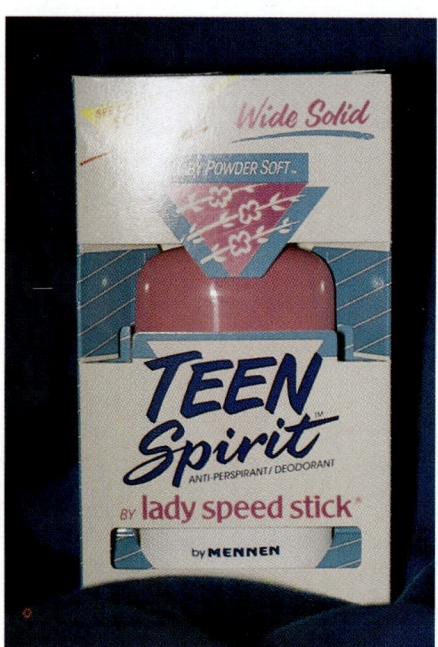

FIGURE 16–1 • Personal care products designed for adolescents utilize the same basic ingredients as those products designed for adults, but come in unique packaging and youthful fragrances.

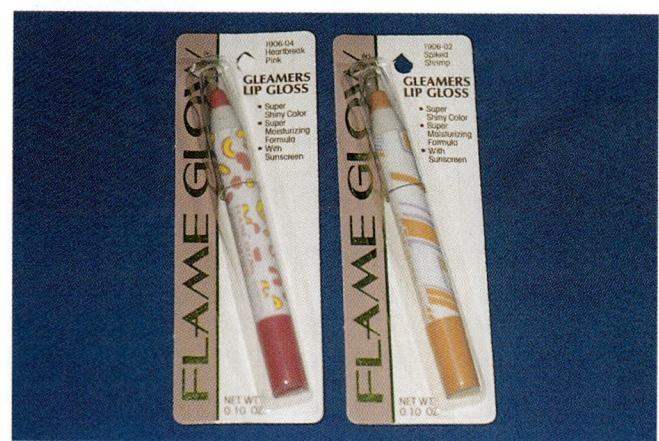

FIGURE 16–3 • Flavored, shiny lip glosses may contribute to perioral comedonal acne in adolescent girls.

17

Cosmetics for Men

Colored cosmetics have been slow to gain popularity in the United States among men. However, great diversity has been seen in skin care and fragrance products marketed to men (Fig. 17–1). There is nothing unique about male skin care and fragrance products except that the packaging and smell are designed to appeal to a masculine image.

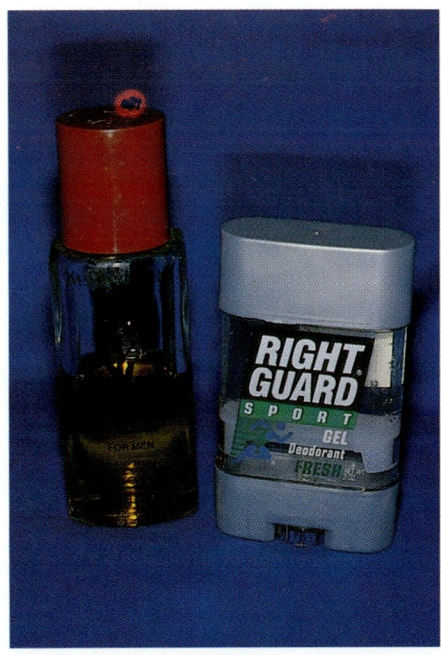

FIGURE 17–1 • Colognes, aftershave products, and deodorants form the largest portion of the consumer market for male skin care products.

18

Cosmetics for Blacks

Some cosmetics are uniquely designed for the physiologic needs of black skin. Compared to Caucasian skin, black skin has subtle structural differences owing to the presence of more mixed apocrine-eccrine sweat glands,[1] increased blood and lymphatic vessels,[2] a predisposition to hyperpigmentation,[3] denser and more compact stratum corneum,[4] increased transepidermal water loss following irritation,[5] and possibly, increased skin sensitivity to irritants.[6,7]

The unique aspect of colored cosmetic formulation for darker skin tones is the blending of pigments with the underlying skin color. Fair-skinned individuals, with little underlying skin pigment, can select a colored cosmetic and expect it to look similar in the packaging and on the skin. However, black individuals can expect the cosmetic to look entirely different in the package than on the skin. For example, a light pink blush that provides cheek highlights in a Caucasian patient, is imperceptible on black skin. Therefore,

cosmetics for blacks generally contain vivid pigments to provide the desired result. Recommended colors for cosmetic selection in black skin are listed in Table 18–1.

1. Facial Foundations

The color diversity of facial foundations for black women must be broader than that for Caucasian skin. It is estimated that there are more than 35 different colors of dark skin, requiring tremendous color selection for complexion matching.[8] This is compared to the seven basic colors of Caucasian skin. Black women traditionally wear facial foundations to blend uneven facial tones, whereas fair-skinned individuals wear facial foundations to add color to the skin (Fig. 18–1). Table 18–2 lists some of the foundations pres-

TABLE 18–1 Cosmetic Colors for Black Skin

Cosmetic	Light Skin	Medium Skin	Dark Skin
Facial foundation	Rose, medium beige, medium peach	Medium beige, bronze	Sun bronze, taupe
Blush and lipstick	Medium coral, medium pink, orange-red	Deep coral, rose, translucent red	Cinnamon, deep translucent rose, true translucent red
Eyebrow pencil and mascara	Dark brown, charcoal, black	Charcoal, black	Black
Eyeliner	Beige, charcoal, black	Beige, charcoal, black	Beige, charcoal, black
Eye shadow	Beige, lavender, aqua, light blue	Beige, deep lavender, medium blue	Deep violet, deep sea-green

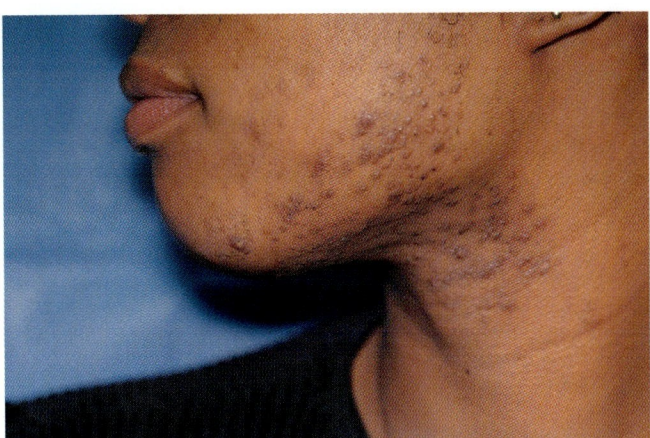

FIGURE 18–1 • Irregular pigmentation, such as postinflammatory hyperpigmentation from acne, is common in black skin, requiring the use of a facial foundation to achieve an acceptable cosmetic appearance.

ently available for black women with various skin types.

2. Eye and Cheek Cosmetics

Colored cosmetics applied to the black face must contain deep pigments. Popular eye shadow colors include deep blue, lilac, wine, gold, or emerald (Fig. 18–2). Facial highlighter and blush colors for facial contouring on black skin include deep plum, bronze, deep orange, coral, and wine or burgundy. The color selected depends upon the skin color shade (e.g., wine or plum blush for jet-black skin; coral or deep orange for brown skin, and pink or peach for light brown skin) (Fig. 18–3).

TABLE 18–2 **Facial Foundations Recommended for Black Skin According to Skin Type**

• • • • • •

Facial Foundations for Black Oily Skin

1. Maquicontrole (Lancôme)
2. Pore Minimizer (Clinique)
3. Stay True (Clinique)
4. Oil-Free Liquid (Fashion Fair)
5. Oil-Free Souflee (Fashion Fair)
6. Demimatte (Estée Lauder)

Facial Foundations for Black Normal Skin

1. Sheer Foundation (Fashion Fair)
2. Balanced Makeup (Clinique)
3. Maquimat Ultra Naturel (Lancôme)

Facial Foundations for Black Dry Skin

1. Maquivelours (Lancôme)
2. Perfect Finish Creme Makeup (Fashion Fair)
3. Maquidouceur (Lancôme)

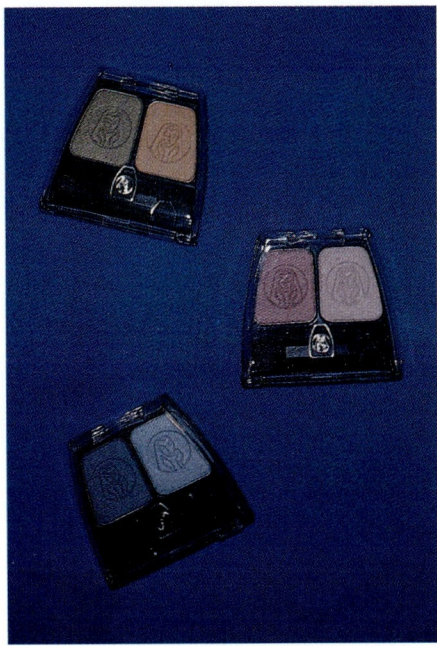

FIGURE 18–2 • Vivid eye shadow colors are appropriate for deeply pigmented skin.

3. Nail Cosmetics

Patients with black skin have a more deeply pigmented nail bed than patients with fair skin. Thus, vivid colors are employed with opaque coverage (Fig. 18–4).

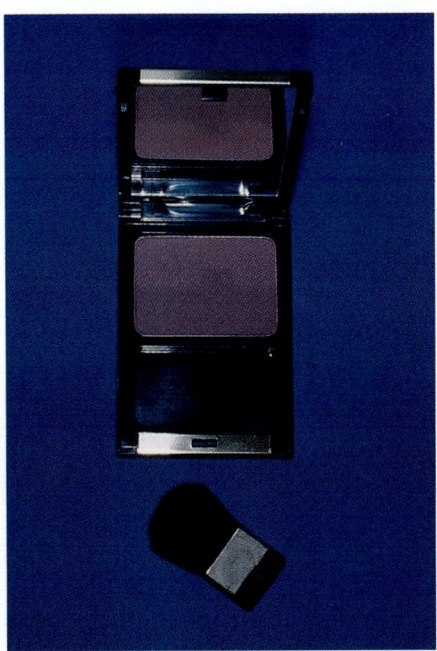

FIGURE 18–3 • Deep plum blush is commonly used on deeply pigmented skin.

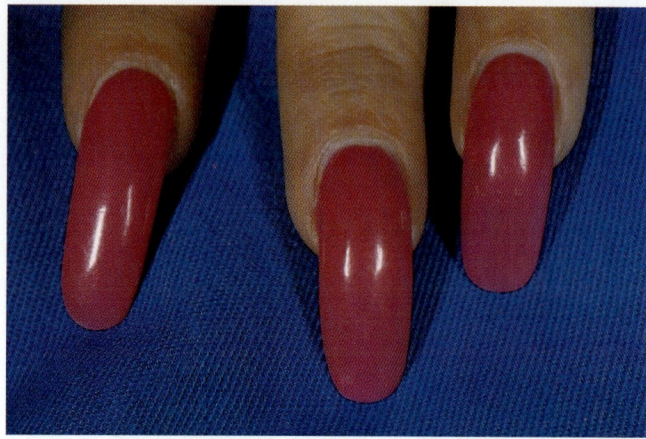

FIGURE 18–4 • Bright pink nail enamel provides an attractive contrast to the deeply pigmented skin on the fingers.

REFERENCES

1. Anderson KE, Maibach HI. African-American and white skin differences. J Am Acad Dermatol 1:276–286, 1979.
2. Montagna W, Carlisle K. The architecture of black and white facial skin. J Am Acad Derm 24:929–937, 1991.
3. McLaurin DI. Unusual patterns of common dermatoses in blacks. Cutis 32:352–360, 1983.
4. Weigand DA, Haygood C, Baylor JR. Cell layers and density of negro and caucasian stratum corneum. J Invest Dermatol 62:563–568, 1974.
5. Wilson D, Berardesca E, Maibach HI. In vitro transepidermal water loss: Differences between black and white human skin. Br J Dermatol 119:647–652, 1988.
6. Stephens TJ, Oresajo C. Ethnic sensitive skin. Cosmet Toiletr 109:75–80, 1994.
7. Berardesca E, Maibach HI. Sensitive and ethnic skin. A need for special skin care agents? Dermatol Clin 9:89–92, 1991.
8. McLaurin CI. Cosmetics for blacks: A medical perspective. Cosmet Toiletr 98:47–53, 1983.

Skin Care Maintenance Products

19

Skin Cleansers

Cleansing is an important part of daily skin hygiene. However, the variety and complexity of cleansing formulations demands organization. Table 19–1 lists the various categories of cleanser, their composition, and currently marketed examples.

1. Soaps and Detergents

In basic chemical terms, soap is a reaction between a fat and an alkali, resulting in a fatty acid salt with detergent properties.[1] Bar and liquid soaps can be divided into three basic types: true soaps, composed of long-chain fatty acid alkali salts with a pH of 9 to 10; combars, composed of alkaline soaps to which surface active agents have been added, with a pH of 9 to 10; and syndets, composed of synthetic detergents and fillers containing less than 10% soap with a pH of 5.5 to 7.0.[2] Specialty additives contribute to the tremendous variety of soaps marketed today (Table 19–2).

Body washes are a special subset of liquid synthetic detergents that combine mild skin cleansing with moisturizing and emollient qualities (Fig. 19–1). They are applied with a puff, which does not support bacterial growth, to break the emulsion through the incorporation of generous amounts of air and water (Fig. 19–2). High amounts of petrolatum can be incorporated in body wash emulsions to improve skin dryness

and hydration (Fig. 19–3). Table 19–3 lists recommended cleansing products for different dermatologic needs.

2. Lipid-free Cleansers

Lipid-free cleansers are liquid products that clean without fats. They are applied to dry or moistened skin, rubbed to produce a lather, and rinsed or wiped away (Fig. 19–4). They leave behind a thin moisturizing film and can be used effectively to remove facial cosmetics and dirt in persons with sensitive or dermatitic skin.[3]

3. Cold Creams

The classic cream for facial cleansing has long been known as cold cream. Cold creams combine the effect of a lipid solvent, such as wax or mineral oil, with detergent action from borax.[4] These products are popular for the removal of cosmetics and for cleansing in patients with dry skin.

4. Astringents and Toners

The terms astringent and toner are synonymous and refer to a fragranced alcohol or propylene glycol

TABLE 19–1 Categories of Cleansing Products

Product Type	Composition	Product Examples
Bar soap	True soap in bar form; pH of 9–10	Ivory Bar Soap (Procter & Gamble), Pure and Natural Bar Soap (Andrew Jergens Corporation)
Syndet bar cleanser	Synthetic detergents; no soap; in bar form pH of 5.5–7	Oil of Olay Bar (Procter & Gamble), Dove Bar (Unilever), Cetaphil Bar (Galderma)
Syndet liquid	Synthetic detergents in liquid form; pH of 5.5–7	Oil of Olay Foaming Fash Wash (Procter & Gamble), Dove Liquid (Unilever)
Combar soap	Combination of true soap and synthetic detergent; pH of 9–10	Dial (Dial Corporation)
Body wash	Emlusion system applied with a puff; allows synthetic detergent cleansing combined with enhanced skin moisturization and emolliency	Oil of Olay Daily Renewal Body Wash (Procter & Gamble)
Lipid-free cleanser	Cleans without fats; may contain glycerin, cetyl alcohol, stearyl alcohol, sodium laurel sulfate, or (occasionally) propylene glycol	Aquanil (Person & Covey), Cetaphil (Galderma)
Cleansing cream	Waxes and mineral oil with detergent action from borax	Noxema (Noxell Corporation)
Astringent/toner	Alcohol-based product that may contain witch hazel, salicylic acid, or glycolic acid	Clarifying Lotion 2, 3, 4 (Clinique)
Moisturizing astringent/toner	Glycerin-based humectant moisturizer	Clarifying Lotion 1 (Clinique)
Exfoliant cleanser	Glycolic or salicylic acid–containing cleanser	Oil-free Acne Face Wash (Neutrogena)
Abrasive cleanser	Polyethylene beads or other small particles within a syndet cleanser	Oil of Olay Age Defying Series Face Wash (Procter & Gamble)
Pore cleaning strips	Cyanoacrylate glue, which adheres to debris at the surface of the follicular ostia	Biore Strips (Andrew Jergens Company)
Face mask	Vinyl-, oatmeal- hydrocolloid, or clay-based masks	Cabot's Face Masks (Cabot Corporation)

TABLE 19–2 Specialty Soap Formulations

Type of Soap	Unique Ingredients
Superfatted soap	Increased oil and fat; fat ratio $\leq 10\%$
Castile soap	Olive oil used as main fat
Deodorant soap	Antibacterial agents
French milled soap	Additives to reduce alkalinity
Floating soap	Extra air trapped during mixing process
Oatmeal soap	Ground oatmeal added (coarsely ground to produce abrasive soap; finely ground for gentle cleanser)
Acne soap	Sulfur, resorcinol, benzoyl peroxide, or salicylic acid added
Facial soap	Smaller bar size; no special ingredients
Bath soap	Larger bar size; no special ingredients
Aloe vera soap	Aloe vera added to soap; no special skin benefit
Vitamin E soap	Vitamin E added, no special skin benefit
Cocoa butter soap	Cocoa butter used as major fat
Nut or fruit oil soap	Nut or fruit oils used as major fat
Transparent soap	Glycerin and sucrose added
Abrasive soap	Pumice, coarse oatmeal, maize meal, ground nut kernels, dried herbs or flowers added
High impact soap	Strong, high-concentration fragrance added to scent skin after cleansing
Soap-free soap	Contains synthetic detergents (syndet bar)

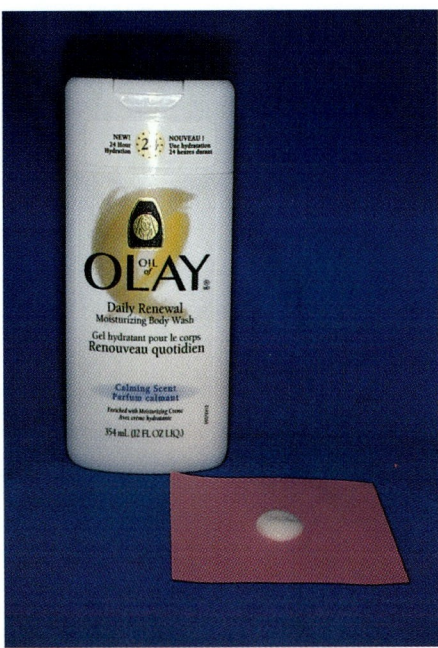

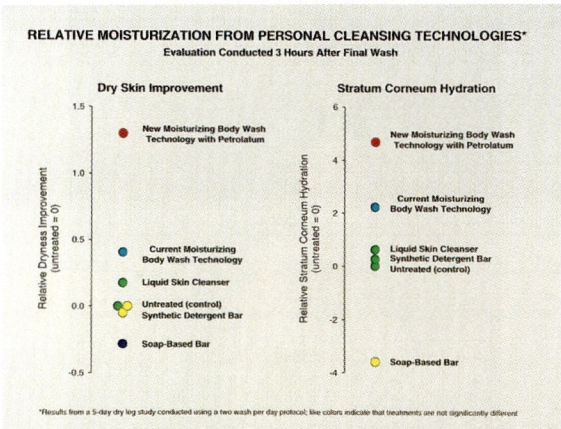

FIGURE 19–3 • Body wash emulsions that contain high concentrations of petrolatum provide greater improvement in skin dryness and stratum corneum hydration than traditional syndet bar soaps.

FIGURE 19–1 • Body washes are concentrated cleansers requiring only a dime-sized amount to cleanse the entire body.

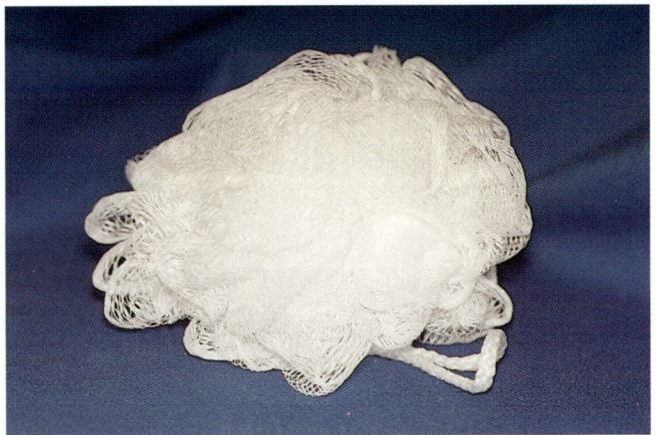

FIGURE 19–2 • A puff is necessary to introduce water and air into the body wash emulsion.

solution used to remove oil and makeup debris following cleansing (Fig. 19–5). They are intended to be applied following use of a lipid-free cleanser, sometimes also called a milky cleanser, or a cold cream to remove any remaining cleanser residue. Many cosmetic cleansing routines recommend use of an astringent after washing with a syndet soap.

Astringents are formulated for all skin types; however, the composition and function varies. Oily skin astringents contain a high concentration of alcohol to remove any remaining sebum following cleansing. Some oily skin/acne treatment astringents may contain salicylic acid, glycolic acid, or witch hazel (Fig. 19–6). Astringents for normal skin contain relatively lower alcohol concentrations, whereas those for dry skin contain largely propylene glycol and water to act as a humectant moisturizer. Soothing agents, such as allantoin, guaiazulene, and Quaternium-19, may also be added.[5]

TABLE 19–3 Recommended Cleansing Products for Dermatologic Needs

Cleansing Area	Skin Type	Recommended Cleanser
Face	Dry	Cetaphil Cleanser (Galderma)
	Normal/Combination	Oil of Olay Sensitive Skin Foaming Face Wash (Procter & Gamble)
	Oily	Purpose Liquid Facial Cleanser (Johnson & Johnson)
Body	Dry	Oil of Olay Daily Renewal Body Wash (Procter & Gamble)
	Normal/Combination	Ivory Moisture Care Bar Soap (Procter & Gamble)
	Oily	Dial (Dial Corporation)

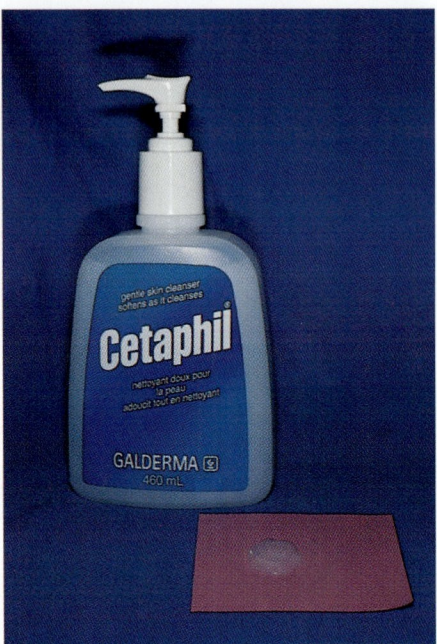

FIGURE 19–4 • Lipid-free cleansers can be used effectively to remove cosmetics.

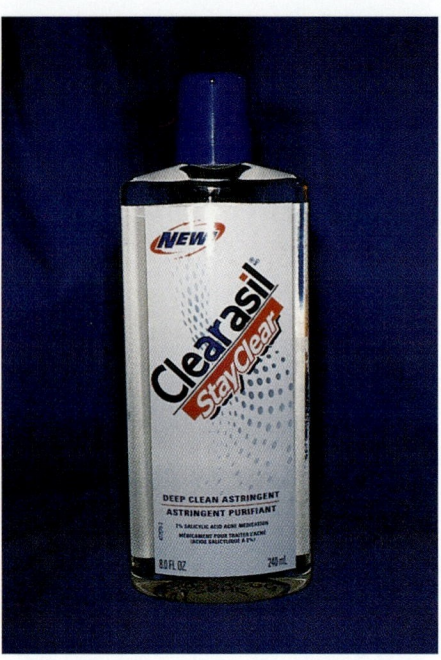

FIGURE 19–6 • Astringents for acne patients may incorporate salicylic acid to facilitate comedolysis.

5. Exfoliant Cleansers

Exfoliant cleansers are basically liquid syndet cleansers to which substances, such as glycolic acid or salicylic acid, have been added to encourage chemical degradation of the intercellular bridges and stratum corneum desquamation (Fig. 19–7). They produce milder exfoliation than an abrasive cleanser.

6. Abrasive Cleansers

Abrasive cleansers are mechanical exfoliants that use particles, such as polyethylene beads, aluminum oxide, ground fruit pits, or sodium tetraborate decahydrate granules, suspended in a liquid synthetic cleanser, to remove skin scale. Aluminum oxide and

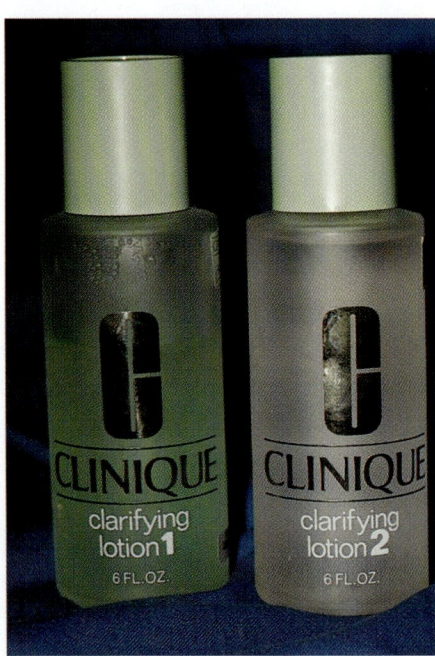

FIGURE 19–5 • Astringents or toners are used to remove sebum, milky cleanser residue, or cleansing cream from the face.

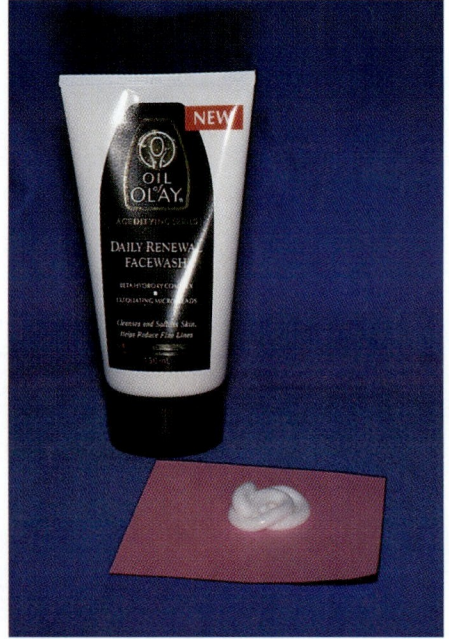

FIGURE 19–7 • This exfoliant cleanser combines salicylic acid and polyethylene beads to provide both chemical and mechanical exfoliation.

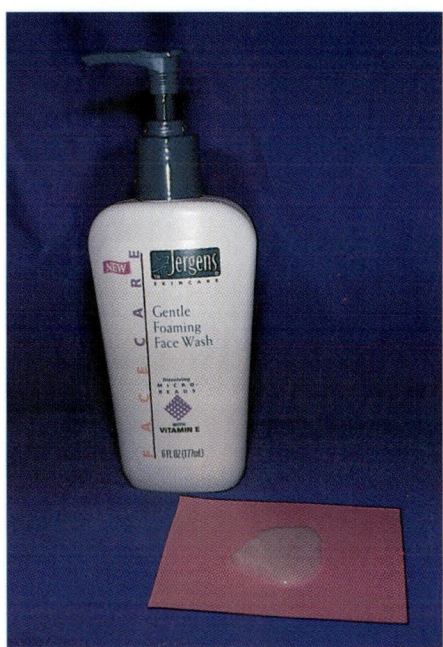

FIGURE 19-8 • Sodium tetraborate decahydrate granules form dissolving cleansing granules that provide mild mechanical exfoliation.

ground fruit pits provide the most abrasive scrub, followed by polyethylene beads, which are softer (Fig. 19-7). Sodium tetraborate decahydrate granules become softer and dissolve during use, providing the least abrasive scrub (Fig. 19-8).

7. Pore Cleansing Strips

Pore cleansing strips are derived from the cyanoacrylate follicular biopsy technique popularized by Albert

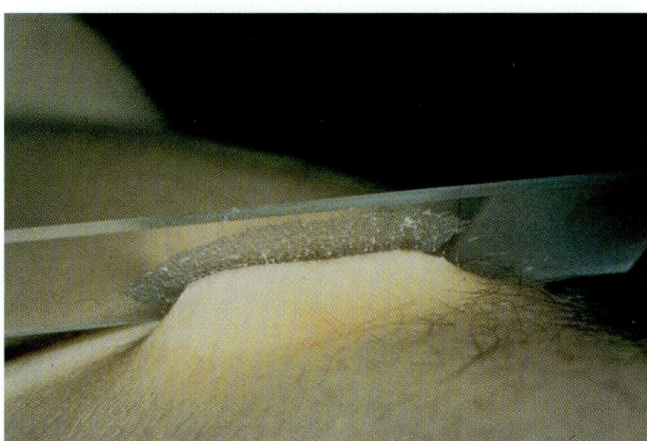

FIGURE 19-9 • Pore strips mimic the effect of cyanoacrylate follicular biopsy performed with methacrylate adhesive applied to a microscope slide. The adhesive is allowed to dry and the microscope slide is subsequently removed from the skin along with follicular debris. (Photo courtesy of Albert Kligman, MD, PhD, Philadelphia, PA.)

Kligman, M.D., Ph.D. (Fig. 19-9). These strips contain an acrylate adhesive that is placed in contact with the skin of the nose or other oily area. The adhesive is allowed to set, and subsequent removal of the strip also removes follicular debris that is adherent to the strip. This technique is a method of mechanical follicular exfoliation.

8. Facial Masks

Facial masks, also known simply as facials, are available in four basic formulations: wax-based, vinyl- or rubber-based, hydrocolloid, and earth-based.

a. WAX FACE MASKS

Wax-based masks are popular among women chiefly for their warm, aesthetically pleasing feel. The masks are composed of beeswax or, more commonly, paraffin wax to which petroleum jelly and cetyl or stearyl alcohols have been added to provide a soft, pliable material for facial application with a soft brush. The wax is heated and may either be applied directly to the face or applied over a thin gauze cloth draped over the face. These face masks are available only in professional salons or spas. Wax-based face masks are most frequently recommended for individuals with dry skin owing to their ability to temporarily impede transepidermal water loss.

b. VINYL- AND RUBBER-BASED MASKS

Vinyl- and rubber-based masks are popular masks for home use, as they are easily applied and removed (Fig. 19-10). Rubber-based masks are usually based on latex, whereas vinyl-based masks are based on film-forming substances, such as polyvinyl alcohol or vinyl acetate. They are squeezed premixed from a tube or pouch and applied with the fingertips to the face. Upon evaporation of the vehicle, a thin, flexible, vinyl or rubber film remains on the face. The mask is generally left in contact with the skin for 10 to 30 minutes and then removed in one sheet by loosening at the edges. Vinyl and rubber masks, which are appropriate for all skin types, temporarily impede transepidermal water loss while in contact with the skin.

c. HYDROCOLLOID MASKS

Hydrocolloid masks are used both in professional salons and at home. Hydrocolloids are substances, such as oatmeal, that are of large molecular weight and thus interfere with transepidermal water loss. These masks are formulated from gums and humectants and enjoy tremendous popularity since many specialty in-

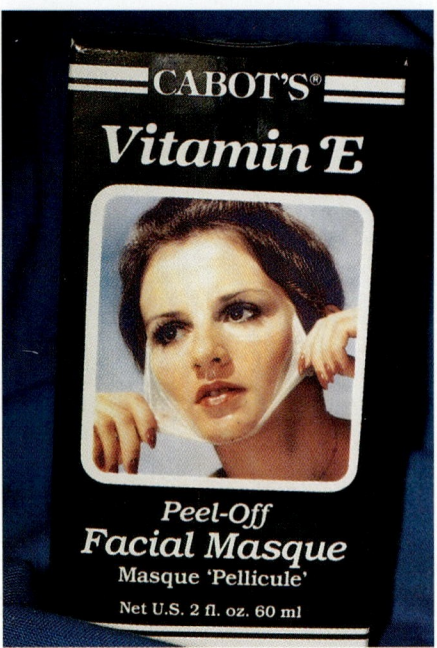

FIGURE 19–10 • Vinyl face masks can be peeled off the face in one complete sheet.

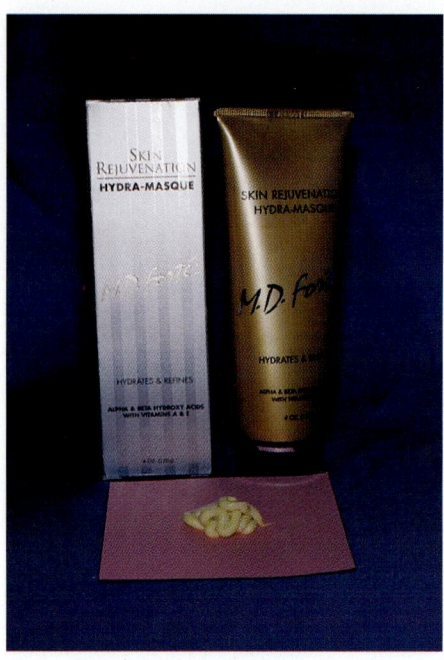

FIGURE 19–12 • Paste-type face masks can be formulated with hydroxy acids to exfoliate the face chemically.

gredients are easily incorporated into their formulation (Fig. 19–11). They are marketed in the form of dry ingredients in a sealed pouch that must be mixed with warm water prior to application. The resulting paste is then smeared over the face and allowed to dry.

Temporary moisturization can occur while the mask is on the skin.

d. EARTH-BASED MASKS

Earth-based masks, also known as paste masks or mud packs, are formulated of absorbent clays, such as bentonite, kaolin, or china clay. The clays produce an astringent effect on the skin, making this mask most appropriate for oily-complected patients. The astringent effect of the mask can be enhanced through the addition of other substances, such as magnesium, zinc oxide, salicylic acid, or others. The versatility of paste masks is tremendous, and the number of possible additives is unlimited. Modern paste-type masks can be squeezed from a tube and usually incorporate an alpha-hydroxy acid (Fig. 19–12).

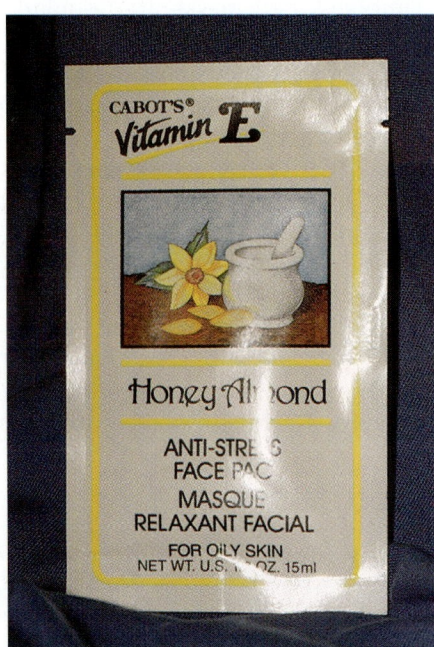

FIGURE 19–11 • Oatmeal face masks are first mixed with water to form a paste and then spread over the face.

REFERENCES

1. Willcox MJ, Crichton WP. The soap market. Cosmet Toiletr 104:61–63, 1989.
2. Wortzman MS, Scott RA, Wong PS, Lowe MJ, et al. Soap and detergent bar rinsability. J Soc Cosmet Chem 37:89–97, 1986.
3. Mills OH, Berger RS, Baker MD. A controlled comparison of skin cleansers in photoaged skin. J Geriatr Dermatol 1:173–179, 1993.
4. Jass HE. Cold creams. In deNaarre MG (ed.). The Chemistry and Manufacture of Cosmetics, Vol. III, 2nd ed. Wheaton, IL: Allured Publishing Corporation, 1975, pp. 237–249.
5. Wilkinson JB, Moore RJ. Astringents and skin toners. In Harry's Cosmeticology, 7th ed. New York: Chemical Publishing, 1982, pp. 74–81.

20

Moisturizers

Moisturizers are products designed to restore and maintain the water content of the skin at normal physiologic levels (between 10% and 30%). However, consumers also require moisturizers to smooth and soften the skin, which are emollient properties, and to reduce irritation, which are skin protectant properties. These objectives are accomplished through the use of four ingredient categories: occlusives, humectants, hydrophilic matrices, and sunscreens.[1,2]

1. INGREDIENT CATEGORIES

a. OCCLUSIVES

There are many different substances that can be utilized to occlude the stratum corneum and reduce transepidermal water loss, the most popular of which are listed in Table 20–1.[3] Each chemical imparts a different feel and thickness to moisturizers (Figs. 20–1 through 20–3).

The most occlusive moisturizing ingredient presently available is petrolatum (Table 20–2).[4] It appears, however, that total occlusion of the stratum corneum is undesirable. Although transepidermal water loss can be completely halted with its use, once the occlusive is removed, water loss proceeds at its preapplication level. Thus, occlusive moisturizers do not allow the stratum corneum to repair its barrier function.[5] However, petrolatum does not appear to function as an impermeable barrier; rather, it permeates throughout the interstices of the stratum corneum, allowing barrier function to be reestablished.[6]

b. HUMECTANTS

Another concept in rehydrating the stratum corneum is the use of humectants. Humectants have been used

TABLE 20–1　Occlusive Moisturizing Ingredients

Chemical Category	Example Ingredients	Comments
Hydrocarbon oils	Petrolatum, mineral oil	Best occlusive agents currently available
Hydrocarbon waxes	Paraffin, squalene	Infrequently utilized in some thick hand creams
Silicones	Dimethicone, cyclomethicone	Basis of oil-free moisturizers; commonly used to decrease the greasiness of oil-containing products
Vegetable oils	Soybean oil, grape seed oil	Commonly combined with petrolatum in ointment moisturizers
Animal fats	Lard	No longer used
Fatty acids	Lanolin acid, stearic acid	Common cream and lotion ingredients
Fatty alcohols	Lanolin alcohol, cetyl alcohol	Common cream and lotion ingredients
Polyhydric alcohols	Propylene glycol	Used in lotions to decrease residue on skin
Wax esters	Lanolin, beeswax, stearyl stearate	Lanolin is rarely used owing to its odor, expense, and allergenicity; stearyl stearate is a common lotion additive
Vegetable waxes	Carnauba wax, candelilla wax	Used in older anhydrous ointment preparations
Phospholipids	Lecithin	Used as a specialty additive
Sterols	Cholesterol	Used as a specialty additive
Polymers	Acrylate	Forms a film over the skin surface

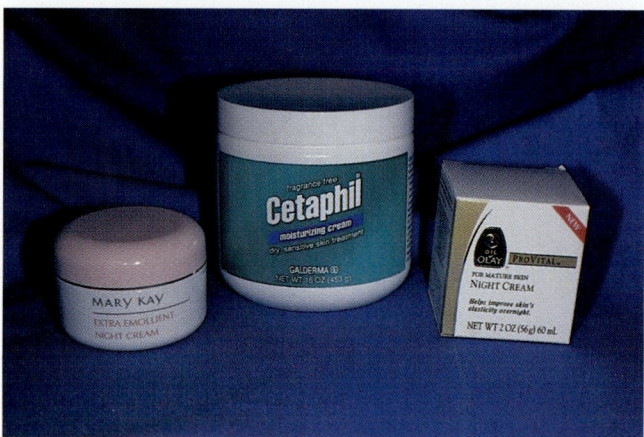

FIGURE 20–1 • These cream formulations contain high concentrations of occlusive moisturizers that significiantly reduce transepidermal water loss.

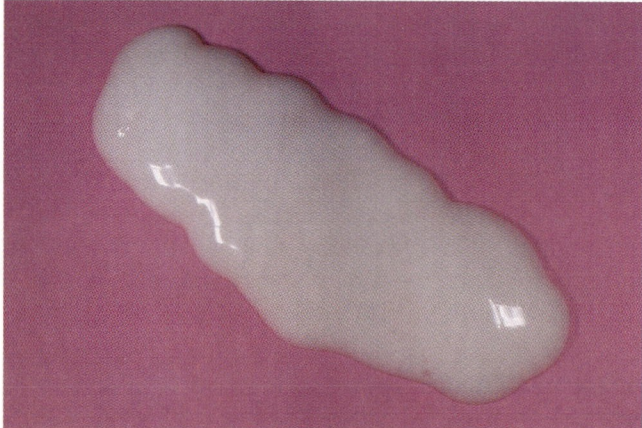

FIGURE 20–2 • Body lotions are generally oil-in-water emulsions containing 10% to 15% oil phase, 5% to 10% humectant, and 75% to 85% water phase.

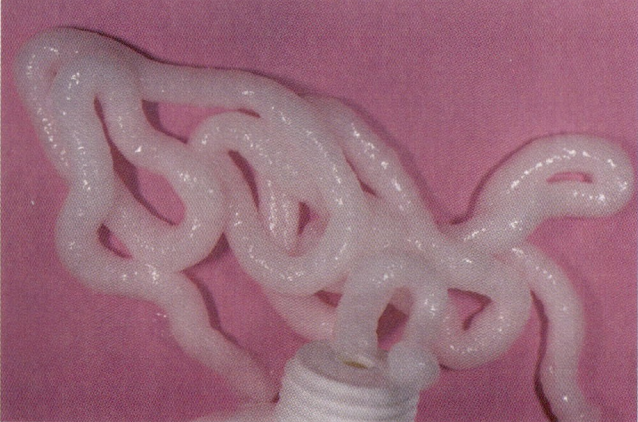

FIGURE 20–3 • Hand creams are oil-in-water emulsions containing 15% to 40% oil phase, 5% to 15% humectant, and 45% to 80% water phase. The addition of silicone derivatives can also render the hand cream water-resistant.

TABLE 20–2 Efficacy of Occlusive Moisturizing Ingredients

Occlusive Moisturizing Agent	% Reduction in TEWL
Petrolatum	99
Lanolin	76
Vegetable or fruit oil	39
Mineral oil	30

TEWL, Transepidermal Water Loss

in cosmetics for many years to increase shelf life by preventing product evaporation and subsequent thickening secondary to variations in temperature and humidity. For example, humectants are a necessary part of all oil-in-water creams, as they maintain the required water content. Table 20–3 lists substances that function as humectant moisturizers.[3,7]

TABLE 20–3 Humectant Moisturizing Ingredients

Humectant Ingredient	Comments
Glycerin	Must be combined with an occlusive agent to prevent increased water loss; can create a humectant reservoir within the stratum corneum
Honey	Used as a specialty additive
Sodium lactate	A form of lactic acid used to decrease corneocyte adhesion and increase the water-retaining capacity of the stratum corneum
Urea	Increases the water-retaining capacity of the skin by disrupting hydrogen bonding and exposing water-binding sites on the corneocytes
Propylene glycol	Also an occlusive agent; commonly used to decrease the oiliness of moisturizers; causes stinging when applied to abraided skin
Sorbitol	Food additive that also functions as a topical humectant
Sodium PCA	The sodium salt of pyrrolidone carboxylic acid, one of the components of the natural moisturizing factor (NMF) thought to be critical for preventing dry skin
Gelatin	Used to thicken and maintain the water content of moisturizer on the shelf
Hyaluronic acid	The most abundant glycosaminoglycan in the dermis; functions as a naturally occurring skin humectant
Vitamins	Vitamins A, C, E, and pantothenic acid (vitamin B complex) can function as humectants if used in sufficient concentrations
Proteins	Hydrolyzed collagen, keratin, and elastin can function as humectants for the skin and hair

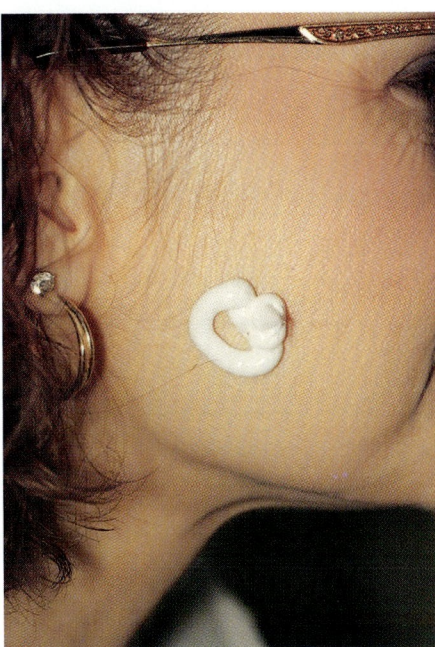

FIGURE 20–4 • It is impossible to tell the efficacy of a moisturizer by appearance alone. Rather, the ingredient label must be read to determine the dermatologic value of the product.

Cosmetic chemists have theorized that humectants can be used to draw water from the environment under conditions in which the ambient humidity exceeds 70%. More commonly, they are used to draw moisture from the deeper epidermal and dermal tissues to rehydrate the stratum corneum. Water that is applied to the skin in the absence of a humectant is rapidly lost to the atmosphere.[8] Humectants may also allow the skin to feel smoother by filling holes in the stratum corneum through swelling.[9] However, under low-humidity conditions, humectants, such as glycerin, will actually draw moisture from the skin and increase transepidermal water loss.[10] Therefore, a good moisturizer should combine both occlusive and humectant properties (Fig. 20–4).

c. HYDROPHILIC MATRICES

Hydrophilic matrices are substances of large molecular size that place a physical barrier over the skin surface. Colloidal oatmeal baths are examples of one such hydropilic formulation. Hyaluronic acid is a hydrophilic matrix found in some moisturizers.

d. SUNSCREENS

Many of the moisturizers that repair and replenish the skin incorporate a chemical or particulate sunscreen to prevent cellular damage, thus preventing cutaneous dehydration. Sunscreens are discussed in further detail, the following chapter (Chapter 20).

2. Emolliency

Emolliency describes the ability of a moisturizer to leave the skin feeling smooth and soft following application. Many emollients also function as humectants or occlusive moisturizers. Emollients function by filling the spaces between the desquamating corneocytes[11] to create a visually and tactilely smooth surface. Table 20–4 lists ingredients that function as emollients.[12] Generally, emollients from several categories are combined to yield the final tactile characteristics of the moisturizer.

3. Formulation

Most moisturizers consist of water, lipids, emulsifiers, preservatives, fragrance, color, and specialty additives. Interestingly enough, water accounts for 60% to 80% of any moisturizer; however, externally applied water does not remoisturize the skin. In fact, the rate of water passage through the skin increases with increased hydration.[13] The water in moisturizers func-

TABLE 20–4 Emollient Ingredients

Emollient Category	Example Ingredients	Comments
Protective emollients	Di-isopropyl dilinoleate, isopropyl isostearate	Leave a long-lasting film on the skin; skin feels smooth immediately upon application
Fatting emollients	Castor oil, propylene glycol, jojoba oil, isostrearyl isostearate, octyl stearate	Leave a long-lasting film on the skin; may feel greasy
Dry emollients	Isopropyl palmitate, decyl oleate, isostearyl alcohol	Confer little skin protection; produce a dry skin feeling
Astringent emollients	Dimethicone, cyclomethicone, octyl octanoate, isopropyl myristate	Minimal greasy residue; can reduce the oily feel of other emollients

TABLE 20–5 Recommended Moisturizer Products for Dermatologic Needs

Body Area to Be Moisturized	Skin Type	Recommended Moisturizer
Face—night application	Dry to Normal	Cetaphil cream (Galderma)
	Normal to Oily	None required
Face—day application	Dry to Normal	Eucerin for Face SPF 25 (Biersdorf)
	Normal to Oily	Oil of Olay Daily UV Complete (Procter & Gamble)
Hands	All	RoC Hand Cream (Johnson & Johnson)
Lips	All	Neutrogena Lip Moisture SPF 15
Body	Dry to Normal	Cetaphil Cream (Galderma)
	Normal to Oily	Moisturel Lotion (Westwood-Squibb)

tions as a diluent, eventually evaporating, leaving the active agents behind. Emulsifiers, which are generally soaps in concentrations of 0.5% or less, function to keep the water and lipids in one continuous phase. Parabens are the most commonly used preservatives in moisturizers and are usually combined with one of the formaldehyde donor preservatives.[14] The variety of specialty additives incorporated into moisturizers is endless, limited only by the imagination of the cosmetic chemist. Table 20–5 lists some of the author's preferred moisturizer formulations.

REFERENCES

1. Baker CG. Moisturization: New methods to support time proven ingredients. Cosmet Toiletr 102:99–102, 1987.
2. Goldner R. Moisturizers: A dermatologist's perspective. J Toxicol Cut Ocul Toxicol 11:193–197, 1992.
3. De Groot AC, Weyland JW, Nater JP. Unwanted Effects of Cosmetics and Drugs Used in Dermatology, 3rd ed. Amsterdam: Elsevier, 1994, pp. 498–500.
4. Friberg SE, Ma Z. Stratum corneum lipids, petrolatum and white oils. Cosmet Toiletr 107:55–59, 1993.
5. Grubauer G, Feingold KR, Elias PM. Relationship of epidermal lipogenesis to cutaneous barrier function. J Lip Res 28:746–752, 1987.
6. Ghadially R, Halkier-Sorensen L, Elias PM. Effects of petrolatum on stratum corneum structure and function. J Am Acad Dermatol 26:387–396, 1992.
7. Spencer TS. Dry skin and skin moisturizers. Clin Dermatol 6:24–28, 1988.
8. Rieger MM, Deem DE. Skin moisturizers. II. The effects of cosmetic ingredients on human stratum corneum. J Soc Cosmet Chem 25:253–262, 1974.
9. Robbins CR, Fernee KM. Some observations on the swelling of human epidermal membrane. J Soc Cosmet Chem 37:21–34, 1983.
10. Idson B. Dry skin: Moisturizing and emolliency. Cosmet Toiletr 107:69–78, 1992.
11. Wehr RF, Krochmal L. Considerations in selecting a moisturizer. Cutis 39:512–515, 1987.
12. Brand HM, Brand-Garnys EE. Practical application of quantitative emolliency. Cosmet Toiletr 107:93–99, 1992.
13. Warner RR, Myers MC, Taylor DA. Electron probe analysis of human skin: Determination of the water concentration profile. J Invest Dermatol 90:218–224, 1988.
14. Jackson EM. Moisturizers: What's in them? How do they work? Am J Contact Dermatitis 3:162–168, 1992.

21

Sunscreens

Sunscreens are an important part of daily skin care to prevent photoaging and carcinogenesis. Modern technology has allowed the development of chemical and physical agents that protect against both ultraviolet B (UVB) and ultraviolet A (UVA) radiation, delivering enhanced sun protection factor (SPF) ratings (Fig. 21–1).

Many substances have been developed for their sun protective capabilities (Table 21–1).[1,2] These substances can be divided into chemical sunscreens and particulate sunblocks. Chemical sunscreens, such as para-aminobenzoic acid (PABA) esters, cinnamates, benzophenones, salicylates, and anthranilates, contain molecules that absorb photons of light energy. They are generally aromatic compounds, based on the benzene ring's ability to transform high-energy ultraviolet radiation into harmless long-wave radiation above the 380-nm range. This phenomenon is accomplished via resonance delocalization, and the long-wave radiation is emitted from the skin as heat.[3] Chemical sunscreens absorb 95% of the UV radiation within wavelengths of 290 to 320 nm, also known as the UVB range.

Some chemical sunscreens absorb in the UVA range of 320 to 400 nm. These substances include the benzophenones (avobenzone, oxybenzone) and the anthranilates (menthyl anthranilate). However, they cannot absorb the shorter-wavelength UVA radiation. This has led to the development of particulate sunblocks, such as micronized titanium dioxide and microfine zinc oxide, which act as physical sunblocks to

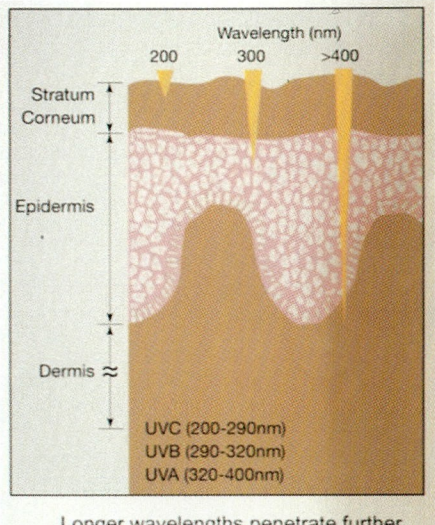

FIGURE 21–1 • The wavelengths and cutaneous penetration of the various components of ultraviolet radiation are shown.

TABLE 21–1 Sunscreening Agents

Chemical UVB Sunscreens

Aminobenzoic acid
Amyl dimethyl PABA
2-Ethoxyethyl *p*-methoxycinnamate
Diethanolamine *p*-methoxycinnamate
Digalloyl trioleate
Ethyl 4-*bis* (hydroxypropyl) aminobenzoate
2-Ethylhexyl-2-cyano-3,3-diphenyl-acrylate
Ethylhexyl *p*-methoxycinnamate
2-Ethylhexyl salicylate
Glyceryl aminobenzoate
Homomenthyl salicylate
Lawsone with dihydroxyacetone
Octyl dimethyl PABA
2-Penylbenzimidazole-5-sulfonic acid
Triethanolamine salicylate

Chemical UVA Sunscreens

Oxybenzone
Sulisobenzone
Dioxybenzone
Avobenzone
Menthyl anthranilate

Particulate Sunblocks

Micronized titanium dioxide
Microfine zinc oxide
Iron oxide
Kaolin
Magnesium silicate
Magnesium oxide

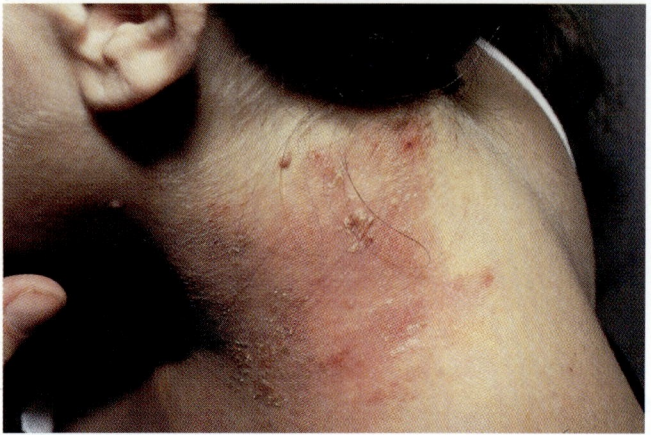

FIGURE 21–2 • Photodermatoses can be minimized by the use of UVA and UVB sunblocks.

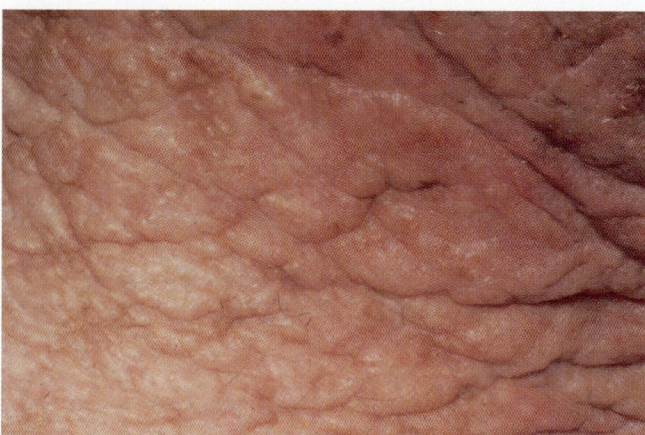

FIGURE 21–5 • Severe end-stage photodamage can be prevented through the use of broad-spectrum sunblocks.

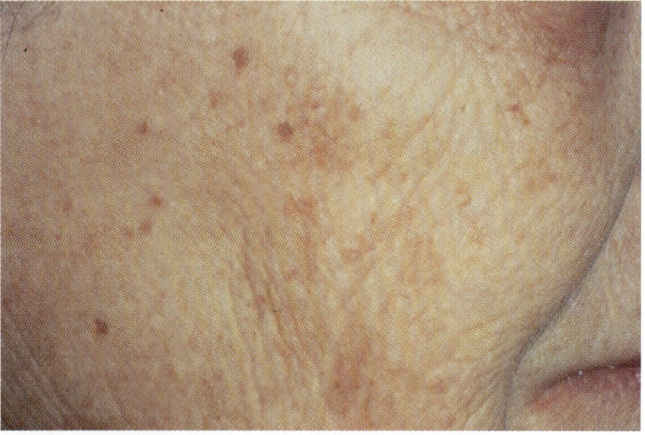

FIGURE 21–3 • Lentigenes are related to UVA radiation, which is not blocked by the majority of the sunscreen formulations currently on the market.

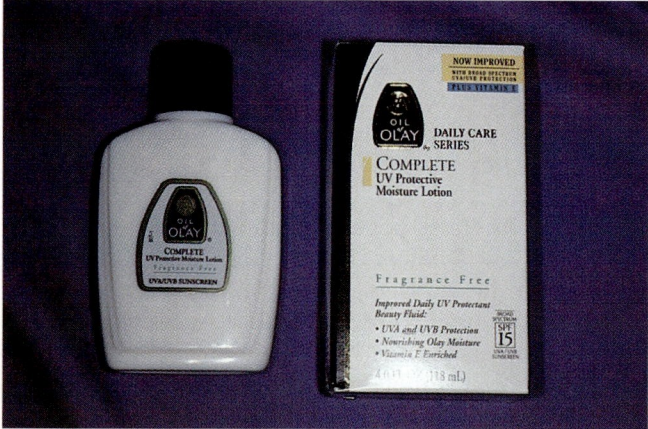

FIGURE 21–6 • The daily application of a moisturizer providing both UVB and UVA protection can minimize dermatoheliosis over a lifetime of use.

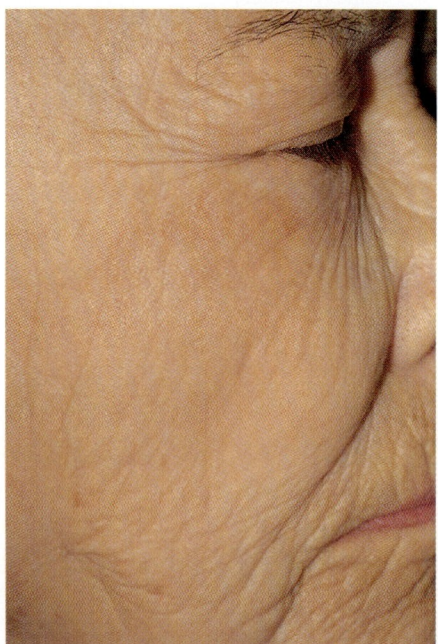

FIGURE 21–4 • Extrinsic aging of the face is largely attributable to UVA exposure. Unfortunately, current SPF ratings are only useful in determining UVB protection.

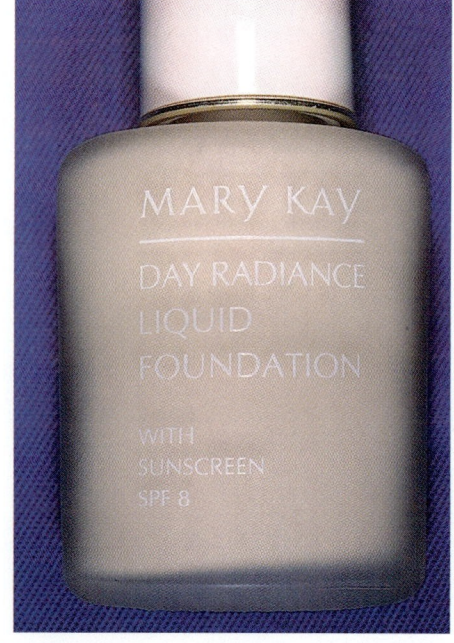

FIGURE 21–7 • Facial foundations that provide sun protection and prevent photoaging can also be applied to the facial skin.

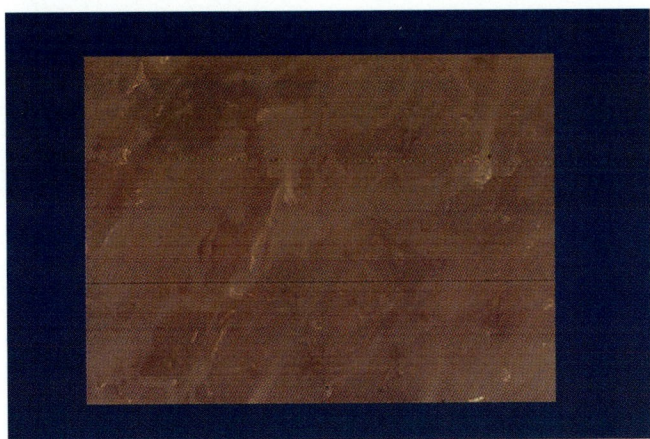

FIGURE 21–8 • This video microscospic image (×400) demonstrates the difficulty encountered in applying some sunscreen formulations to the skin in a uniform layer. The skipped areas shown leave the skin unprotected.

reflect and scatter light energy, but may also operate through resonance delocalization.[4] The use of these particulate sunblocks is valuable in patients with photosensitive dermatoses and signs of photoaging (Figs. 21–2 through 21–5).

Many cosmetic companies are now incorporating the cinnamate sunscreens in their facial foundations to improve the SPF from 2 to 3, based on the titanium dioxide in the formulation, to at least 8 (Fig. 21–6). Sunscreen-containing moisturizers are an excellent method of obtaining patient compliance with sun protection (Fig. 21–7). However, any sunscreen-containing formulation must leave an even film on the skin to provide consistent protection (Fig. 21–8).

REFERENCES

1. Murphy EG. Regulatory aspects of sunscreens in the United States. In Lowe NJ, Shaath NA (eds.). Sunscreens Development, Evaluation and Regulatory Aspects. New York: Marcel Dekker, 1990, pp. 127–130.
2. Lowe NJ. Sun protection factors: Comparative techniques and selection of ultraviolet sources. In Lowe NJ (ed.). Physician's Guide to Sunscreens. New York: Marcel Dekker, 1991, pp. 161–165.
3. Shaath NA. The chemistry of sunscreens. In Lowe NJ, Shaath NA (eds.). Sunscreens Development, Evaluation and Regulatory aspects. New York: Marcel Dekker, 1990, pp. 223–225.
4. Sayre RM, Hughes SNG. Sun protective apparel: Advancements in sun protection. Skin Cancer J February–March, 1993.

22

Topical Hydroxy Acid Products

Topical hydroxy acids provide antiaging, skin-smoothing effects through their ability to induce exfoliation of corneocytes (Fig. 22–1). Several hydroxy acid varieties are available for consumer purchase: alpha hydroxy acids (AHAs), triple hydroxy acids (THAs), beta hydroxy acid (BHA), combination hydroxy acids (CHAs), and polyhydroxy acids (PHAs).[1]

1. Alpha Hydroxy Acids

This group of organic carboxylic acids is distinguished by a hydroxy group in the alpha position (Fig. 22–2). The linear, aliphatic nature of the AHA structure accounts for its water solubility. The three subcategories of the AHAs consist of monocarboxylic acids, such as glycolic acid and lactic acid, dicarboxylic acids, such as malic acid, and tricarboxylic acids, such as citric acid. AHAs are thought to induce exfoliation by interfering with the ionic bonding between corneocytes.

2. Triple Hydroxy Acids

THAs are combinations of AHAs, one monocarboxylic acid, one dicarboxylic acid, and one tricarboxylic acid, to yield a hydroxy acid cocktail. These combinations are thought to offer exfoliation benefits identical to the single AHA formulations. It is doubtful that the individual AHA entities can be distinguished in the final formulation.

3. Beta Hydroxy Acid

Salicylic acid, the only BHA, is an organic, aromatic, carboxylic acid with a hydroxy group in the beta position (see Fig. 22–2). This phenolic, oil-soluble compound is chemically unrelated to the AHAs. Salicylic acid is unique among the hydroxy acids, as it can enter the milieu of the sebaceous unit, inducing exfoliation in the pores and on the skin surface (Figs. 22–3 and 22–4). Salicylic acid is thought to function through solubilization of intercellular cement, thereby reducing corneocyte adhesion.

4. Combination Hydroxy Acids

CHA formulations generally combine glycolic and salicylic acid. Unfortunately, it is impossible to optimize the free acid levels of glycolic and salicylic acid in the same formulation. The optimum free acid level is

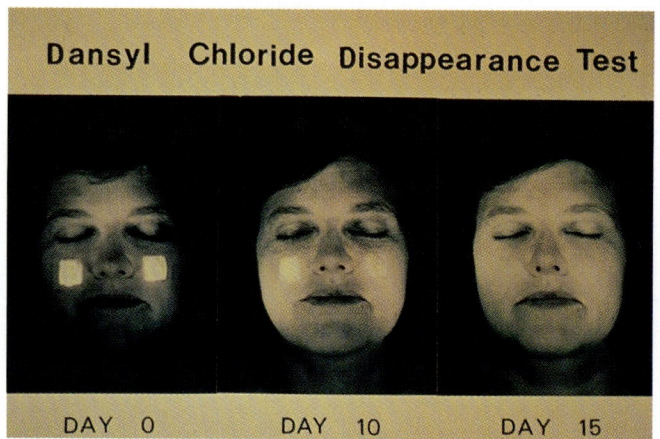

Dansyl Chloride Disappearance Test

DAY 0   DAY 10   DAY 15

FIGURE 22–1 • The ability of a hydroxy acid to exfoliate the skin can be measured by the dansyl chloride disappearance test. Dansyl chloride is applied to the stratum corneum in a petrolatum vehicle to stain the corneocytes. It is colorless under visible light, but becomes fluorescent when viewed with a Wood's light. The fluorescence decreases as the corneocytes are sloughed. (Photo courtesy of Albert Kligman, MD, PhD, Philadelphia, PA.)

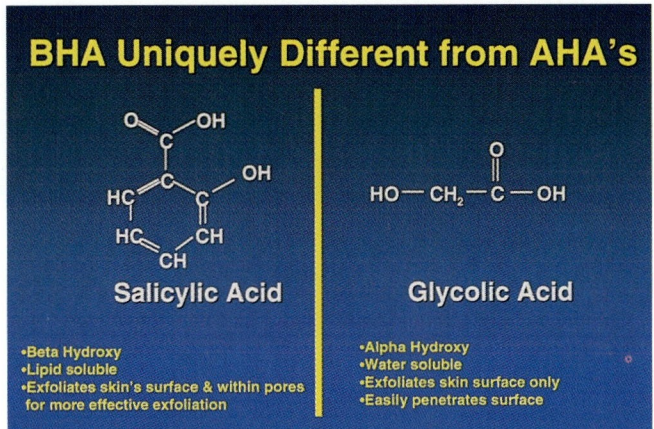

FIGURE 22–2 • Alpha hydroxy acids are linear, water-soluble substances, whereas beta hydroxy acid (salicylic acid) is a phenolic, oil-soluble substance.

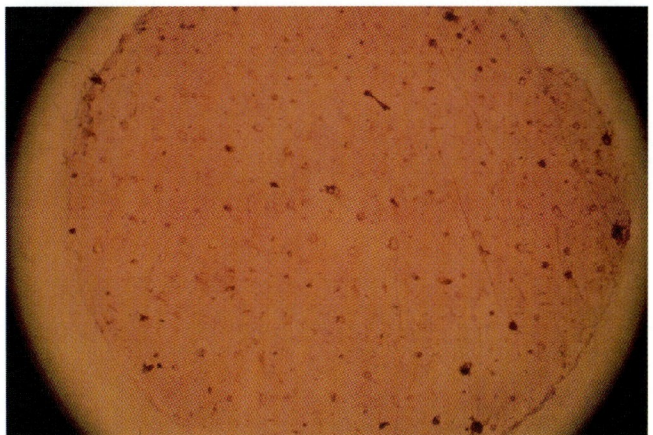

FIGURE 22–4 • This follicular biopsy specimen shows reduced follicular debris following exfoliation induced by salicylic acid (Photo courtesy of Albert Kligman, MD, PhD, Philadelphia, PA.)

obtained at the pKa of the substance, and these substances have different pKa levels. The pKa of salicylic acid is 2.98, whereas the pKa of glycolic acid is 3.8 (Fig. 22–5). Thus, one ingredient must be selected of primary importance to dominate the formulation. Combination hydroxy acid formulations do not offer the maximum benefits of both AHA and BHA ingredients.

5. Polyhydroxy Acids

PHAs are chemically similar to AHAs, but are substances of greater molecular weight (e.g., gluconolactone), intended to limit dermal penetration.[2] The decreased dermal penetration theoretically means that there will be less stinging, burning, and irritation.

6. Considerations in Hydroxy Acid Formulation

Optimal product selection depends on formulation. Issues to be considered include concentration, pH, and vehicle effects.

a. CONCENTRATION AND pH

All hydroxy acids perform better at low pH levels, but the optimal pH for a given formulation is determined by the pKa of the active ingredient, as discussed previously. One method of controlling pH is by altering the concentration of the hydroxy acid (Fig. 22–6). For example, 10% glycolic acid is four times more acidic than 1% glycolic acid, with the acidity being deter-

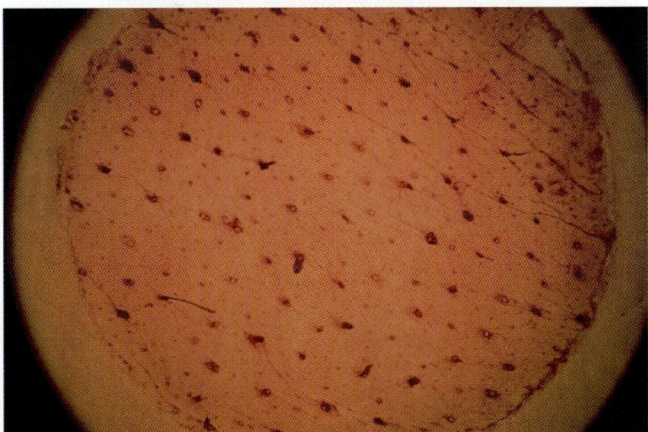

FIGURE 22–3 • The results of a follicular biopsy taken with cyanoacrylate glue prior to skin treatment with salicylic acid. A large amount of follicular debris is present. (Photo courtesy of Albert Kligman, MD, PhD, Philadelphia, PA.)

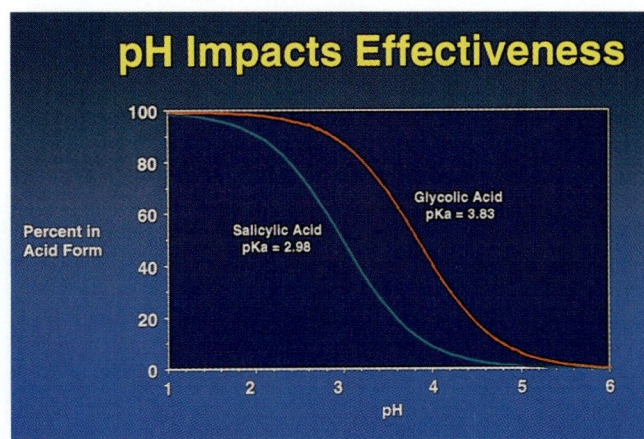

FIGURE 22–5 • The differing pKa levels of alpha hydroxy acids and salicylic acid do not allow optimization of both ingredients in a single formulation.

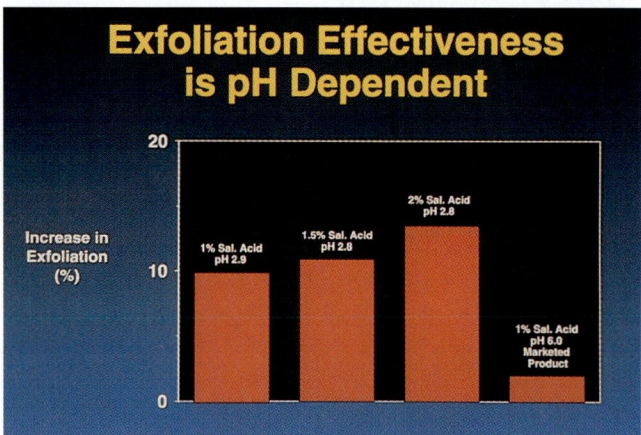

ACIDIC MATERIAL	pH	CELL RENEWAL	IRRITATION
4% GA	3	35	2.8
	5	24	2.1
	7	13	1.2
0.5% TCA	3	54	5+
	5	40	4.5
	7	14	1.7

FIGURE 22–6 • Deceasing the pH of glycolic acid (GA) preparations increases exfoliation and irritation. Stronger acids, such as 0.5% trichloroacetic acid (TCA), produce even more dramatic exfoliation and irritation as the pH decreases.

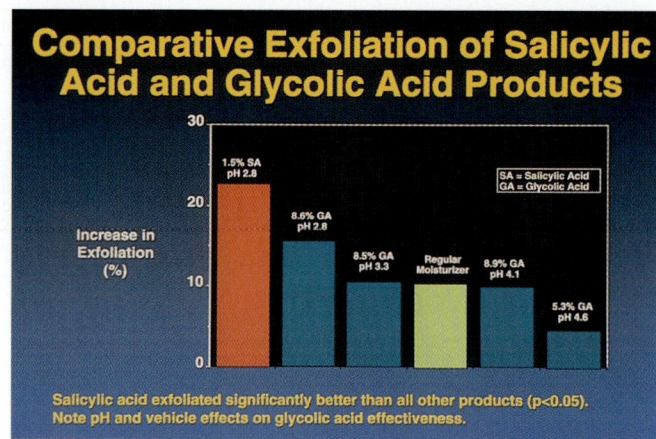

Comparative Exfoliation of Salicylic Acid and Glycolic Acid Products

Salicylic acid exfoliated significantly better than all other products ($p < 0.05$). Note pH and vehicle effects on glycolic acid effectiveness.

FIGURE 22–9 • The product's formulation determines the degree of exfoliation with hydroxy acid preparations. Some high-concentration glycolic acid preparations formulated at a pH exceeding 4 produce no greater exfoliation than a bland moisturizer.

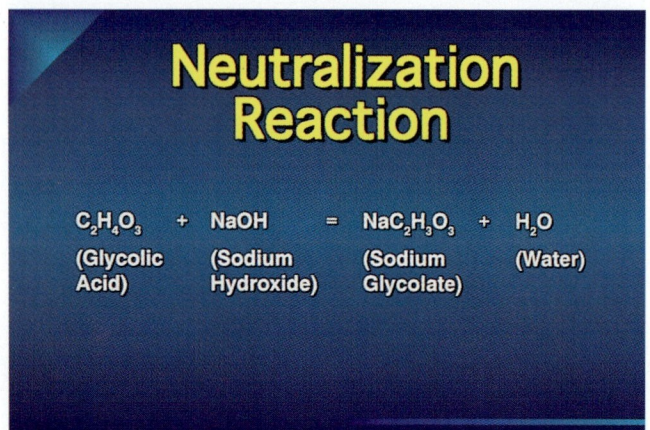

Exfoliation Effectiveness is pH Dependent

FIGURE 22–7 • Completely neutralized salicylic preparations at a pH of 6 produce little increase in exfoliation.

mined by electrostatic, inductive, and steric effects, as well as hydrogen bonding. Figure 22–7 demonstrates the relationship between salicylic acid concentration and pH in terms of exfoliation.

The pH and free acid content of hydroxy acid preparations can be changed by buffering the product or through neutralization. Hydroxy acids can be neutralized with an inorganic alkali or organic base to raise the product's pH (Fig. 22–8). Glycolic acid preparations are frequently neutralized with sodium hydrox-

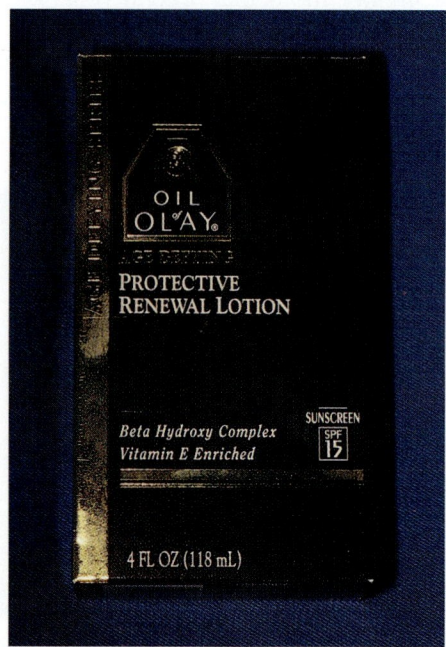

FIGURE 22–10 • Sun protection is recommended in daytime hydroxy acid formulations to prevent the development of sunburn cells in the newly exfoliated skin.

Neutralization Reaction

$$C_2H_4O_3 + NaOH = NaC_2H_3O_3 + H_2O$$

(Glycolic Acid) + (Sodium Hydroxide) = (Sodium Glycolate) + (Water)

FIGURE 22–8 • This neutralization reaction is used to minimize the irritation associated with low-pH glycolic acid preparations.

ide, resulting in decreased cutaneous irritation. Completely neutralized glycolic acid, however, with a pH exceeding 4.8, contains mostly sodium glycolate, which has no anti-aging exfoliant properties.

b. VEHICLE EFFECTS

The vehicle of delivery can increase the in-use aesthetics of the product, resulting in improved patient compliance. It is important to discern which enhanced skin benefits are attributable to the vehicle and which are attributable to the active agent (Fig. 22–9). The vehicle can also deliver sun protection to the exfoliated skin (Fig. 22–10).

REFERENCES

1. Draelos ZD. Hydroxy acids for the treatment of aging skin. J Geriatric Dermatol 5:236–240, 1997.
2. Draelos ZD. Hydroxy acid update, Cosmet Dermatol 7:27, 1998.

23

Hydroxy Acid Peels

Hydroxy acid peels are low-pH solutions that are applied to the skin surface, under the direction of a dermatologist, to enhance exfoliation. Peels can be supplemented with hydroxy acid moisturizers (see Chapter 20) to maintain a smooth skin surface.

The author's guidelines for peel selection are listed in Table 23–1. The equipment used for the peel is shown in Figure 23–1.

1. Alpha Hydroxy Acid Peels

The alpha hydroxy acid the author prefers to use in peel solutions is glycolic acid. It is readily available in a 70% aqueous stock solution and can easily be diluted owing to its hydrophilic properties. However, it can also be purchased as a patented preparation (Fig. 23–2). The author prefers to prepare her own glycolic

acid peels in strengths of 20%, 30%, 40%, 50%, 60%, and 70%, as demonstrated in Table 23–2. These are unneutralized and unbuffered peels, which induce noticeable exfoliation. The different strengths are necessary to tailor the peel results to the patient's skin type and desired degree of exfoliation.

Glycolic acid peels must be neutralized with copious amounts of ice water to completely remove the acid from the skin. Any acid that is inadvertently left on the skin surface will be absorbed into the dermis and produce continued stinging and burning. Whether this dermal absorption is valuable remains controversial. The exfoliant effect of the peel is epidermal; however, some dermatologists believe that dermal penetration leads to wrinkle reduction through the synthesis of glycosaminoglycans, such as hyaluronic acid. The author believes that the dermal effects are attributable to nonspecific irritation and should be avoided to pre-

TABLE 23–1 Selection Criteria for Hydroxy Acid Peels

Type and Concentration of Peel Solution	Expected Results
20%, 30% Glycolic acid	Produces minimal exfoliation with 20–30 minutes of erythema; resembles an aggressive facial; good in heavily retinized patients
40%, 50% Glycolic acid	Produces mild exfoliation with 4 hours of erythema; good maintenance peel for most patients if repeated every 10–12 weeks
60%, 70% Glycolic acid	Produces moderate exfoliation with 8 hours of erythema; good lightening of epidermal pigmentation when repeated every 3 weeks for six treatments
10% Salicylic acid	Produces minimal exfoliation with 20–30 minutes of erythema; effective in younger patients with comedonal acne to initiate comedolysis; also appropriate for patients with rosacea or sensitive skin
20%, 30% Salicylic acid	Produces mild to moderate exfoliation with 1 hour of erythema; good peel for patients with acne and dyspigmentation when repeated every 10–12 weeks
40%, 50% Salicylic acid	Produces moderate exfoliation with 2 hours of erythema; good peel for patients with pronounced photoaging when repeated every 3 weeks for five treatments
Jessner's solution (combination hydroxy acid)	Produces moderate to dramatic exfoliation in the retinized patient with 12 hours of erythema; preferred peel for lightening epidermal pigmentation without frequent peel repetition

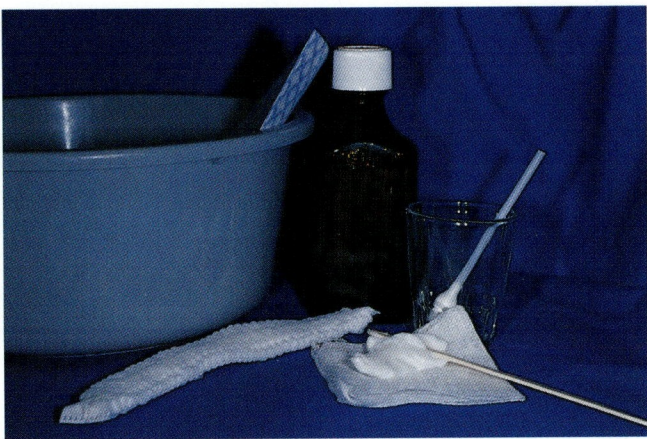

FIGURE 23–1 • The surgical tray the author uses for peels includes a basin filled with ice cubes and ice water, several diposable towels, a disposable hairnet, a bottle of the peel solution of choice, a short, rayon-tipped applicator, a small glass, and a bland cream moisturizer.

TABLE 23–2 Glycolic Acid Peel Recipe

Glycolic Acid Peel Percentage (%)	Volume of 70% Glycolic Acid Stock Liquid (cc)	Amount of Water (cc)
20	29	71
30	43	57
40	57	43
50	71	29
60	86	14
70	100	0

TABLE 23–3 Salicylic Acid Peel Recipe

Salicylic Acid Peel Percentage (%)	Weight of Salicylic Acid Powder (g)	Amount of Ethyl Alcohol 95% (cc)
10	10	100
20	20	100
30	30	100
40	40	100
50	50	100

vent damaging the skin. Therefore, rinsing of the skin with water should continue until all burning and stinging has resolved.

2. Beta Hydroxy Acid Peels

Beta hydroxy acid peels are formulated from salicylic acid powder and 95% ethyl alcohol (Everclear). The author mixes these peels in strengths of 10%, 20%, 30%, 40%, and 50%, as demonstrated in Table 23–3. Salicylic acid peels of 30% and greater are suspensions, which require shaking immediately prior to application to ensure accurate concentration and even distribution of the salicylic acid (Fig. 23–3). The author's guidelines for peel selection are listed in Table 23–1; the appearance of the skin following a 20%

salicylic acid peel is shown in Figure 23–4. The salicylic acid crystallizes on all the equipment used, necessitating washing in detergent and water (Fig. 23–5).

Beta hydroxy acid peels differ from glycolic acid peels in that the salicylic acid also crystallizes on the skin surface, leaving a white film (Fig. 23–6). This is not to be confused with the acetowhitening achieved

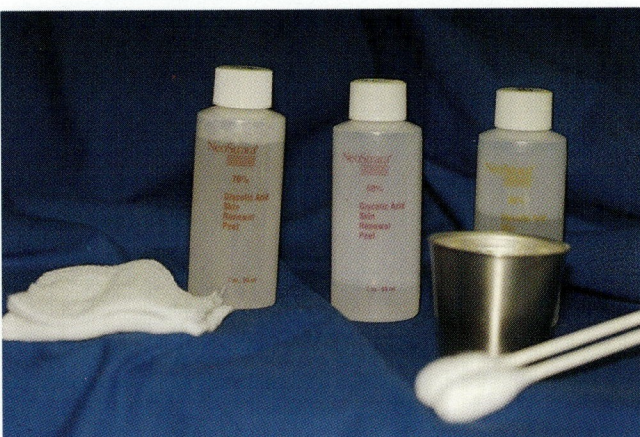

FIGURE 23–2 • Patented glycolic acid peel solutions can be purchased for use in the dermatologist's office.

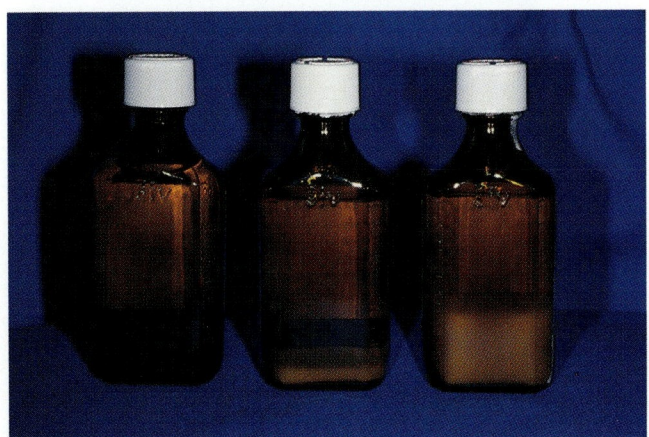

FIGURE 23–3 • These bottles contain from left to right salicylic acid peels in concentrations of 20%, 30%, and 40%. Salicylic acid peels in strengths of 30% or more are suspensions, and require shaking immediately prior to application.

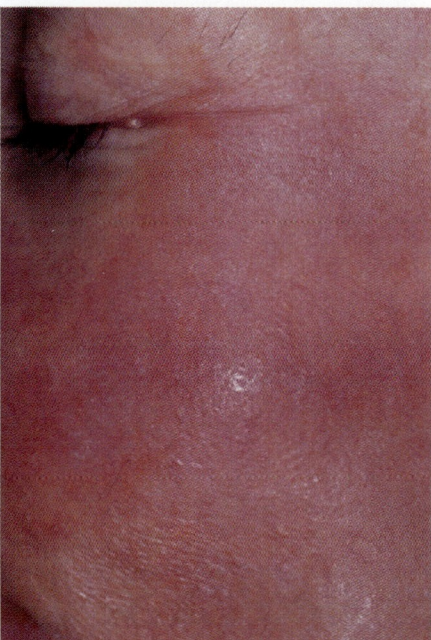

FIGURE 23–4 • Whitish salicylic acid crystals and mild frosting can be seen on the lower cheek of this patient following a 40% salicylic acid peel for dermatoheliosis.

with trichloroacetic acid peels. The crystallized material is easily wiped away with water. Small amounts of the crystallized salicylic acid will remain in the follicular ostia, however, accounting for the ability of this peel to induce comedolysis. This peel is actually self-

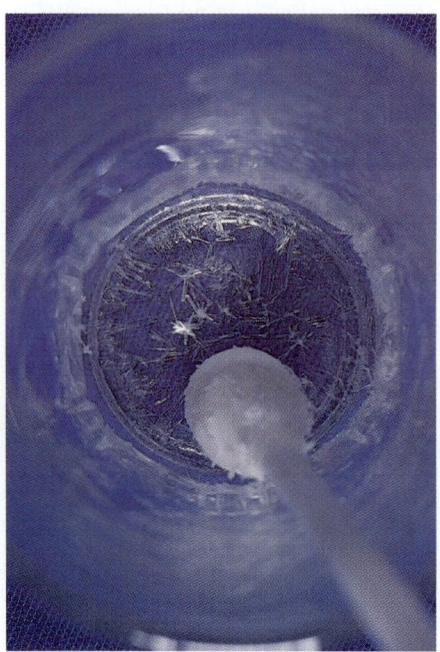

FIGURE 23–5 • Salicylic acid crystallizes on all of the equipment used during the peel, necessitating removal with detergent and water.

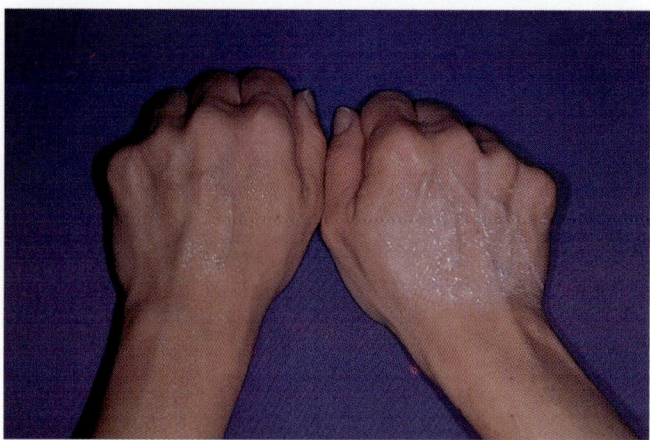

FIGURE 23–6 • Glycolic acid has been applied to the left hand, whereas salicylic acid has been applied to the right hand. Glycolic acid requires rinsing with water to remove the excess peel solution from the skin. Salicylic acid crystallizes on the skin surface and self-neutralizes.

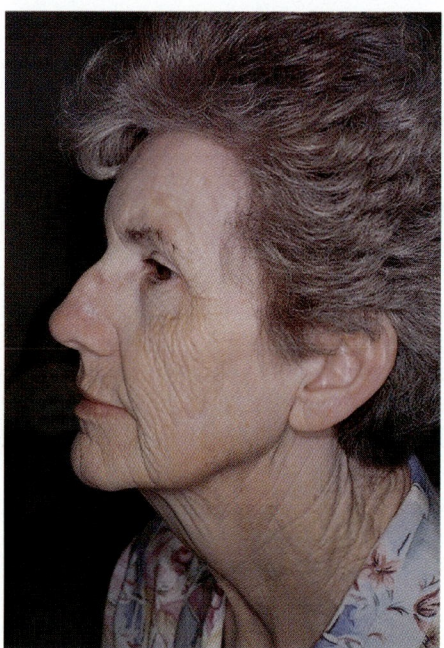

FIGURE 23–7 • Patients with prominent dermatoheliosis will experience only minimal improvement from a glycolic acid or salicylic acid peel alone. A combination peel tends to yield more dramatic results.

TABLE 23–4 Combination Hydroxy Acid Peel or Jessner's Peel Recipe

Ingredient	Amount
Lactic acid liquid	14 mL
Salicylic acid powder	14 g
Resorcinol powder	14 g
Ethyl alcohol 95%	Enough to make a solution totaling 100 cc in volume

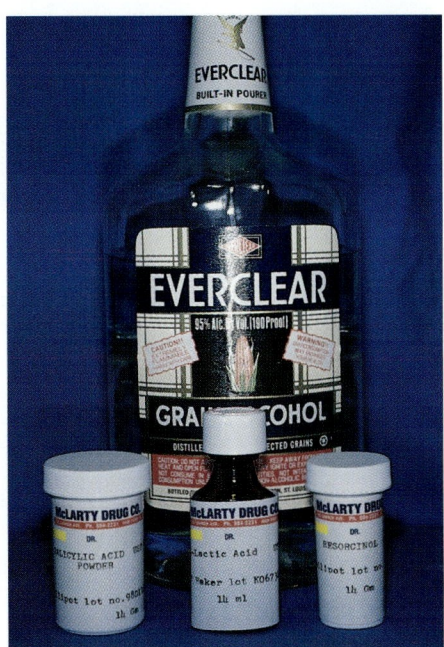

FIGURE 23–8 • The author prepares the Jessner's peel solution with Everclear and premeasured portions of resorcinol, lactic acid, and salicylic acid.

neutalizing owing to the crystallization. The crystallization also minimizes dermal penetration of the salicylic acid, making this the preferred peel for patients with rosacea and sensitive skin.

3. Combination Hydroxy Acid Peels (Jessner's Solution Peels)

For patients who wish to have a deeper peel, or for those who smoke or exhibit moderate photoaging, pure glycolic or salicylic acid peels induce little exfoliation (Fig. 23–7). These patients achieve better results with a combination hydroxy acid peel, also known as the Jessner's peel (see Table 23–2). These peels contain both lactic and salicylic acid, combined with resorcinol and ethyl alcohol (Table 23–4, Fig. 23–8). The peel is applied in the same manner as a pure salicylic acid peel, except more intense frosting is achieved. For patients who wish to have a surgical peel, the Jessner's peel should be combined with trichloroacetic acid. A full discussion of deeper surgical peels is beyond the scope of this text.

24

Cellulite Treatments

Cellulite is a cosmetic problem of medical interest that afflicts most postpubertal women. The exact nature of cellulite is unknown; however, current thinking revolves around the theory that cellulite represents an inflammatory process secondary to decreased circulation. The new data available have resulted from ultrasound evaluation of the upper thighs. The initial change leading to cellulite formation is the deterioration of the dermal vasculature, particularly loss of the capillary networks. As a result, excess fluid is retained within the dermal and subcutaneous tissues. This loss of the capillary network is thought to be attributable to engorged fat cells clumping together and inhibiting venous return. The fat deposition is hormonally mediated, accounting for the higher number of women than men affected by cellulite and the propensity for upper/outer thigh involvement.[1]

Once the capillary networks have been damaged, vascular changes begin to occur within the dermis, resulting in decreased protein synthesis and an inability to repair tissue damage. Clumps of protein are deposited around the fatty deposits beneath the skin, giving the skin an "orange peel" appearance when it is pinched between the thumb and forefinger (Fig. 24–1). At this stage, however, there is no visual evidence of cellulite.

The characteristic appearance of cellulite is only seen after hard nodules, composed of fat surrounded by hard reticular protein, form within the dermis (Fig. 24–2). At this stage, ultrasound imaging of skin affected by cellulite reveals thinning of the dermis, with subcutaneous fat pushing upward. This translates into the rumpled skin known as cellulite (Fig. 24–3). Inflammation is also operative in the process.

Current methods for improving the appearance of cellulite include herbal supplements, methylxanthines, and manipulation.[2] Herbal treatments for cellulite abound, and usually contain a complex mixture of numerous extracts, such as those listed in Table 24–1. These extracts contain xanthine derivatives, which are thought to act as tissue decongestants by improving lymphatic drainage and minimizing peripheral edema.[3] Well-controlled medical studies are lacking, however.

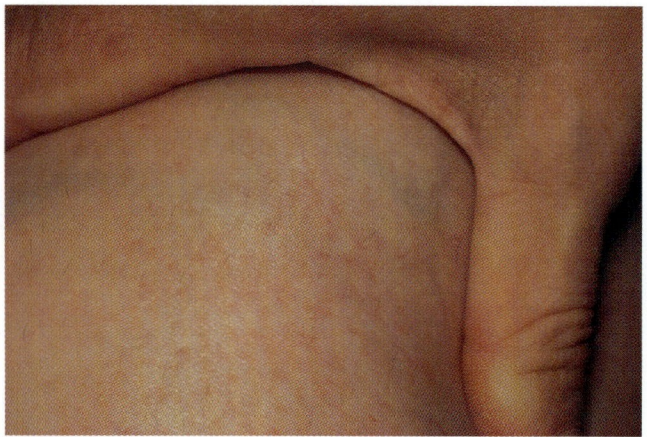

FIGURE 24–1 • Early cellulite is characterized by a dimpling of the skin surface. Note the varicosed vein that is also present, probably contributing to the vascular damage that is thought to give rise to cellulite.

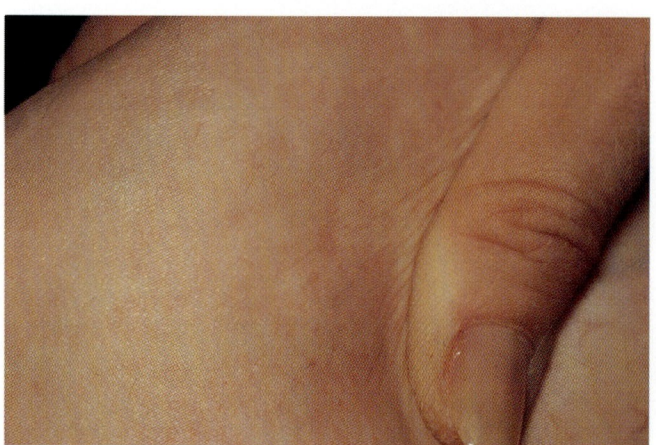

FIGURE 24–2 • Large, clumped nodules, indicative of intermediate-stage cellulite, are present on the upper thighs of this patient.

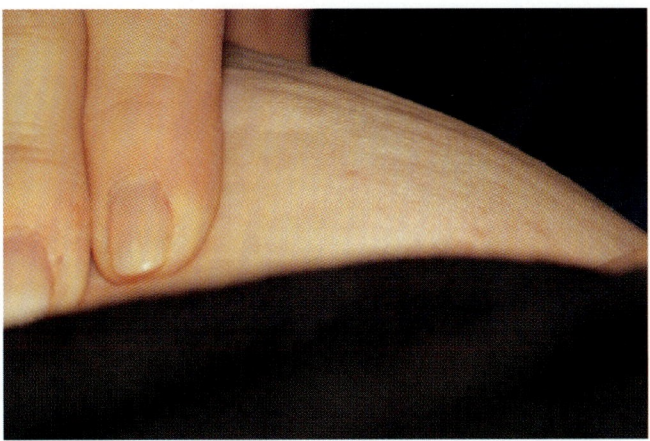

FIGURE 24–3 • With side lighting, the characteristic dimples of the final stage of cellulite can be visualized.

TABLE 24–1 Herbal Extracts Used in Topical Cellulite Treatments

Botanical Extract	Common Name
Aloysia triphylla	Verbena
Camellia japonica	Green tea
Citrus limon	Lemon
Cola acuminata	Kola nut
Foeniculum officinale	Fennel
Fucus vesiculosus	Algae
Hedera helix	Ivy
Hordeum	Barley
Mitchella repens	Strawberry
Origanum vulgare	Marjoram
Trifolium subterraneum	Sweet clover

Another approach to the treatment of cellulite is enhanced lipolysis via topical methylxanthines, such as caffeine and theophylline. Methylxanthines promote lipolysis by inhibiting phosphodiesterase, which transforms cyclic adenosine monophosphate (cAMP) into adenosine monophosphate (AMP), leading to the conversion of triglycerides into free fatty acids and glycerol. Any improvement in cellulite occurs over a period of months, and continued methylxanthine application is required.

Skin kneading, also known as endermologie (LPG; Fort Lauderdale, Florida), is a cellulite treatment technique based on the use of a patented machine.[4] The treatment involves rubbing of the skin with an electrically powered, hand-held box containing two rollers. The skin is sucked between the rollers and kneaded. A technician moves the machine over the hips, stomach, legs, and buttocks, which are covered with a nylon stocking to decrease friction. Each treatment lasts 35 to 45 minutes. Initially, 15 treatments are ad-

ministered, followed by monthly maintenance treatment sessions. The company's literature is careful to state that mechanized skin kneading does not remove the cellulite, but rather reduces its appearance, probably by decreasing tissue edema.

Cellulite treatments are included here for completeness. However, they currently represent cosmetic rather than medical treatments.

REFERENCES

1. Smith WP. Cellulite treatments: Snake oils or skin science? Cosmet Toiletr 110:61–70, 1995.
2. Di Salvo RM. Controlling the appearance of cellulite. Cosmet Toiletr 110:50–59, 1995.
3. Bascaglia DA, Conte ET, McCain W, Frideman S. The treatment of cellulite with methylxanthine and herbal extract–based cream: An ultrasonographic analysis. Cosmet Dermatol 9:30–40, 1996.
4. Vergereau R. Use of mechanical skin fold rolling in cosmetic medicine. J Cosmet Med Dermatol Surg (French) 85:49–53, 1995.

25

Evaluating Skin Care Product Lines for Dispensing

Dispensing of cosmetics and skin care products is currently a controversial area within dermatology. Dermatologists have traditionally provided medical advice, rather than products, to their patients. In most states, physicians cannot dispense prescriptions, but can sell over-the-counter products through their offices (Figs. 25–1 and 25–2). These products can be manufactured either in the United States or abroad. It is interesting to note that dispensing dermatologists are more numerous in California, New York, and Florida than in other areas of the United States. The Midwest is an area where dispensing is less common.

Dermatologists must be extremely careful in how they develop the practice of dispensing within their office. It is always sad when a patient enters my office and inquires about the value of two jars of cream she has purchased for $100 from a dermatologist in a

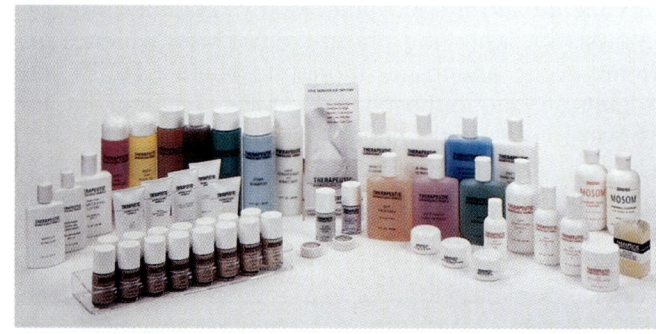

FIGURE 25–2 • Some product lines incorporate a tremendous variety of products for dispensing.

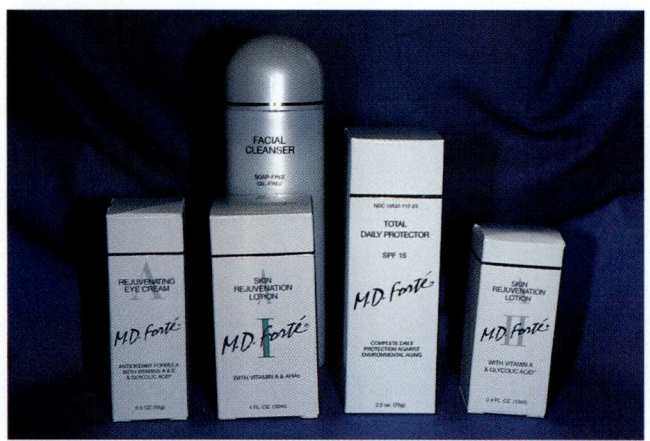

FIGURE 25–1 • This product line was one of the first alpha hydroxy acid formulations available for physician dispensing.

neighboring community. The patient always asks if the creams are worth the money and if the products will provide the benefit she desires. To be honest, there is no jar of over-the-counter cream on the market today that contains substances worth more than $35, excluding the cost of the jar and the packaging. However, the jar and the packaging provide no skin benefit. Certainly, research and development costs must be recouped, but still there is no nonprescription cream that the author has encountered that is worth $50 per jar in terms of medical benefit. It is difficult to put a price on aesthetic benefits, however.

Clearly, there is a need for some guidelines governing dermatologist dispensing, and the author has organized these guidelines in three tables. First, there are some general guidelines to be followed by the dispensing dermatologist (Table 25–1). The dermatologist who dispenses must be much better informed than the nonmedically trained salesperson at the cosmetic counter. The dermatologist should understand

TABLE 25–1 General Guidelines for the Dispensing Dermatologist

• • • • •

1. Personally use every product you dispense for 1 month.
2. Understand the purpose and effect of every ingredient contained in the dispensed formulations.
3. Define the medically established skin benefit(s) of each product dispensed.
4. Do not claim to have personally developed the product line unless this statement is factually true.
5. Obtain a business license and sales tax number in compliance with the laws of your state.

TABLE 25–2 Product Selection Guidelines for Dispensing

• • • • •

1. Select a product that has an established reputation in the dermatologic community.
2. The price point of the product should not be excessive for the area in which the dermatologist practices.
3. The product should be dated to reduce the risk of dispensing spoiled materials.
4. The product should be sealed to avoid dispensing of contaminated materials.
5. A physician hotline number, provided by the manufacturer, should be available for answering questions and discussing problems.
6. Data that meet current standards of scientific accuracy should be provided to support the product line.
7. Patch test materials should be readily available from the manufacturer.
8. Product lines with untested novel ingredients should not be selected.
9. The product line should be formulated with a minimum of ingredients, potential allergens, and potential irritants.
10. The product line should be manufactured in the United States where FDA guidelines are enforced.

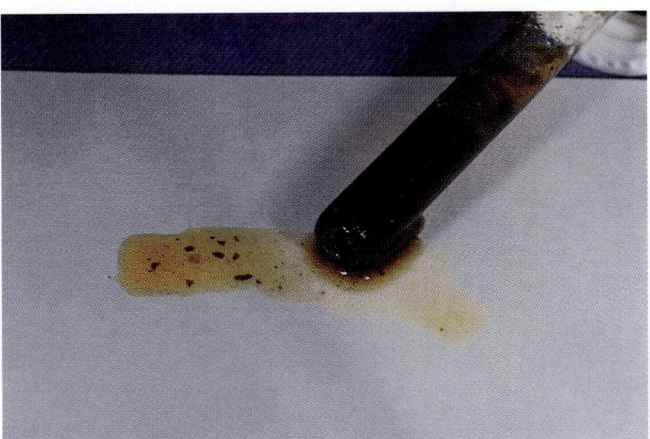

FIGURE 25–3 • A vitamin C product available for physician dispensing was examined after storage on a temperature-controlled shelf for 3 months. The brown color and irregular appearance of the product indicate that the ascorbic acid oxidized, rendering the product inactive.

the function of each and every ingredient in the formulation and be able to offer the patient a concrete description of the expected skin benefits. Products that have no medically established skin benefit should not be dispensed. Products that are not accompanied by scientific data generated according to current scientific study guidelines also should not be dispensed. Moreover, in the author's opinion, dermatologists should use all products dispensed for at least 1 month. Products that do not perform on the dermatologist's face cannot be expected to perform on a patient's face.

Second, there are criteria that should be applied to products selected for dispensing. Many, many products are available for physician dispensing. One can be assured that the company is making more money off of the products dispensed than the dermatologist, hence the fierce competition. Any product selected for dispensing should meet all of the guidelines listed in Table 25–2, or the dermatologist may experience difficulties related to liability issues (Fig. 25–3). Many dermatologists are not aware that some of the products they are asked to dispense are not manufactured

TABLE 25–3 Guidelines for Ethical Dispensing

• • • • •

1. The final product purchase price should cover wholesale cost, shipping, and office overhead only.
2. The medical portion of the office should be separate from the dispensing showcase.
3. Patients should not be required to walk by the dispensing showcase to exit the office.
4. Products should not be dispensed in the examination room. The medical portion of the visit should remain separate from any dispensing activities.
5. Unused products that are returned by the patient should be refunded in cash.
6. The identity and manufacturer of the products should be revealed to the patient.
7. Ingredient lists for purchased products should be provided to all patients. (*Note:* This is not a requirement for professional products.)
8. Patients who purchase products should be shown no favoritism over patients who do not purchase products.
9. Patients should not be given a discount on a product purchase based on referred sales from other patients.
10. False claims regarding the efficacy of products must not be made. If no scientific data exist to support product efficacy, the patient must be so informed.
11. Patients should not be told that dermatologist-dispensed products are better than those sold in the mass market, unless scientific data exist to support that claim.
12. Patients should not be encouraged to purchase products they do not need to meet accepted skin care standards.
13. Bonuses based on product sales should not be paid to the medical office staff.

in the United States. Products that are imported do not have to meet FDA guidelines for plant cleanliness, manufacturing procedures, raw materials, etc. These products may contain substances that are not appropriate for patient use.

Lastly, the dermatologist must practice ethical dispensing, guidelines for which are included in Table 25–3. It is important to separate the medical aspects of a visit to a dermatologist from the product sales. Patients should feel like they are coming to visit a physician, not visiting the cosmetic counter at the local mall. Physicians are valued highly in our society for their professionalism, knowledge, and intellect. Patients share experiences and concerns with physicians that they would not relate to anyone else. Dermatologists are a privileged few who have received the training to heal problems related to the skin, hair, and nails. We are in jeopardy of losing this privilege if we do not carefully consider the important aspects of product dispensing.

PART

·
·
·
·
·
·
·
·
·
·
·
·
·
·
·
·
·

HAIR
CARE

26

Hair Care Implements

Hair care involves the use of a variety of implements designed to groom, style, shape, and alter the configuration of the hair shafts into an aesthetically pleasing appearance, dictated by individual preference and fashion trends. A discussion of these implements is important to the dermatologist, as the improper selection of hair care devices can lead to hair loss or accentuate the effect of medically induced alopecia. The altas format of this text lends itself to the visual presentation of guidelines to share with patients regarding hair care. Table 26–1 can be used as a patient instruction sheet, summarizing the material presented below.

1. Combs

Combs are the most common grooming implement used by men and women to arrange the hair shafts in a parallel, orderly manner. Selection of a comb that does not fracture the hair shaft is especially important in dermatologic patients with hair loss. Figure 26–1 demonstrates the ideal comb for hair loss patients. The comb should have broadly spaced teeth with rounded tips and sides to prevent tearing the hair shafts. Ideally, a handle should be present to allow the comb to be gradually drawn through the hair without undue force or friction. Soft, molded plastic combs are preferred over wood or metal combs owing to the rounded and smoothed teeth. Other specialty combs are manufactured for hair cutting purposes (Fig. 26–2).

Excessive trauma from combing contributes to weathering, or damage to the cuticle of the hair shaft. Figure 26–3 shows an undamaged hair shaft, with even overlapping of the cuticular scale. Contrast this image with Figure 26–4, in which the cuticular scale is irregular and even missing in certain areas (Fig. 26–5). Loss of cuticular scale is accentuated by vigorous combing and by combing the hair when it is wet. However, the most damage occurs when the hair is combed opposite to the direction of cuticular scale overlap, in other words, from the distal to proximal hair shaft (Fig. 26–6). This grooming technique, known as "teasing," should be avoided to minimize hair shaft damage and ultimate loss.

2. Brushes

Similar advice applies to the selection of brushes. They, too, should have broadly spaced teeth with rounded tips, and ideally, should be made out of a pliable plastic material (Fig. 26–7). Brushes used during the hair drying process should have vents to prevent heat build-up along the brush, which can denature hair protein. If the hair is severely tangled, it should be combed first and then brushed. Some tangles can only be removed by combing or brushing the hair in small segments beginning at the distal hair shaft and working toward the scalp.

TABLE 26–1 **Grooming Guidelines for Patients with Hair Loss**

1. Never comb or brush the hair while it is wet.
2. Allow the hair to air dry.
3. Always use the lowest temperature setting for heated hair appliances.
4. Select a wide-toothed, flexible, plastic comb to use for gentle grooming.
5. Comb, rather than brush, the hair whenever possible.
6. Select a plastic, rounded-tip, coarse brush, if required.
7. Avoid the use of tight hair clasps or rubber bands.
8. Vary the part line and hair style frequently.
9. Select hair styles that place minimal tension on the hair and the scalp.
10. Groom the hair only when necessary, keeping manipulation of the hair to a minimum.
11. Avoid exposing the hair to wind and sun.
12. Handle the hair like a fine silk blouse.

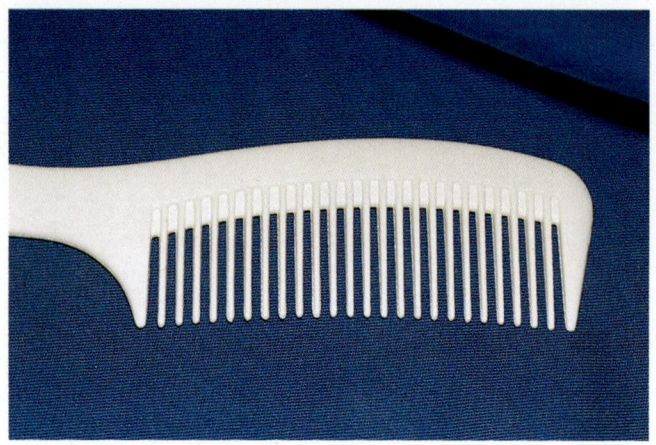

FIGURE 26–1 • Combs with smooth, widely spaced teeth should be selected.

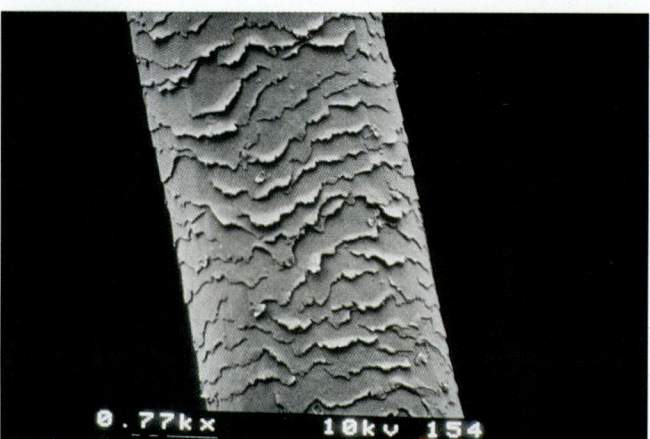

FIGURE 26–4 • Early damage to the hair shaft results in a lifting of the cuticular scale.

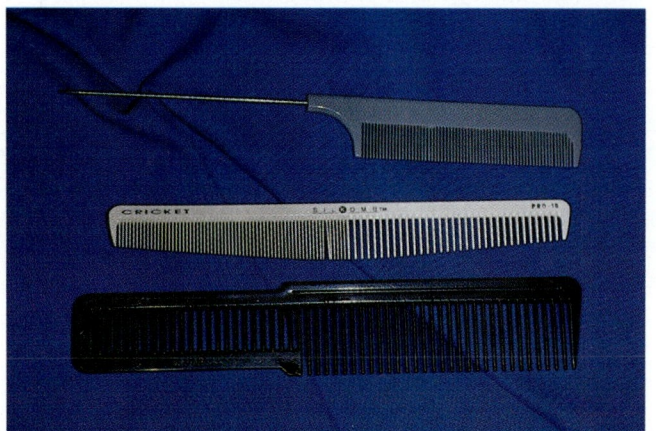

FIGURE 26–2 • These specialty fine-toothed combs are used to smooth and even the hair for cutting.

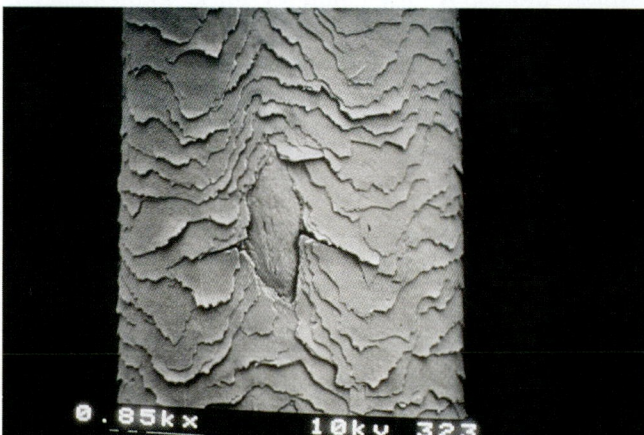

FIGURE 26–5 • Severe damage results in loss of the cuticular scale.

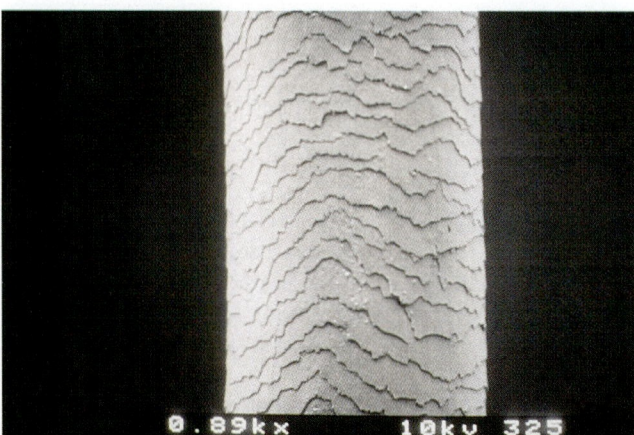

FIGURE 26–3 • A healthy hair shaft has an evenly overlapping, intact cuticle.

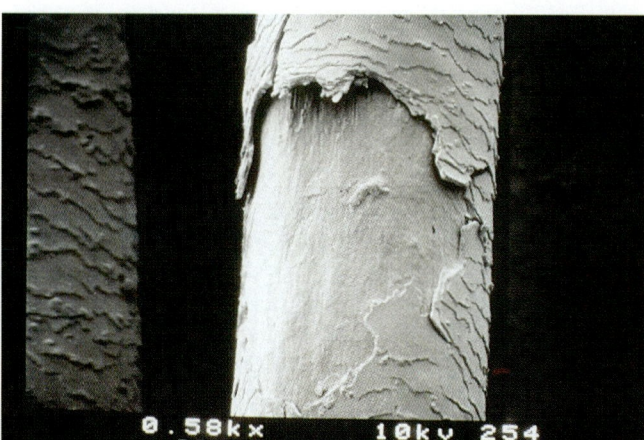

FIGURE 26–6 • Loss of large areas of the cuticle weakens the hair shaft and lessens its cosmetic value.

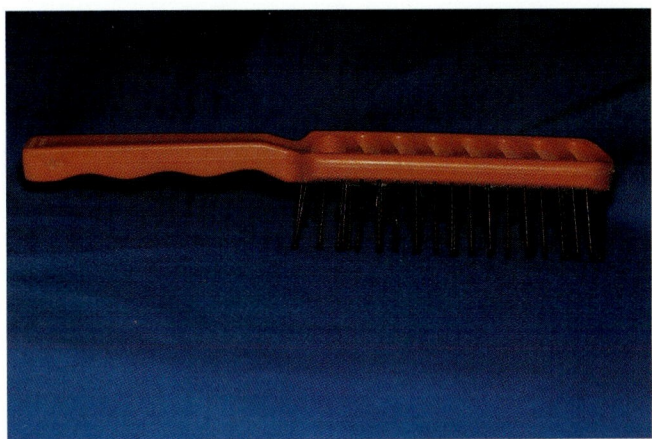

FIGURE 26–7 • A vented, wide-toothed, ball-tipped brush is essential for drying and styling the hair with minimal damage.

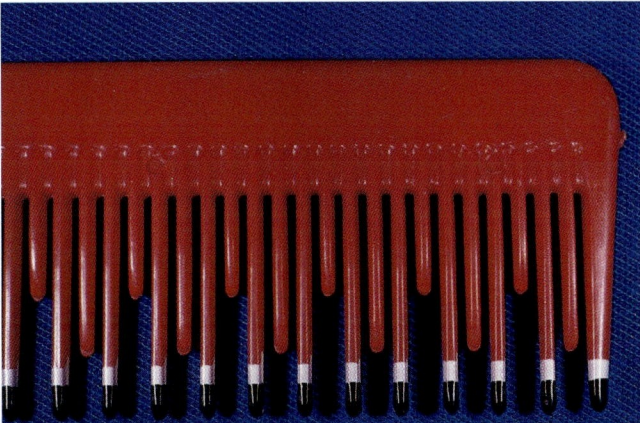

FIGURE 26–9 • This teasing comb is used to comb the hair from the distal hair shaft to the proximal hair shaft, resulting in tangles of hair that create the illusion of fullness.

Proper selection of brushes may be ensured by stroking the brush across the palm of the hand. If the bristles feel rough, they are more likely to fracture the hair shaft. Figure 26–8 demonstrates a poor brush design for patients with hair loss.

3. Styling Combs

A variety of specialty combs have been developed to finish the hair styling process. Two are worthy of mention: teasing combs (Fig. 26–9) and hair picks (Fig. 26–10). Teasing combs contain closely spaced teeth of different lengths which are designed to create tangles in the hair, known in hair dressing circles as "rats." Teasing combs are sometimes referred to as "rat combs" for this reason. These tangles (Fig. 26–11) create the illusion of fullness by allowing the hair to stand away from the scalp. However, this backcomb-

ing is extremely damaging to the hair shafts owing to the cuticular disruption mentioned earlier. The tangles are also difficult to remove and eventually result in hair breakage.

Hair picks are combs on a handle with broadly spaced long teeth. They are used for several purposes. In straight hair that has been teased, the pick is used to smooth and arrange the tangles into a finished hair style prior to setting with hair spray. These combs are also used in kinky hair for basic grooming, since combing is impossible.

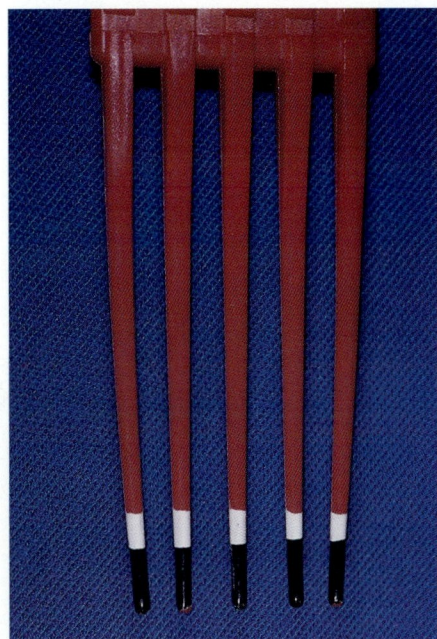

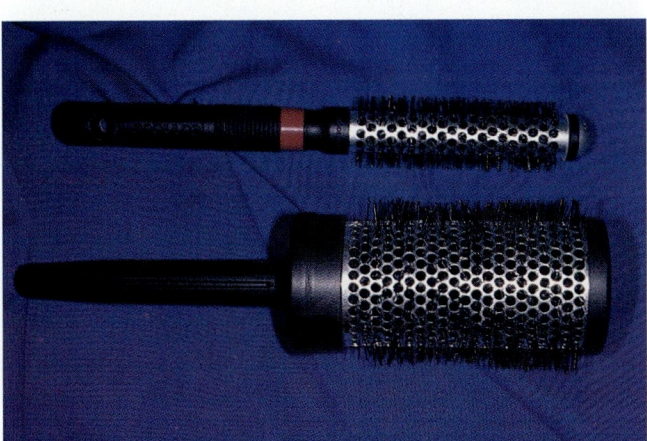

FIGURE 26–8 • These brushes easily catch and tear the hair shaft.

FIGURE 26–10 • This broad-toothed comb is known as a pick. It is used to arrange and smooth the tangles created by teasing, as the hair can no longer be combed.

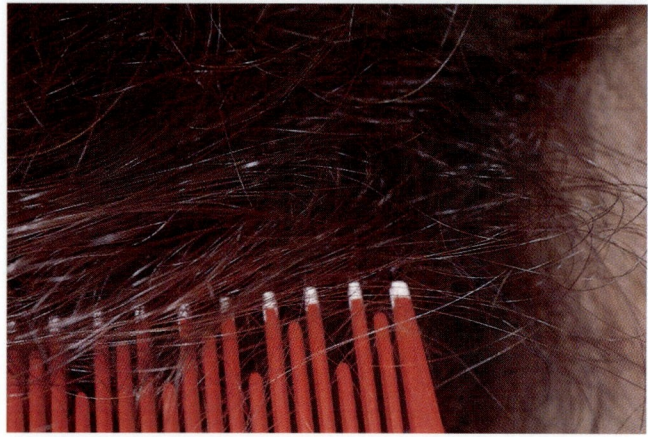

FIGURE 26–11 • Teasing of the hair purposefully creates tangles, resulting in hair breakage and irreversible damage to the cuticle.

4. Clasps and Adornments

The number of combs, barrettes, clasps, bands, clips, bows, pins, and ties available to style the hair is extensive. This section focuses on hair clasps and adornment selection in patients with easily fractured hair shafts. Selection should be made based on the concept that hair should not be tightly squeezed, since this precipitates hair loss. Figure 26–12 demonstrates bands and clasps used to hold the hair into a pony tail on the back of the head. These barrettes will cause the hair to fracture if used repeatedly in the same place on the scalp. Patients using these clasps may state that their hair is no longer growing when, in

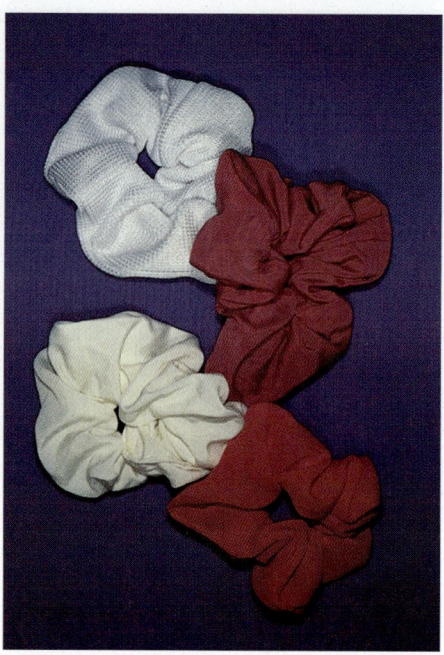

FIGURE 26–13 • Cloth-covered, loose-fitting bands prevent hair breakage.

fact, the hair shafts are breaking off at a rate quicker than new growth. Preferred hair clasps are shown in Figure 26–13.

5. Rollers and Hair Curling Aids

Rollers and hair curling aids should also be selected to minimize hair breakage. For example, sleeping in brush rollers or toothed rollers is likely to result in substantial hair breakage over time (Figs. 26–14

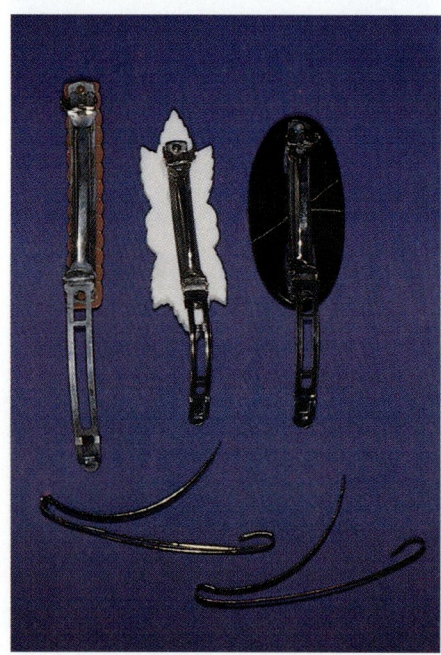

FIGURE 26–12 • Tight hair clasps can fracture the hair shaft.

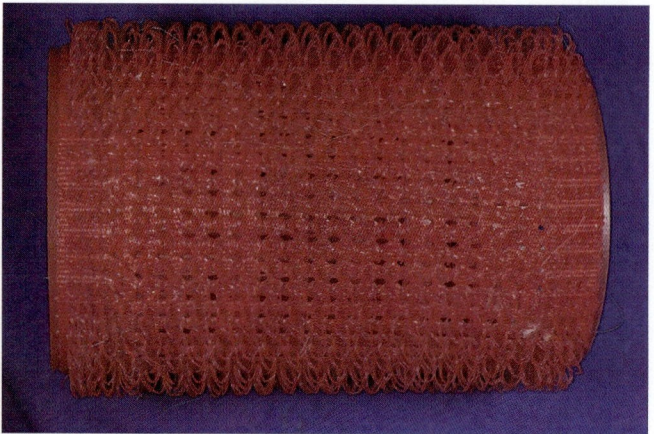

FIGURE 26–14 • Brush rollers are preferred by hairdressers because they securely hold the hair shafts. However, hair breakage is common.

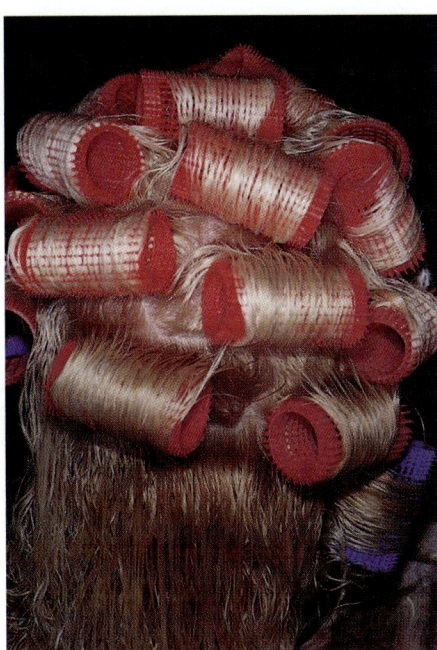

FIGURE 26–15 • This is a typical roller set, as might be done in a hair salon.

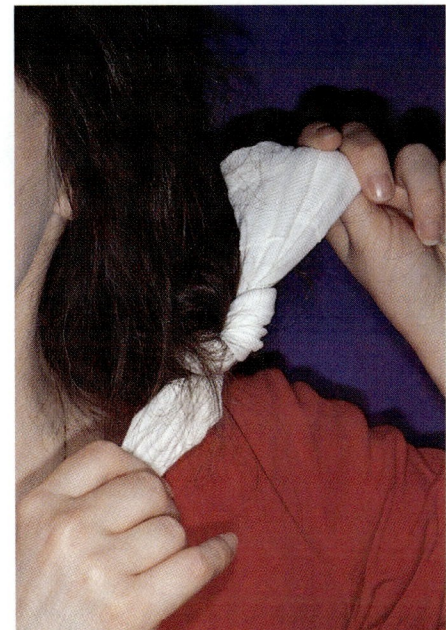

FIGURE 26–17 • Nylon stocking that have been torn in strips are a minimally traumatic method of curling the hair.

through 26–16). Ideally, the hair should be allowed to flow freely while sleeping. However, some elderly patients prefer to maintain their hair styles overnight. This can be accomplished by placing a fine hairnet over the hair. If the patient insists on curling their hair at night, the use of old nylon stockings, instead of the more traditional pin curls, may be advantageous. The nylon stockings are cut into strips and the hair is wrapped around the stocking and secured by tying (Fig. 26–17). This provides an inexpensive, effective method of curling the hair while minimizing hair breakage.

6. Dryers

Heat drying of the hair can also be extremely damaging. Bubbles, leading to longitudinal fractures in the hair shaft, occur when the hair is exposed to high temperatures (Fig. 26–18). This damage is irreversible and ultimately results in hair breakage. For this reason, the hair should be air dried, when possible. If heat drying is required, the low temperature setting

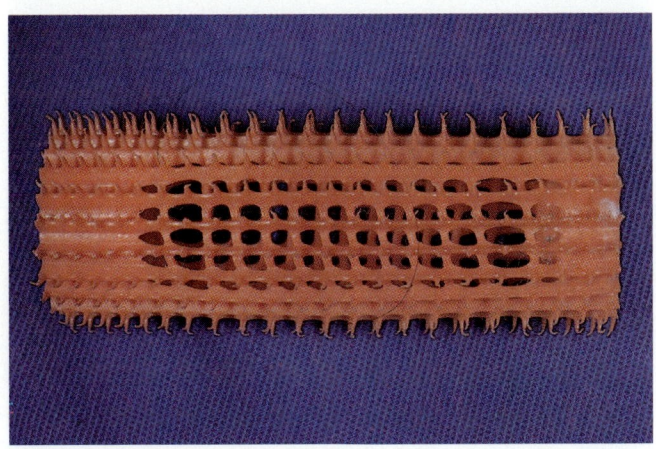

FIGURE 26–16 • Toothed rollers can also tear the hair shaft.

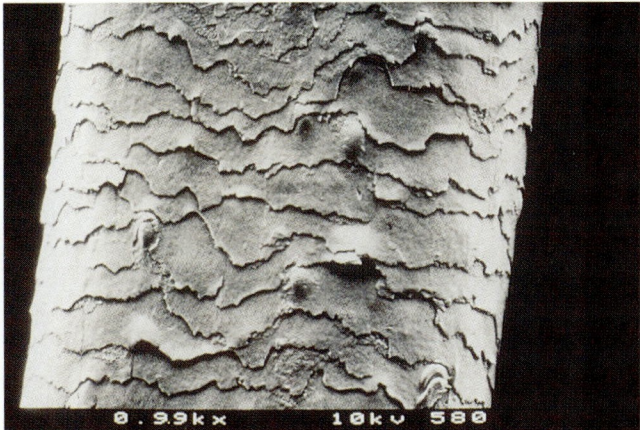

FIGURE 26–18 • Exposure of the hair shaft to high temperature results in the formation of bubbles within the hair shaft, which permanently weaken its strength.

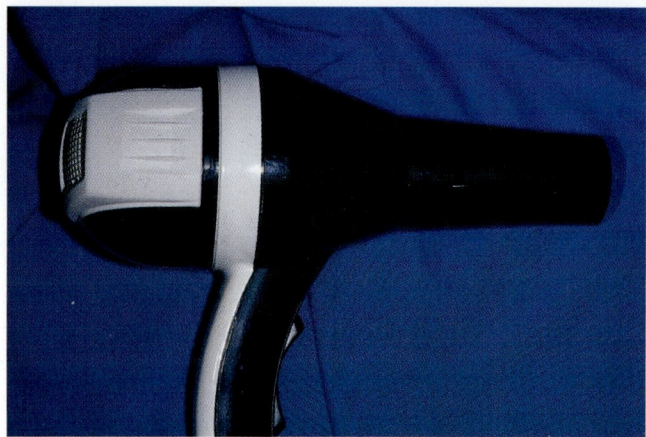

FIGURE 26–19 • Hand-held hair dryers are preferred to hooded hair dryers, yet they must be used on a low heat setting to avoid permanent hair shaft damage.

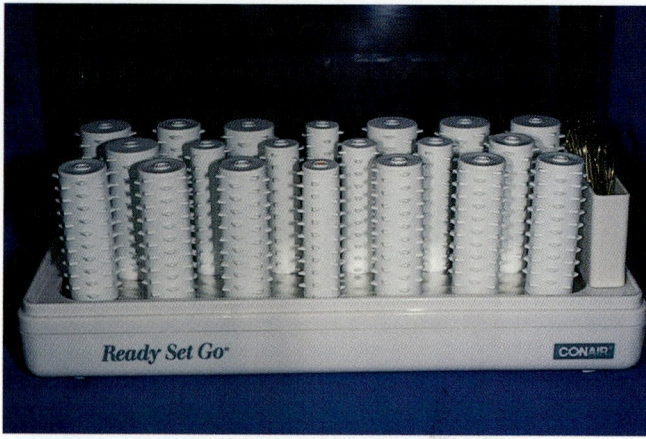

FIGURE 26–21 • Heated curlers should be used on a low heat setting or allowed to cool a few minutes after heating prior to wrapping the hair.

should be selected and the dryer held at least 12 inches from the hair (Figs. 26–19 and 26–20). Damage can also be minimized by selecting a brush with vents to prevent heat build-up during drying, as mentioned previously (see Fig. 26–7).

7. Electric Styling Devices

Electric styling devices, such as heated curlers (Fig. 26–21) and curling irons (Fig. 26–22), are even more

damaging to the hair than blow dryers, since the heat is applied directly to the hair shaft. These appliances operate at temperatures ranging from 100° C to 170° C. In the temperature range of 50° to 120° C, removal of water from the hair shaft occurs, decreasing its plasticity.[1] This means that the hair shaft will fracture more readily when pulled. It also renders the hair shaft more susceptible to static electricity, ultimately decreasing manageability. Heat-altered hair also requires increased combing force, which also promotes hair breakage.

Longer applications of direct heat to the hair shaft, such as is the case with curling irons, can result in destabilization of the alpha helical component of the hair shaft. This structural change renders the hair shaft extremely weak. Decomposition of cysteine and tyrosine, as well as oxidation of trytophan to kynurenine,

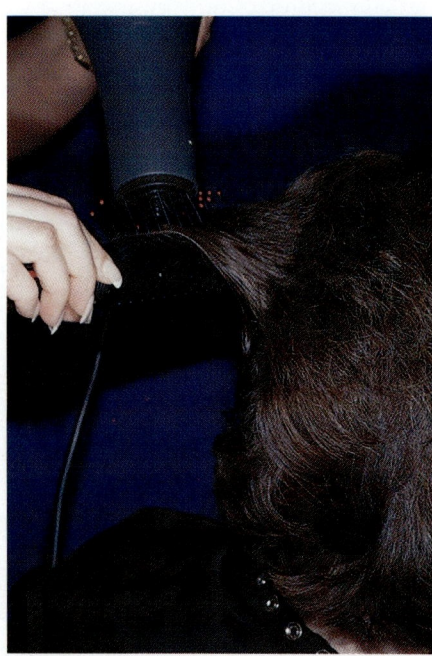

FIGURE 26–20 • Holding the blow dryer directly over the hair shafts will result in permanent heat damage. At least 12 inches should be allowed between the dryer nozzle and the hair shaft.

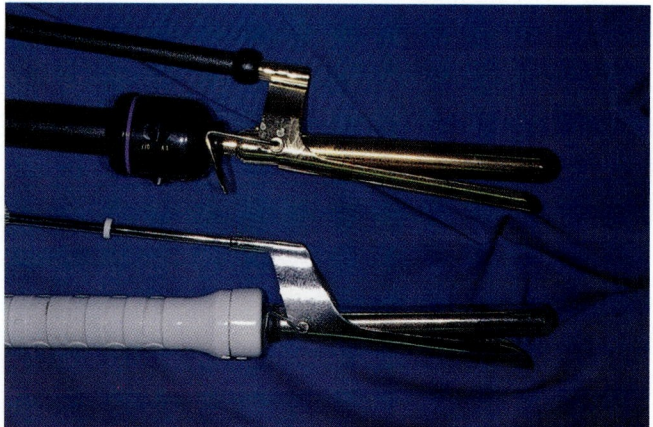

FIGURE 26–22 • Curling irons are major sources heat-induced damage to the hair shaft. Prior to use on the hair, they should be cooled by wrapping the hot iron in a moist bath towel.

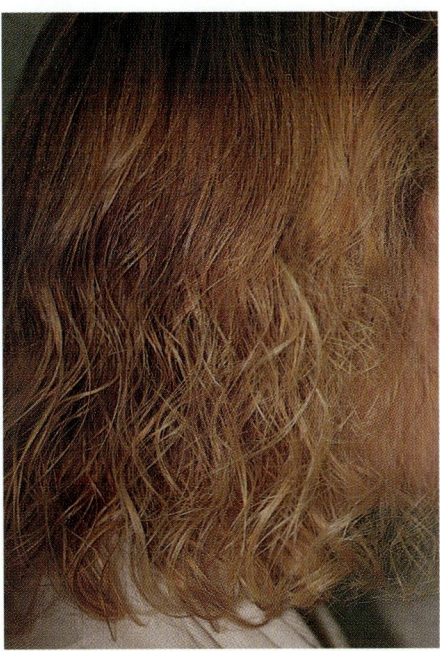

FIGURE 26–23 • An example of the yellowing of blond hair due to prolonged heat damage.

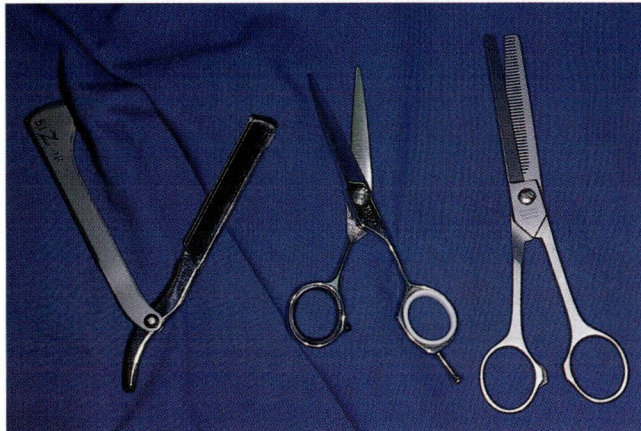

FIGURE 26–25 • Three hair cutting tools are demonstrated: a razor for razor cuts (far left), a straight hair cutting scissor (center), and a pair of toothed, thinning shears for extra-thick hair (far right).

also can result in yellowing of the hair shaft. This color change is especially noticeable in bleached hair, blonde hair, and light brown hair (Fig. 26–23).[2]

The heat causes bubbling, splitting, and protein denaturation that is permanent. Many patients are amazed at the second-degree burns they develop when the skin is accidentally momentarily touched with a curling iron. This is the same heat to which the hair is exposed during the curling process. Again, it is important to use the heated styling devices on the low heat setting. It is also desirable to cool down the devices prior to use by touching the heated surface to a moist towel. This will remove any excess heat and minimize damaging the hair shaft.

8. Scissors

A variety of scissors are available for trimming the hair. A quality pair of sharp scissors will cut the hair shaft with one clean cut, minimizing trauma to the cut edge (Fig. 26–24). Specialty scissors, such as the thinning shears shown in Figure 26–25, are useful for thinning and layering thick hair, but should not be used on fine hair. A good haircut can enhance the appearance of patients with alopecia.

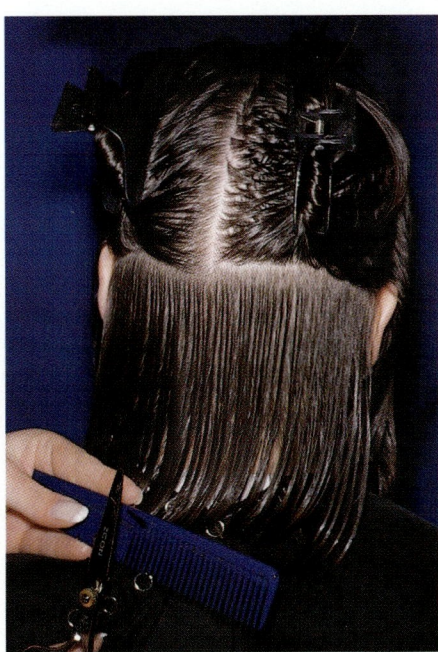

FIGURE 26–24 • Sharp scissors are essential for cutting the hair with a clean, even edge.

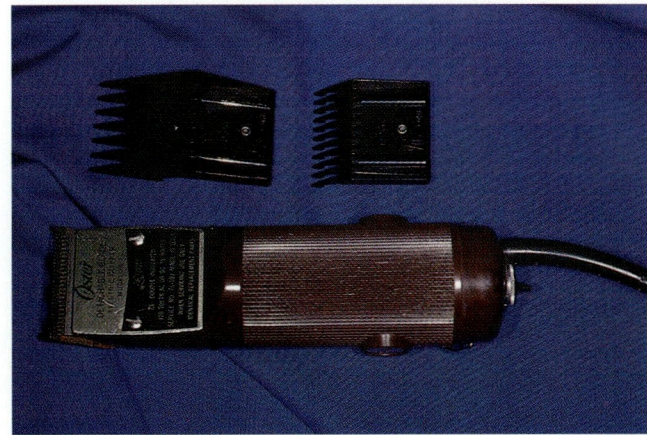

FIGURE 26–26 • Clippers with a sterilized blade guide should be used on patients with acne nuchae keloidalis.

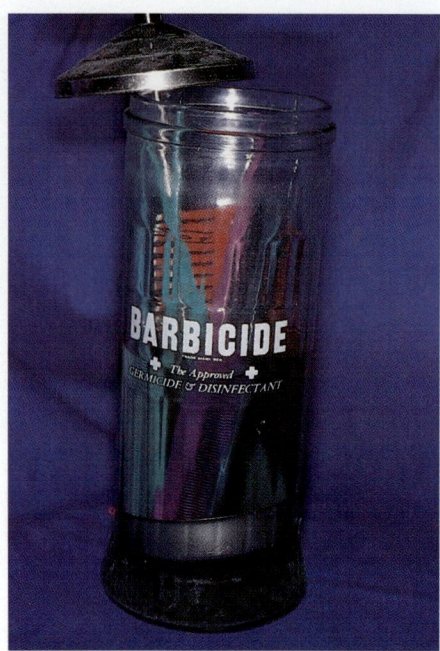

FIGURE 26–27 • This is the typical method used for sterilizing hair cutting equipment in salons; however, it may be inadequate, as demonstrated here. Notice that the combs are not completely submerged in sterilant.

9. Clippers

Clippers are the other hair cutting device, besides scissors, that are used to shorten and groom the hair (Fig. 26–26). Clippers are used to cut the hair close to the skin on the neck and scalp in men. Sharp, sanitized blades are essential to preventing pseudofolliculitis barbae and acne nuchae keloidalis (Fig. 26–27). Patients who suffer from these conditions can greatly benefit from the use of a blade guide on the clippers that prevents the hair from being cut too close to the skin surface (see Fig. 26–26). The blade guides come in a variety of lengths, depending on the desired length of the hair. Leaving the hairs longer can prevent the reentry of hairs into the skin that is responsible for a variety of inflammatory skin conditions.

REFERENCES

1. Milczarek P. Zielinski M. Garcia M. The mechanism and stability of thermal transition in hair keratin. Colloid Polym Sci 270:1106, 1992.
2. McMullen R, Jachowicz J. Thermal degradation of hair. I. Effect of curling irons. J Cosmet Sci 49:223–244, 1998.

27

Hair Prostheses

The patient who is experiencing hair loss from exogenous or endogenous causes may be one of the most difficult to treat. Occasionally, the need arises for temporary or permanent solutions to thinning hair. This section pictorially demonstrates the use of hairpieces, hair additions, and hair forms to camouflage dermatologic hair conditions, also briefly discussing side effects related to their use.

1. Hairpieces

Hairpieces can restore a positive self-image in patients who experience temporary or permanent hair loss. Standard hairpieces, which may be purchased at wig salons, are available in several varieties, as listed in Table 27–1 (Figs. 27–1 through 27–8). Custom-made hairpieces for individuals with special needs can also

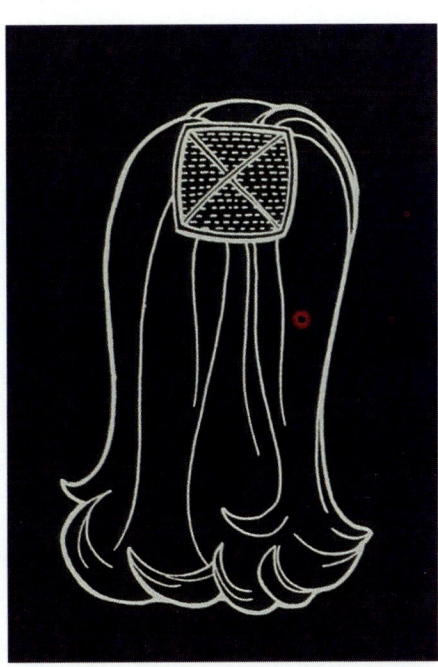

FIGURE 27–1 • A fall consists of long locks of hair attached to a firm, contoured mesh that is designed to rest on the scalp vertex.

be created. Figures 27–9 through 27–14 demonstrate the steps required to fit, manufacture, and customize a vacuum-attached hairpiece for a patient with alopecia universalis. Unique hairpieces can also be designed for patients with special needs (e.g., localized hair loss secondary to radiation therapy) (Figs. 27–15 through 27–18). Hair integration systems can aid the patient with androgenetic alopecia by supplementing existing hair (Figs. 27–19 and 27–20).

Hairpieces may be made of either synthetic fibers or natural human hair. Synthetic hairpieces are easiest to maintain, as the fibers are more resistant to breakage and can be curled permanently, thus eliminating the need for styling. Care for a hairpiece is relatively simple. To wash it, the hairpiece is turned inside out

TABLE 27–1 Standard Types of Hairpieces

Type of Hairpiece	Description
Wig	Covers entire scalp
Fall	Long locks of hair attached to the scalp vertex
Cascade	Curled locks or a bun attached to the posterior scalp
Toupee	Covers the top of the head in men
Demiwig	Covers the entire scalp except the anterior hairline
Wiglet	Localized hairpiece designed to create bangs, add fullness at the top of the scalp, or create the illusion of increased hair length
Switch	Long strands of hair in the form of braids or ponytails
Hair integration system	A coarse meshwork through which existing hair is pulled to increase fullness

113

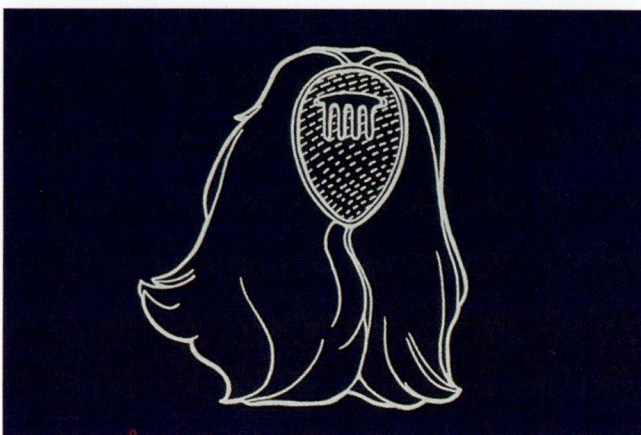

FIGURE 27–2 • A cascade consists of curled locks or a bun attached to a firm, oblong, contoured base that rests on the posterior scalp.

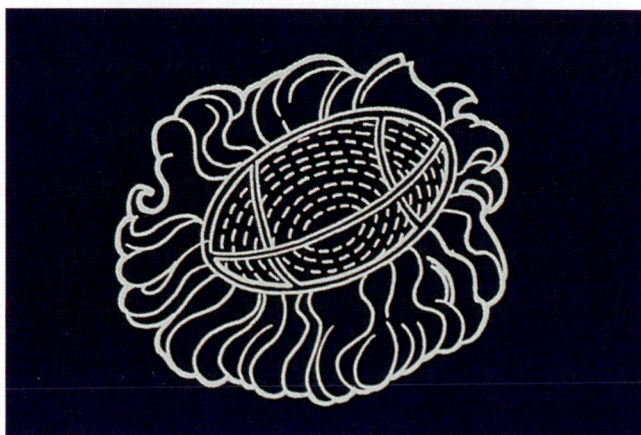

FIGURE 27–3 • A demiwig consists of a flexible, cap-shaped mesh that is designed to cover the entire scalp except the anterior hairline.

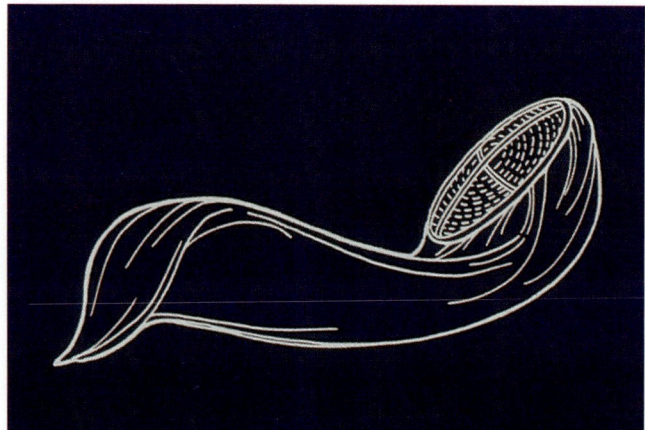

FIGURE 27–4 • A wiglet consists of long lengths of hair attached to a flexible mesh and is intended to create the illusion of long hair.

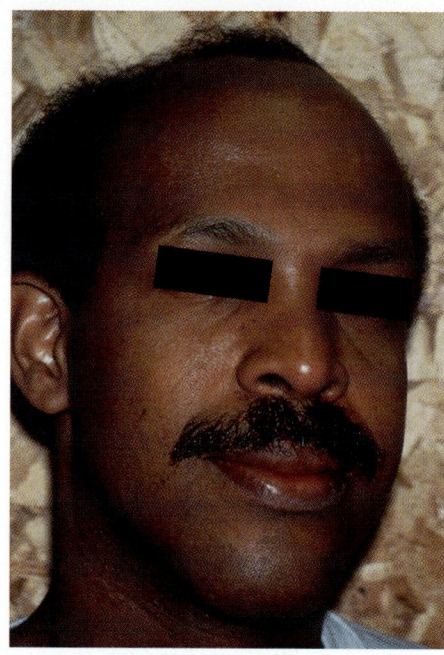

FIGURE 27–5 • A male patient with moderately severe androgenetic alopecia.

and a drop of mild shampoo is placed in the center and gently agitated under a stream of warm water. Once the shampoo is completely removed, a drop of instant conditioner is placed—in natural human hair wigs only—and the hairpiece is again rinsed. The

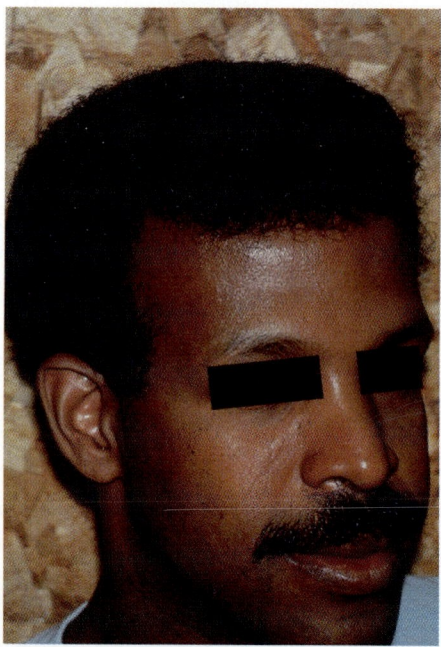

FIGURE 27–6 • The same male patient as in Figure 27–5 is shown wearing a toupee.

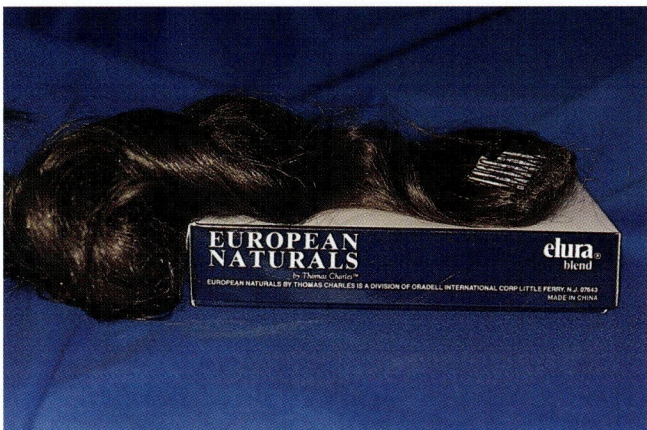

FIGURE 27–7 • A small wiglet designed to be attached to the existing hair with one comb. This might be used to camouflage crown hair loss in women with female pattern hair loss.

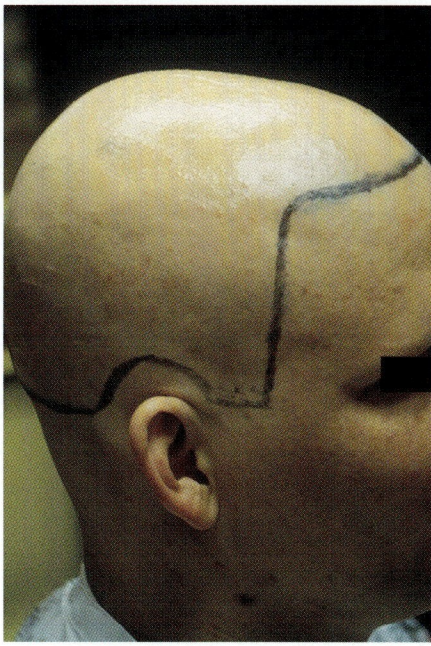

FIGURE 27–9 • The scalp is marked to designate the area where the vacuum prosthesis is to rest.

hairpiece is allowed to air dry while inside out by attaching it with a clothespin to an indoor clothesline. Once dry, the hairpiece may be styled, if required, with a specially designed wig brush.

It is recommended that the patient select a hairpiece prior to complete hair loss, if possible. This allows the patient to adjust emotionally to the prospect of wearing a hairpiece and also aids in selecting a hairpiece that mimics the patient's natural hair color and style. If this is not possible, a picture of the patient prior to hair loss may be extremely helpful.

The biggest problem associated with the use of hairpieces is the method of attachment to the scalp. When the head is completely devoid of hair, vacuum prostheses work well with the aid of an attachment gel. However, if hair remains on the scalp, this tech-

nique cannot be used. Wigs that cover the entire scalp generally are attached to a flexible mesh that stretches to conform to the scalp and can be worn much like a cap. Smaller hairpieces utilize clips as the most common type of attachment (Figs. 27–21 and 27–22). These clips can cause traction alopecia and hair breakage (Fig. 27–23). To prevent this unwanted side effect, some salons have tried implanting clips into the scalp, which ultimately causes even greater problems, such as infection and permanent scarring

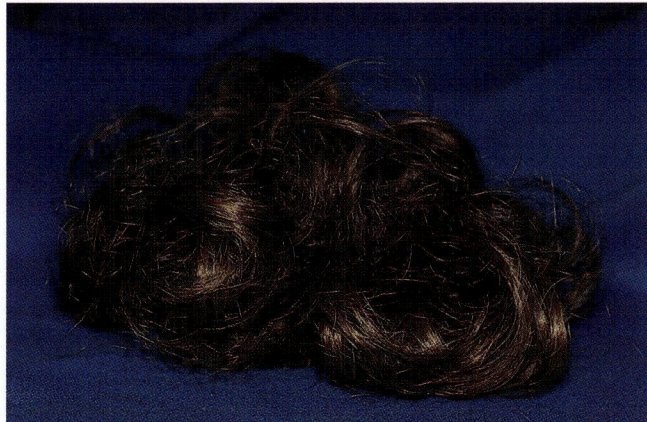

FIGURE 27–8 • This wiglet, known as a hair thickener, is designed to rest on top of the scalp with a loose meshwork through which the patient can pull existing hair. This hairpiece is designed to cover hair loss on top of the scalp in patients with female pattern hair loss.

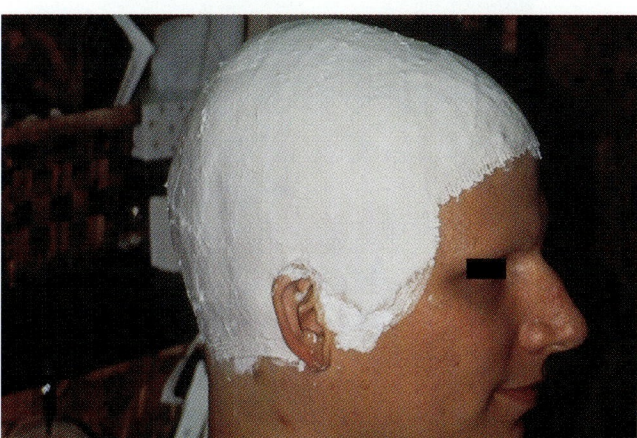

FIGURE 27–10 • A plaster mold is made of the scalp to ensure an exact fit.

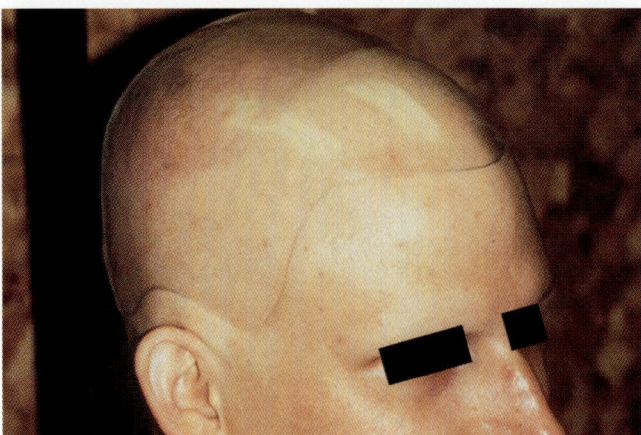

FIGURE 27–11 • From the plaster mold, a form is made to which the hair will eventually be attached. The form must be checked for a proper fit prior to application of the synthetic or human hair.

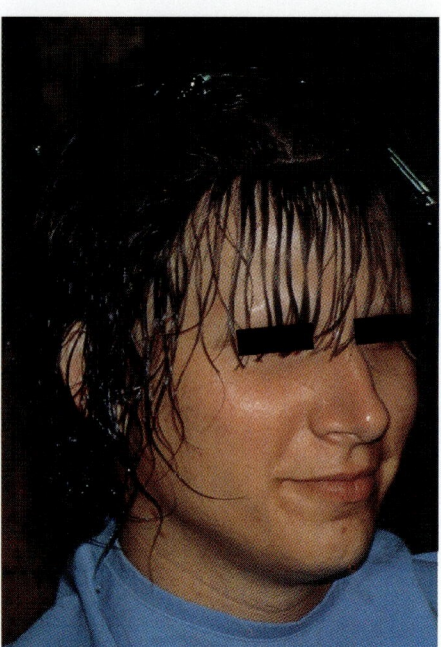

FIGURE 27–13 • The patient then takes the prosthesis to his hairdresser and the hair fibers are styled according to the patient's wishes.

hair loss (Figs. 27–24 and 27–25). The need for secure hairpiece attachment has led to the popularity of hair additions.

2. Hair Additions

With hair additions, existing scalp hair is used to anchor synthetic or natural human hair fibers. Synthetic hair fibers are more popular than natural fibers because they are less expensive, easier to maintain, and lighter in weight. The added fibers may be affixed by braiding, sewing, bonding, or glueing. The attachment method selected depends on the amount of natural hair and the number or length of fibers to be added.

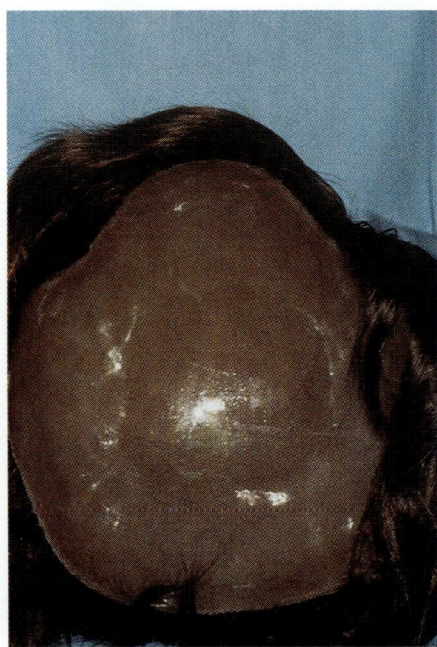

FIGURE 27–12 • The hair is attached to the form and the vacuum prosthesis is completed.

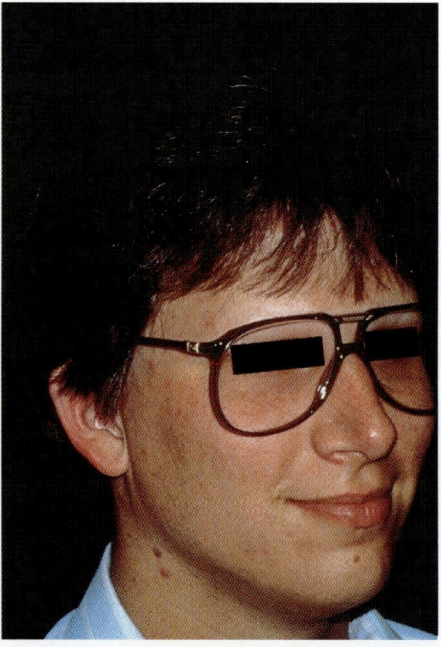

FIGURE 27–14 • The final appearance of a patient with alopecia universalis wearing a vacuum hair prosthesis.

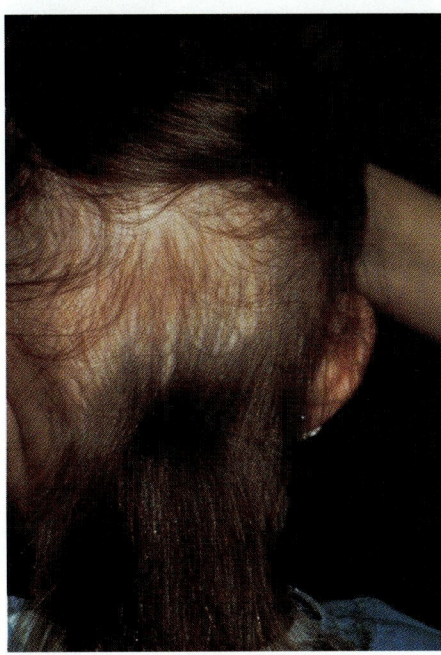

FIGURE 27–15 • A patient with focal hair loss on the posterior scalp secondary to radiation therapy.

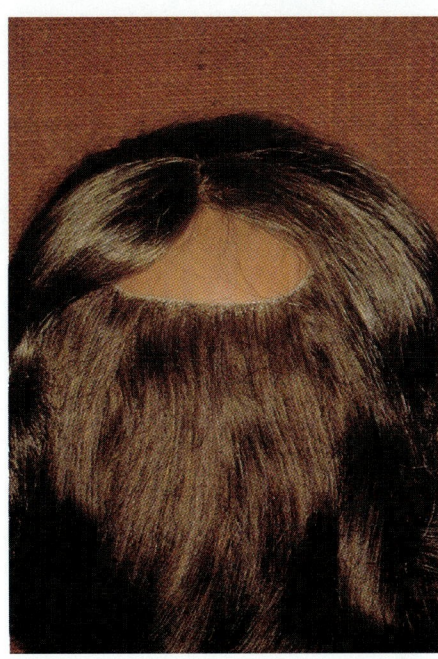

FIGURE 27–17 • The hole in the custom hairpiece allows the patient to pull her existing hair through the hairpiece, imparting a more natural look while anchoring the hairpiece to the scalp.

a. BRAIDING ON THE SCALP

The most popular method of hair additions employs braiding on the scalp, adapted from the black hair style known as "cornrows." Cornrows are plaited on the scalp in geometric designs, with tension applied to the hair shafts exposing scalp between the braids (Figs. 27–26 through 27–28). This is a popular hairstyle among black individuals, as it allows for organization of tightly kinked hair. Individual hair fibers can be woven into the braids to either thicken their ap-

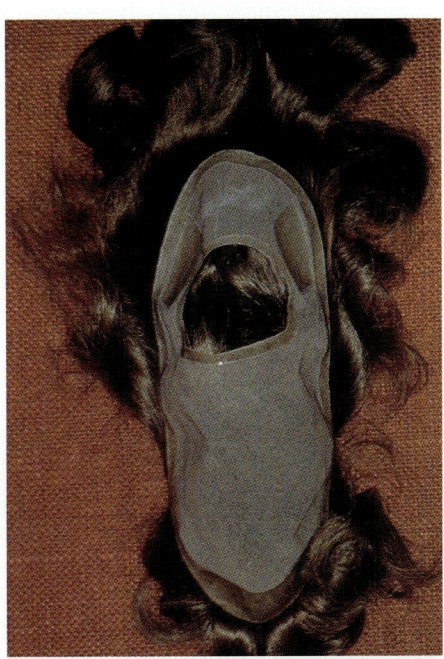

FIGURE 27–16 • A custom hairpiece is designed for the patient in Figure 27–15 to supplement her existing hair while covering the area of loss.

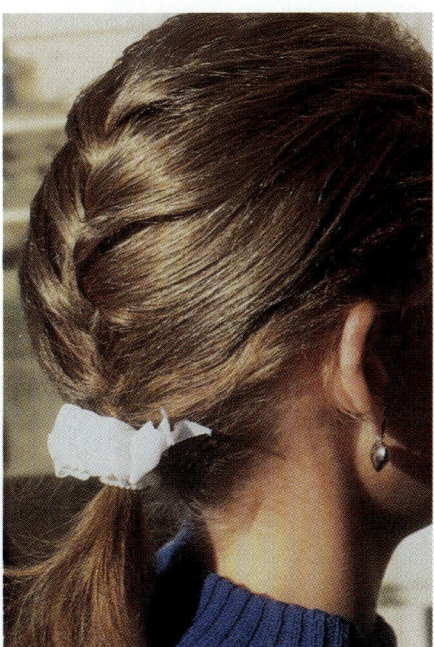

FIGURE 27–18 • The appearance of the same patient as in Figure 27–16 after completion of the unique hairpiece.

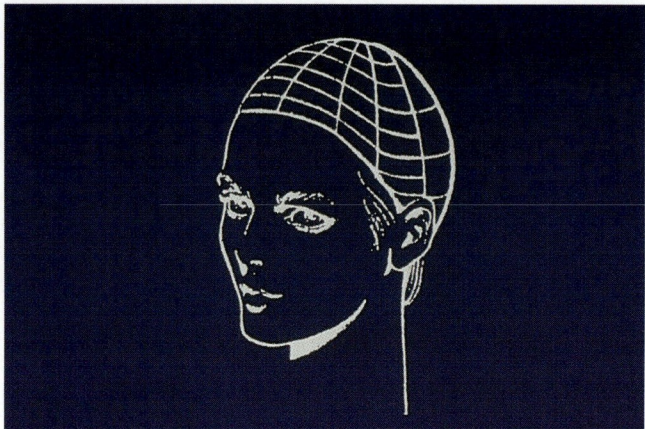

FIGURE 27–19 • In a hair integration system, a loose mesh, to which hair fibers can be attached, is fashioned.

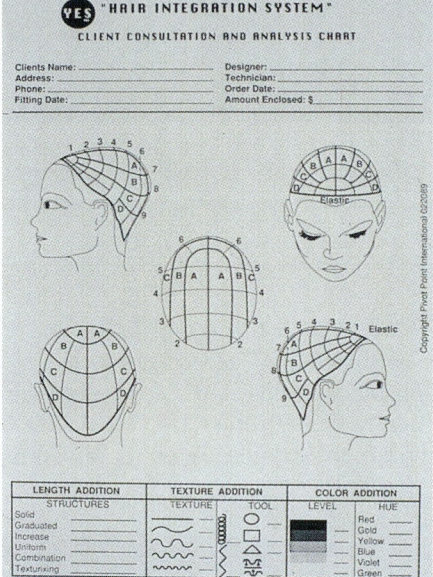

FIGURE 27–20 • This hair integration template allows the patient to designate the color, amount, and curl of the hair fibers to be woven into each part of the hairpiece. The integration system is designed so that the patient pulls her own hair through the loose mesh, anchoring the prosthesis in place and giving a more natural appearance.

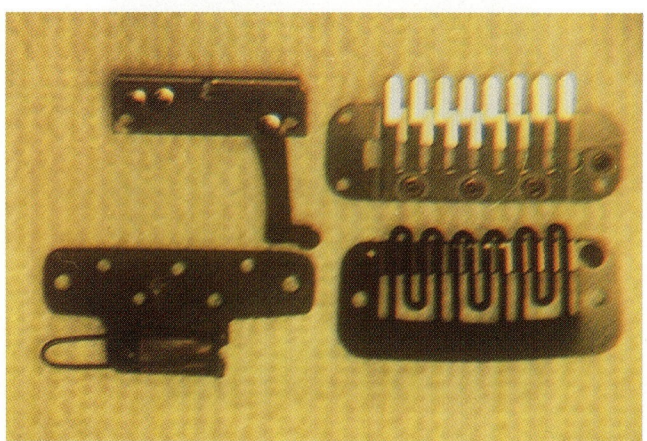

FIGURE 27–21 • These are a few styles of clips that are used to attach hairpieces to existing scalp hair.

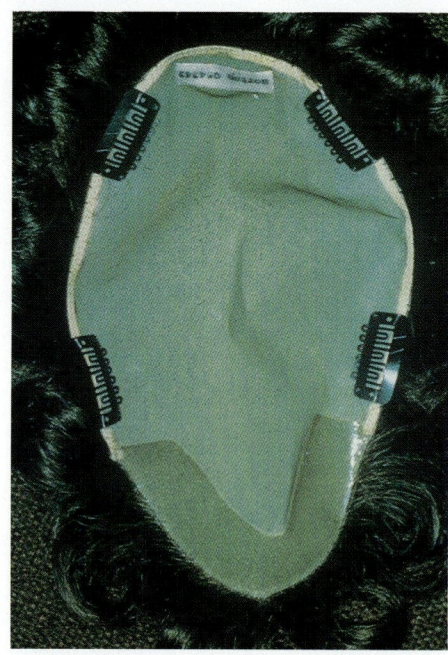

FIGURE 27–22 • Clips are sewn into toupees in order to attach the hairpiece to the existing hair on the sides of the scalp.

pearance or, more commonly, to add length (Fig. 27–29). Wefted hair, or hair fibers sewn together in a strip, can be sewn with a needle and thread to the cornrows to quickly add large amounts of hair (Fig. 27–30).

b. BRAIDING OFF THE SCALP

Braiding off the scalp employs a standard plaiting technique to which individual hair fibers are added.

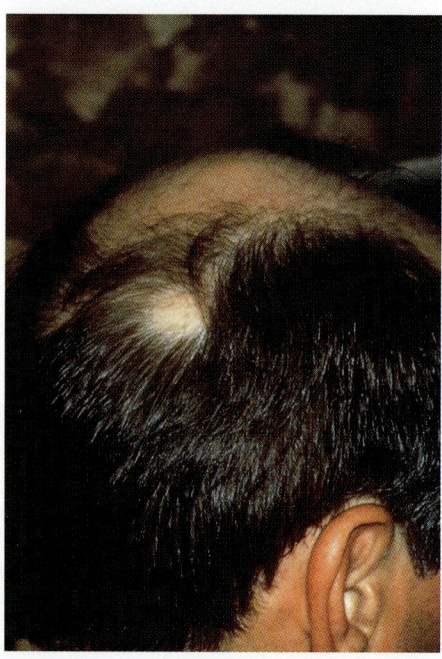

FIGURE 27–23 • Prolonged use of clips to attach hairpieces results in hair breakage, hair loss, and eventually, traction alopecia.

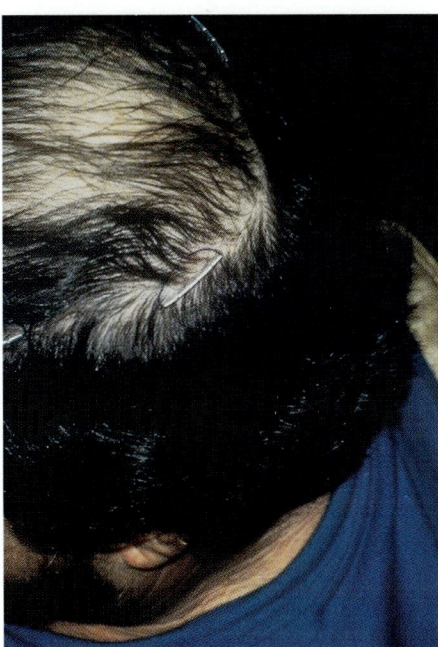

FIGURE 27–24 • Some hair studios implant clips into the scalp for hairpiece attachment purposes. However, this may result in scarring and infection.

Fibers are attached by working them securely into the braids and leaving the loose ends for curling and styling (Fig. 27–31). This technique is popular among individuals with short, kinky hair who wish to have long straight hair.

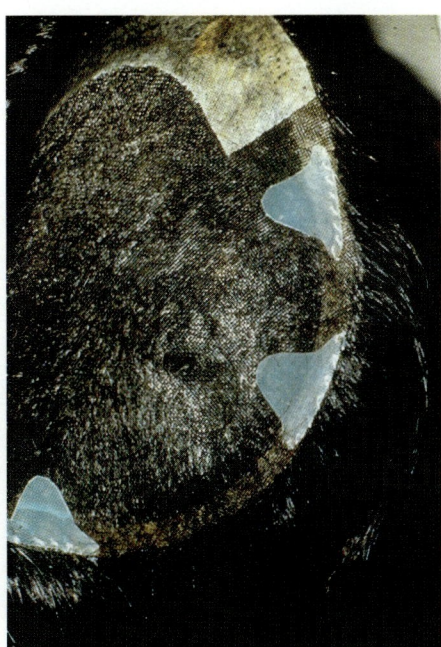

FIGURE 27–25 • This hairpiece is designed to be worn with implanted hooks in the scalp. Reputable hair salons do not recommend this attachment technique.

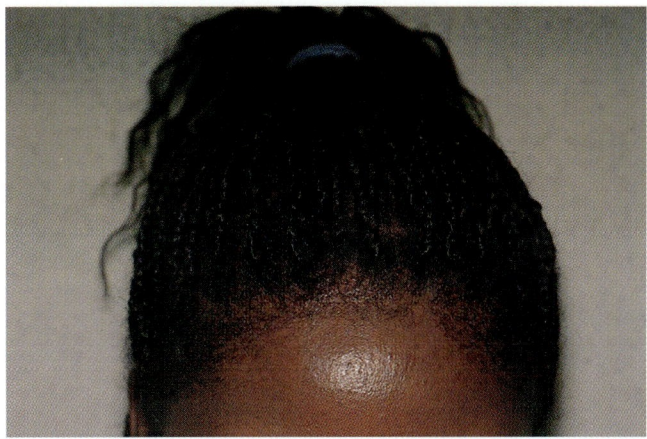

FIGURE 27–26 • An example of braiding on the scalp, whereby the patient's own hair is combined with synthetic hair fibers to create the illusion of long hair.

c. ADHESIVES

This hair addition technique utilizes adhesives to attach the hair to the scalp. Either groups of synthetic hair fibers can be bonded to existing hair shafts or, more commonly, the hair piece is glued to a prepared site on the scalp. Figures 27–32 through 27–37 demonstrate how adhesives are used to attach a toupee to a male patient's scalp. This form of attachment allows the hairpiece to be worn while sleeping, bathing, swimming, and other strenuous physical activity.

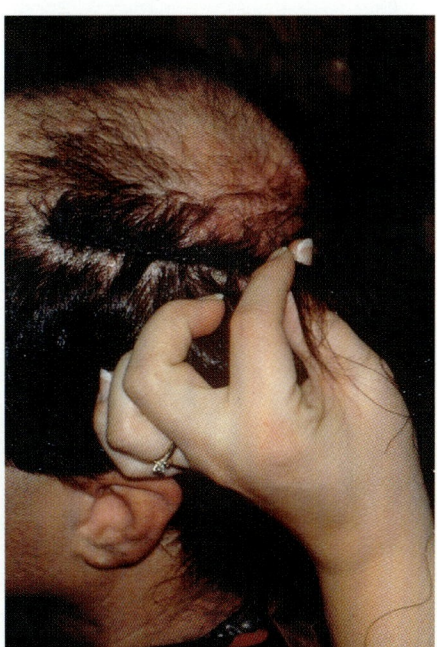

FIGURE 27–27 • Braiding on the scalp can also provide a track for the attachment of toupees in men.

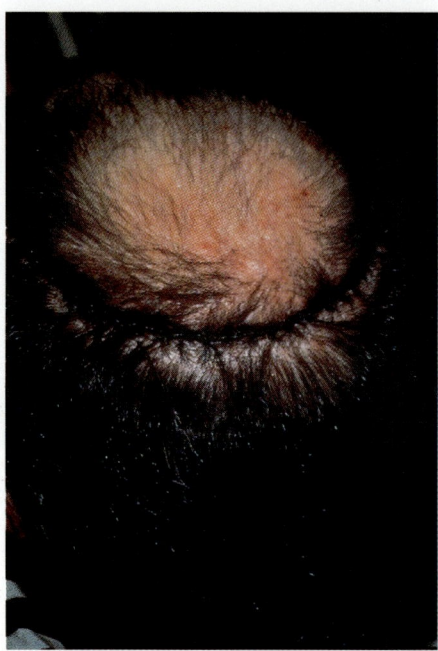

FIGURE 27–28 • The toupee is attached by sewing the hairpiece with needle and thread to the cornrow track on the scalp.

d. CARE AND COMPLICATIONS

Hair additions are worn continually for a period of 8 weeks or less, at which time they must be removed. Individuals with slowly growing hair may wear the

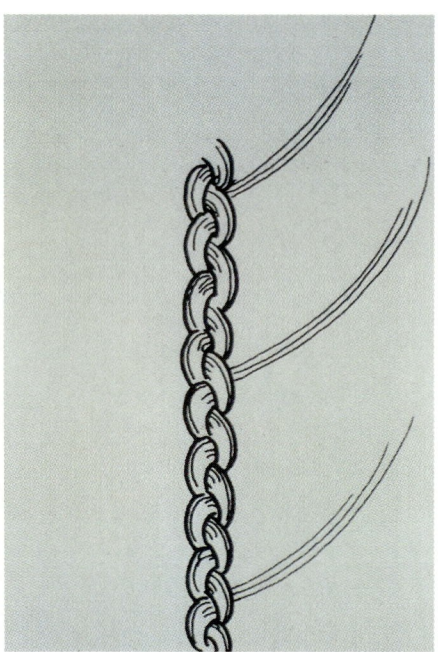

FIGURE 27–29 • Braiding can be done with added hair fibers, which are allowed to exit the braid periodically, creating the illusion of length and fullness.

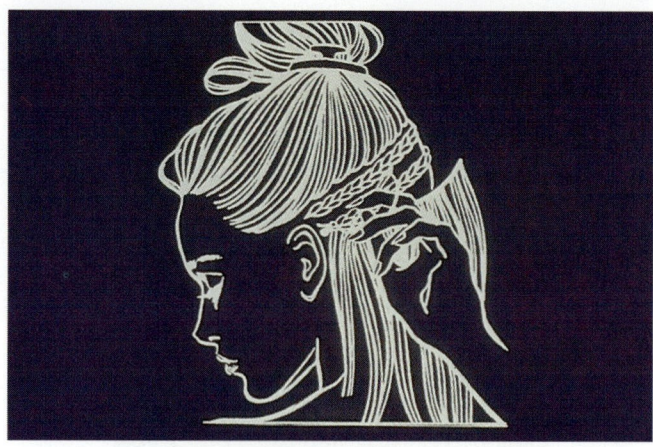

FIGURE 27–30 • Braiding on the scalp can create tracks to which wefted or sewn bands of hair can be attached.

hairstyle longer, whereas those with rapidly growing hair will notice that the added hair fibers loosen more quickly. The additions are shampooed along with the individual's existing hair using the same cleansing products and cleansing frequency. Many individuals are afraid to wash the additions as they fear loosening will occur, but good hygiene is important (Fig. 27–38).

The additions should be removed after 8 weeks to avoid hygiene problems and other complications, such as traction alopecia. If the hair and scalp have been cleansed properly, hair additions begin to loosen and look ungroomed at 8 weeks. Removal of braided additions simply requires undoing the braid and removing the added strands of hair, which may be reused in later procedures. Bonded additions are removed by melting the glue attachments and pulling out the

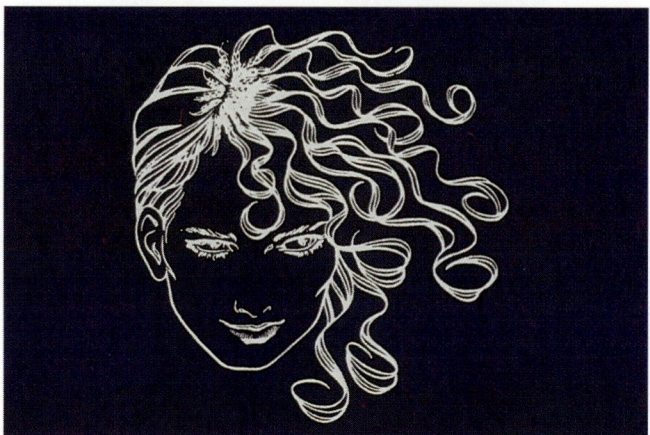

FIGURE 27–31 • Synthetic or natural hair fibers can be braided to the patient's own hair to create hair extensions and the illusion of length and fullness.

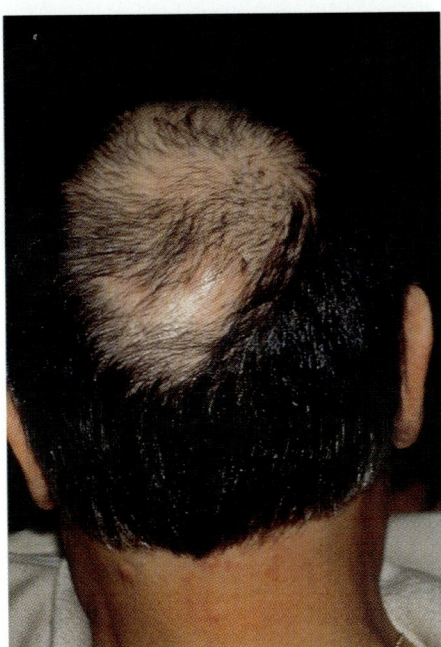

FIGURE 27–32 • This patient's hair has been clipped close to the scalp to allow a hairpiece to be glued in place.

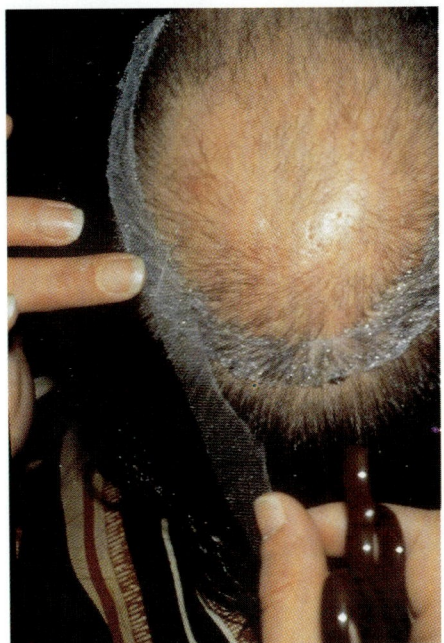

FIGURE 27–34 • Meshwork is embedded in the glue to allow hairpiece attachment.

added hair fibers. Peanut oil is then rubbed through the scalp to facilitate removal of any remaining material. Latex-based glue is removed with a specially designed solvent. Lastly, sewn additions can be removed by cutting the attachment thread.

Successful use of hair additions requires the aid of a hairstylist who is trained in the technique and a client who will put forth the effort to maintain the added hair. Braided and sewn hair additions pose the least problem as no adhesives are used; however the added hair fibers put increased pull on existing scalp hair, augmenting the pull already exerted by the tight braids. For these reasons, traction alopecia can be a problem in individuals who continually wear hair additions (Fig. 27–39). The traction alopecia is identical

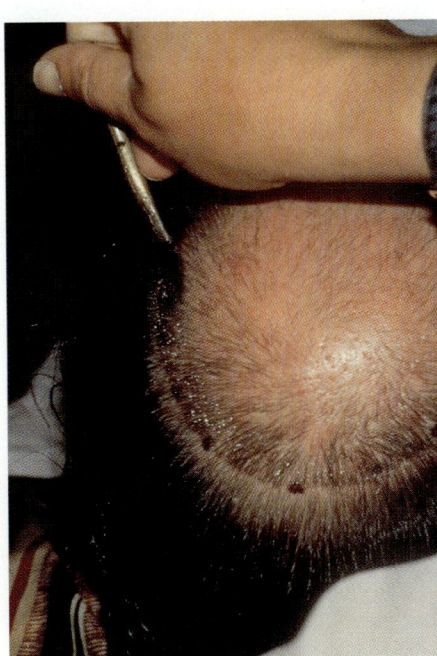

FIGURE 27–33 • Glue is then applied to the scalp where the hairpiece is to rest.

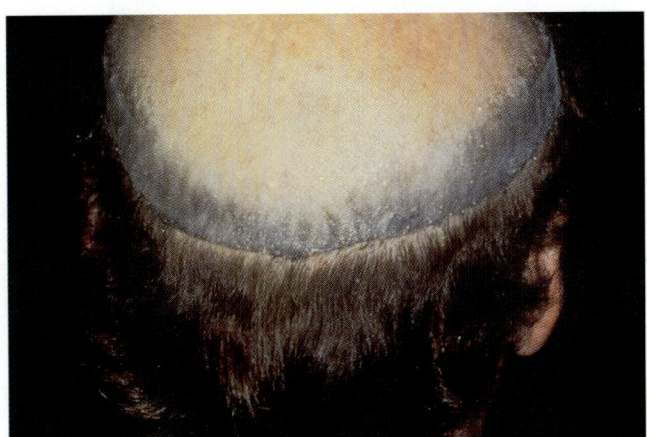

FIGURE 27–35 • The gluing and scalp attachment is now complete.

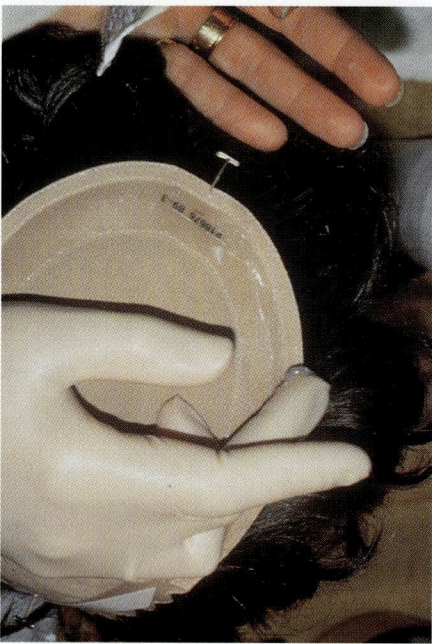

FIGURE 27–36 • This is the toupee that will be attached to the patient's scalp.

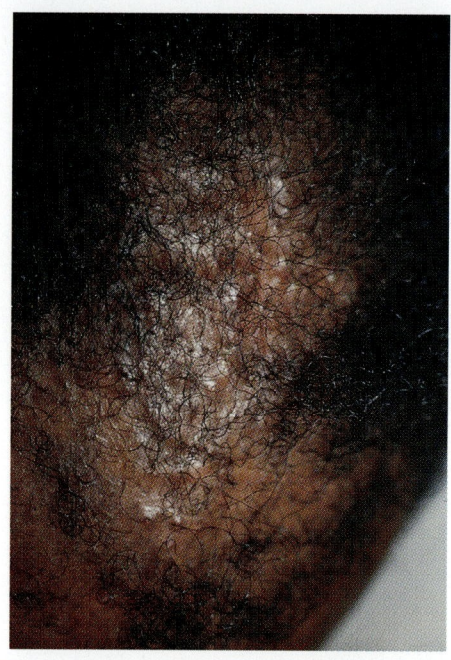

FIGURE 27–38 • Infection is a serious complication of hair additions.

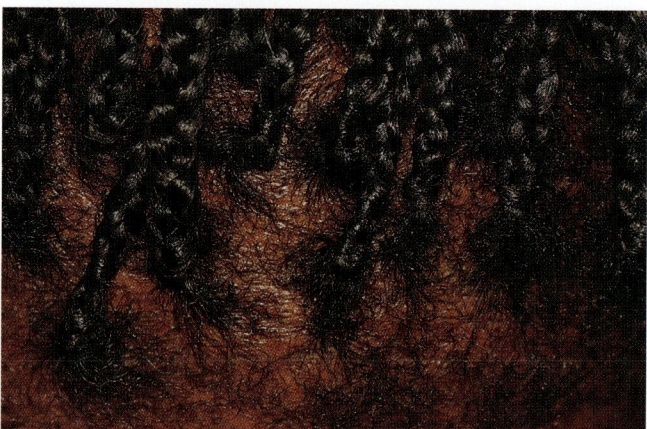

FIGURE 27–39 • Traction alopecia is the most common complication of hair additions.

to that seen in black patients who wear tightly pulled hair styles. Initially, only loss of the hair shaft is observed, but with continued traction, the process can result in loss of the follicular ostia and permanent alopecia (Figs. 27–40 through 27–42). Extensive traction alopecia eventually precludes the use of hair ad-

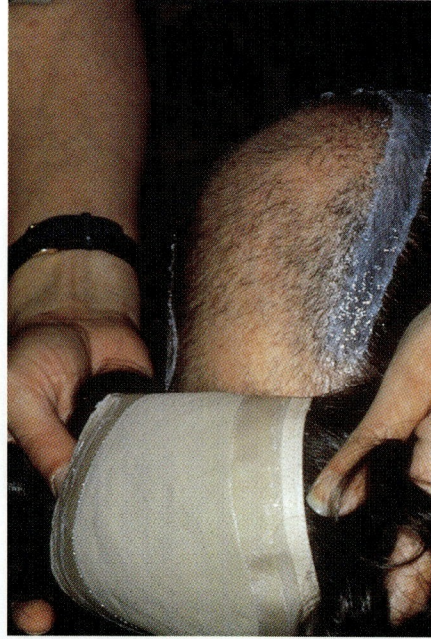

FIGURE 27–37 • The toupee is attached to the patient's scalp and can be worn continuously for 4 to 8 weeks.

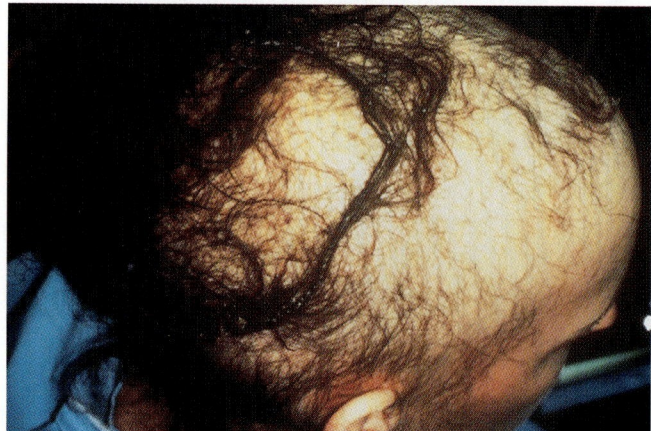

FIGURE 27–40 • Patients who have worn hair additions for a prolonged period of time can develop severe traction alopecia that may prevent them from continuing to use the hair addition technique.

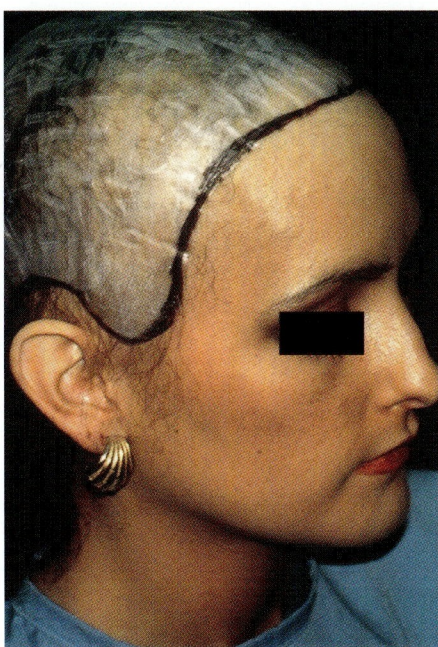

FIGURE 27–41 • This patient developed such severe traction alopecia that she had to resort to a custom hairpiece, as insufficient scalp hair remained for any other type of prosthesis.

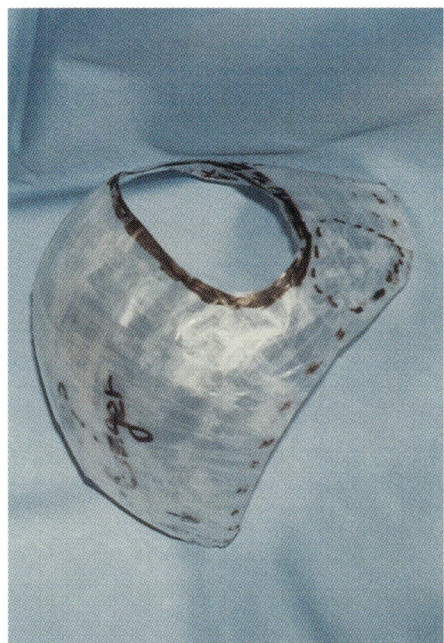

FIGURE 27–42 • This form provides a template for the custom prosthesis. It is hoped that some of the patient's natural hair will regrow while she is wearing the hairpiece.

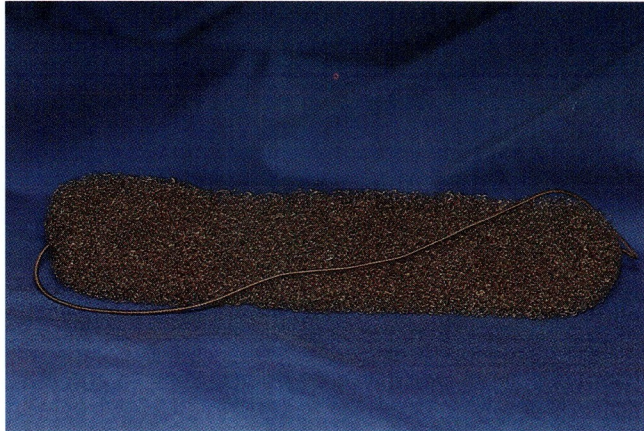

FIGURE 27–43 • A hair form used to create the illusion of fullness on the posterior scalp when wearing a French roll.

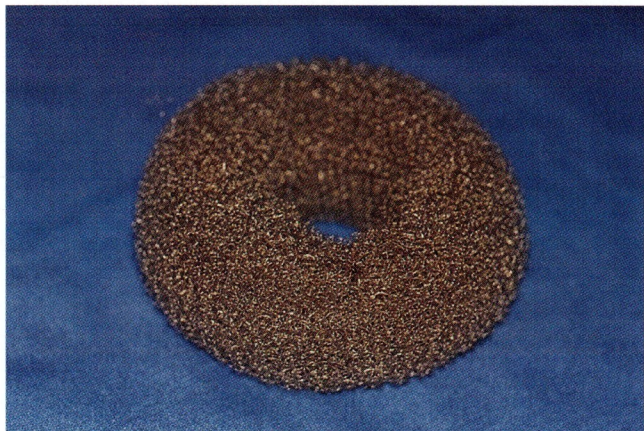

FIGURE 27–44 • A hair form that may be used to create the illusion of fullness when styling the hair as a bun.

ditions, as no existing scalp hair will be available to anchor added hair.

3. Hair Forms

Hair forms are synthetic woven meshes over which hair can be placed to achieve the illusion of fullness. In Figure 27–43, the form is placed beneath a French roll on the posterior of the scalp to yield a larger hair mass. In Figure 27–44, the form is used to create the illusion of a fuller bun on the top of the head. These forms are available in a variety of shapes, sizes, and colors to camouflage thinning hair.

28

Hair Removal Techniques

Hair removal is an important aspect of grooming for men and women. A variety of hair removal techniques are available; however, this section will focus on the more useful methods, including shaving, plucking, epilating, waxing, depilatories, electrolysis, and laser treatments. A comparison of these techniques is presented in Table 28–1.

1. Shaving

Shaving is the most widespread method of hair removal owing to its rapid speed, effectiveness, and low expense. Shaving is the preferred hair removal technique for facial hair in men and underarm or leg hair in women. A major limitation of this technique is the rapid, bristly regrowth that is due to a hair shaft now devoid of a naturally tapered tip (Fig. 28–1).[1,2] It is this loss of the tapered tip that creates the coarse feel of the hair shaft when regrowth occurs following shaving (Fig. 28–2).

Wet shaving involves the use of a manual razor blade and shaving cream applied to moistened hair. Shaving cream is used to soften the beard, through hair shaft swelling, and to lubricate the skin, thereby reducing razor drag.[3] The swelling is actually due to the entraining of water into the hair shaft, which reduces the force required to cut the hair shafts, minimizing razor burn. Shaving gels, which foam on the skin following application, have a higher viscosity and seem to prevent surface trauma more efficiently than do shaving creams (Fig. 28–3). However, shaving gel

TABLE 28–1 Methods of Hair Removal

Technique	Equipment	Cost	Regrowth Period	Suitable Body Sites	Advantages	Disadvantages
Shaving	Razor or shaver	+	Days	Face, arms, legs, axilla	Fast, easy	Irritating, rapid regrowth
Plucking	Tweezers	+	Weeks	Eye-brows, facial hair	Longer regrowth period	Painful, slow
Epilating	Epilator	+	Weeks	Arms, legs	Longer regrowth period, fast	Painful, irritating
Waxing	Wax and melting pot	++	Weeks	Face, eyebrows, groin	Longer regrowth period	Painful, slow
Depilatories	Depilatory	++	Days	Legs, groin	Quick	Irritating
Electrolysis	Trained professional, electrolysis machine	+++++	May be permanent	All	May be permanent	Painful, time-consuming, expensive
Laser treatment	Trained professional, laser	+++++++++	May be permanent	All	May be permanent	Expensive, painful, possible scarring

Cost key: +=$2–$4; ++=$4–$5; +++=$5–$10; +++++=$30–$60; +++++++++=$200. This cost represents the average cost per hair removal session.

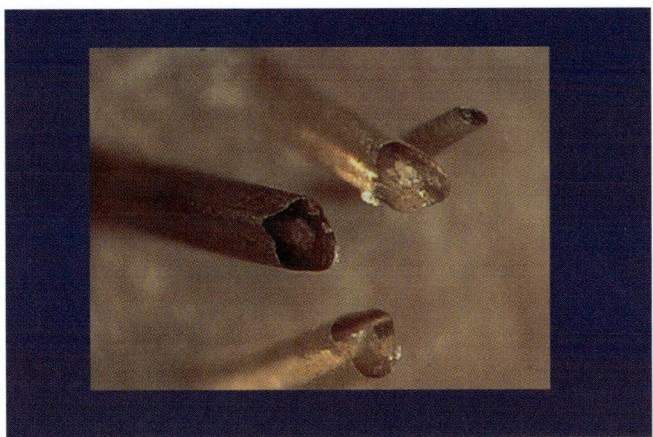

FIGURE 28–1 • Following shaving, the hairs feel coarse owing to the sharp corners that are demonstrated by video microscope (X400).

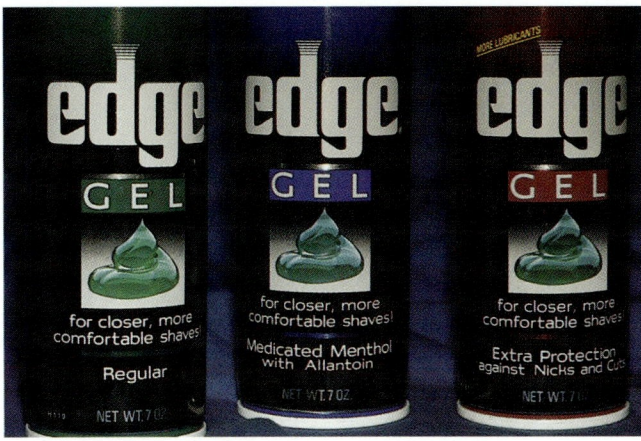

FIGURE 28–3 • Shaving gels foam when rubbed into the skin surface. They provide less drag between the razor blade and the skin surface, minimizing razor burn.

must be left in contact with the hair and skin for at least 4 minutes to diminish razor burn and prolong razor blade life (Fig. 28–4).

The main advantage of wet shaving is that it allows the hair to be cut closely at the skin surface (Fig. 28–5). It is an excellent hair removal technique for large, well-keratinized body surfaces, such as the legs in women and the face of men, where rapid regrowth and a coarse skin texture are not a problem. Females who have keratosis pilaris on the upper outer thighs should use wet shaving over dry shaving, as shaving cream can soften the perifollicular keratotic material, thus minimizing skin trauma. Selection of a razor designed with the appropriate angle for shaving the female body is also important (Fig. 28–6).

By contrast, dry shaving involves the use of an electric shaver without moisture or shaving cream. The electric shaver contains blades that rotate or vibrate,

thereby cutting the hair shaft. In general, an electric shaver cannot cut the hairs as close to the skin surface as a razor, but skin abrasion is not as great a problem (Fig. 28–7). Skin irritation and the spread of cutaneous infections may still occur (Fig. 28–8).[4]

2. Plucking

Plucking of the hair is a method of removing the entire hair shaft, including the bulb, using a pair of tweezers.[5] It is an easy, inexpensive method of hair removal requiring minimal equipment, but it is tedious and mildly uncomfortable. Plucking does not encourage rapid regrowth. Removal of hair from large areas is not feasible, but plucking is effective for removal of stray eyebrow hairs or isolated coarse hairs on the chin (Fig. 28–9). Only terminal hairs can be effi-

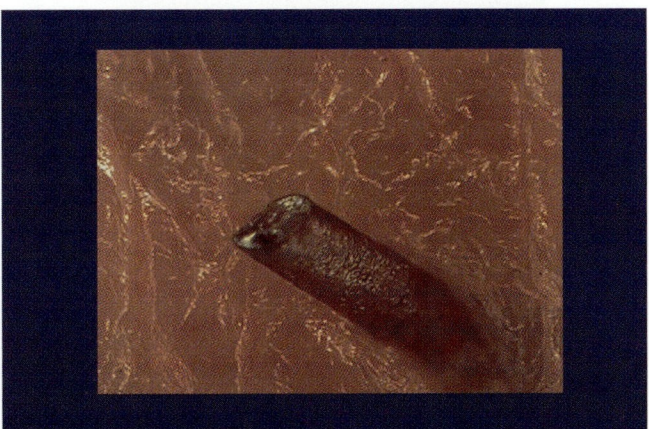

FIGURE 28–2 • This is the video microscopic appearance of a male beard hair 24 hours after shaving with a blade and shaving cream (X400).

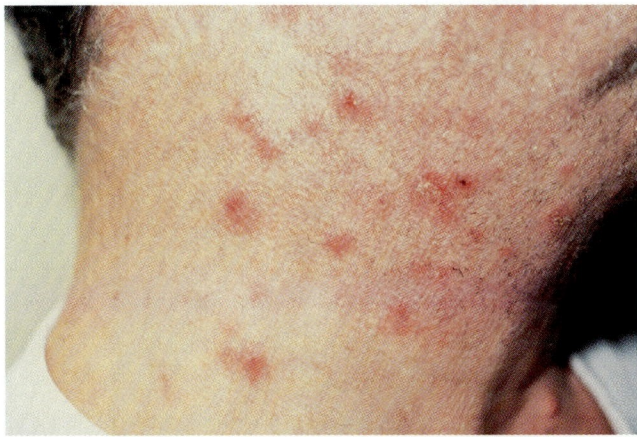

FIGURE 28–4 • Razor burn can be a troublesome condition in transitional areas of hair growth, such as the neck.

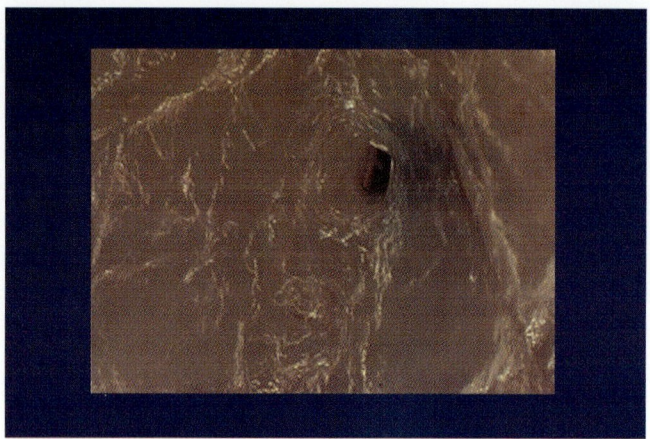

FIGURE 28–5 • Immediately following wet shaving with a double blade, the cut hair can be visualized beneath the skin surface, yielding a smooth shave (X400).

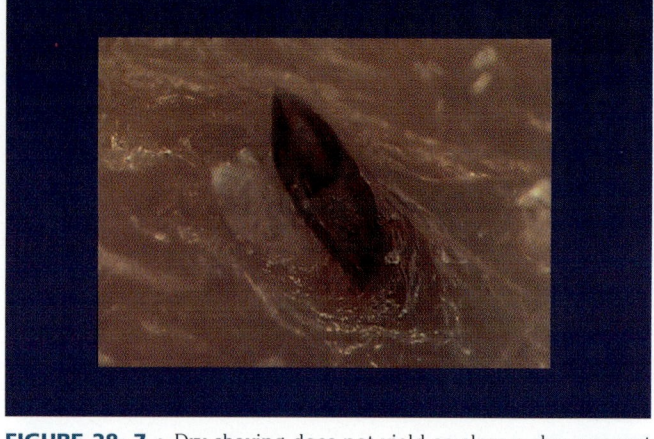

FIGURE 28–7 • Dry shaving does not yield as close a shave as wet shaving, as demonstrated on this video microscopic image (X400). The hair has not been cut beneath the skin surface.

ciently plucked, as vellus hairs usually break close to the skin surface.

3. Epilating

Epilating has now come to refer to a mechanized method of plucking hair.[6] Most electric, hand-held epilating devices are stroked over the skin, much like an electric shaver. These devices consist of a rotating, tightly coiled spring that traps the hair and pulls it out at the level of the hair bulb (Fig. 28–10). This efficient hair plucking provides a long regrowth period, but is

somewhat painful. Additionally, the device functions poorly on curved surfaces, such as the underarms, and can do considerable damage to body areas with thin skin, such as the face.

Epilating is best used on large flat surfaces, such as the arms and legs, but the hair must be of sufficient length for entrapment in the coiled spring. Follicular disruption is a problem that can result in ingrown or coiled hairs beneath the skin surface.[7,8] Infection may also be a problem, so use of an antibacterial agent prior to and following hair removal is recommended. If the epilator is pressed too firmly against the skin, purpura may result.

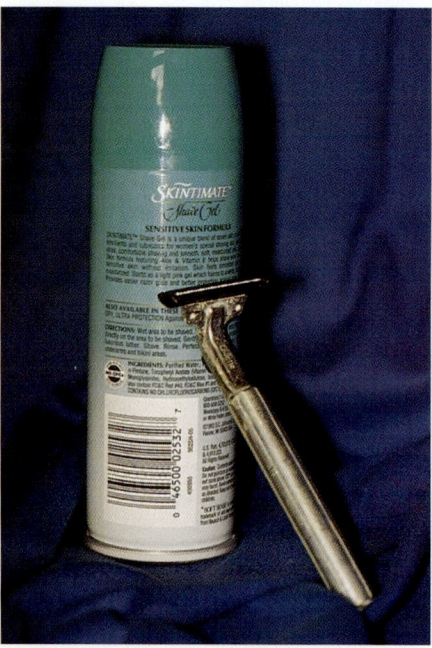

FIGURE 28–6 • This razor handle is designed for the male face. Females should select razor handles and blades that are specifically designed for women.

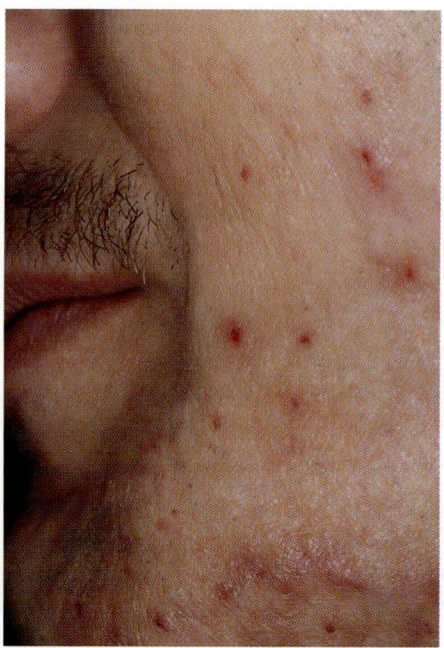

FIGURE 28–8 • Skin irritation can occur following dry shaving if the shaver is pressed too firmly against the skin surface or if the blades are dull.

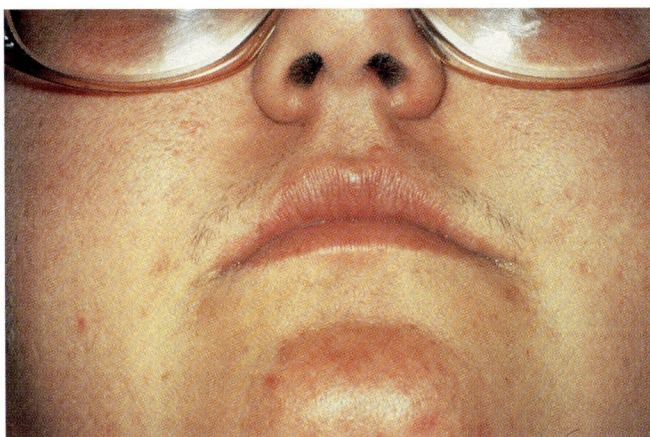

FIGURE 28–9 • Tweezer-assisted plucking is the recommended method of hair removal in women with small amounts of coarse facial hair on the upper lip or chin.

4. Waxing

Waxing is another variation on plucking of the hair. Hot wax is composed of rosin, beeswax, paraffin wax, petrolatum, and mineral or vegetable oil. Some products are mentholated. The wax is melted in a double boiler or professional wax pot and applied to the hairs with a wooden spatula (Figs. 28–11 and 28–12). Hair becomes embedded within the wax, which is allowed to cool and harden. The hair is then pulled out at the level of the hair bulb as the wax is ripped from the skin (Fig. 28–13). Care must be taken not to burn the skin.

Waxing has the advantage of adequate removal of both terminal and vellus hairs. This is important on

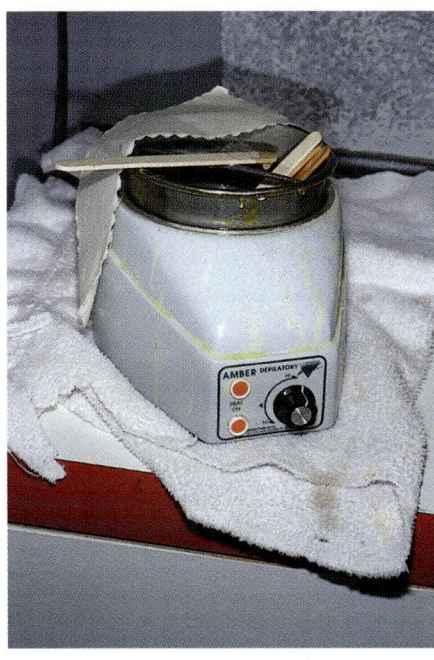

FIGURE 28–11 • Hot wax may be applied, using the sticks shown, to unwanted eyebrow hairs. A strip of muslin cloth is then pressed over the area where the hair is to be removed.

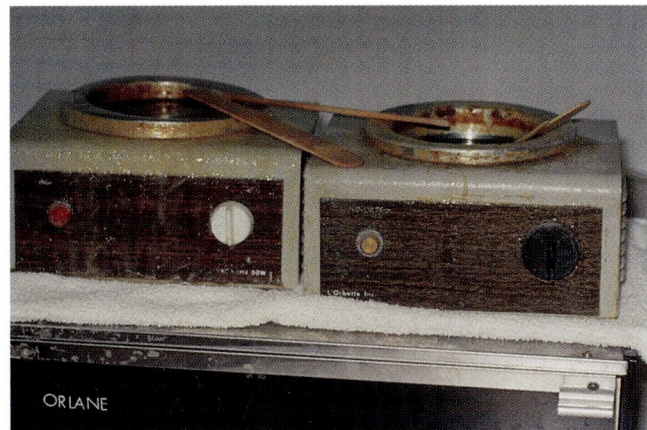

FIGURE 28–12 • Larger wax pots, such as these shown here, are used to wax larger body areas, such as the bikini line and legs.

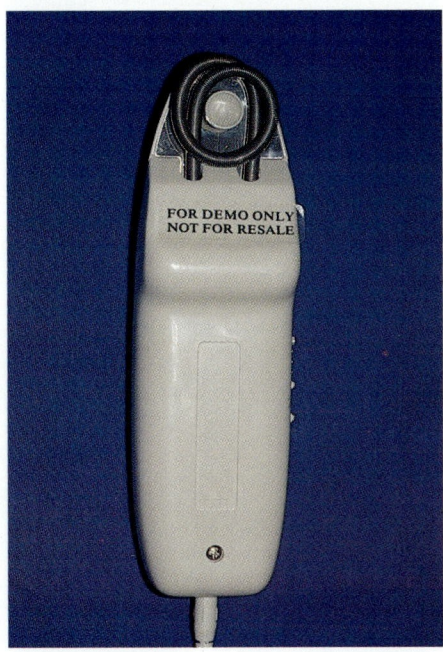

FIGURE 28–10 • An example of one type of rotating coil mechanical epilator.

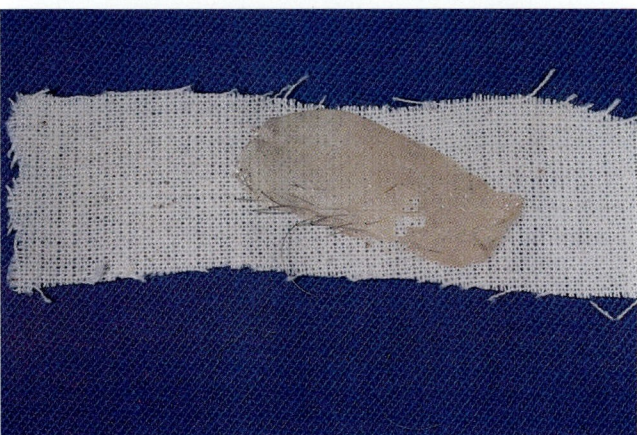

FIGURE 28–13 • The wax, with the adherent removed hairs, is shown attached to the muslin strip.

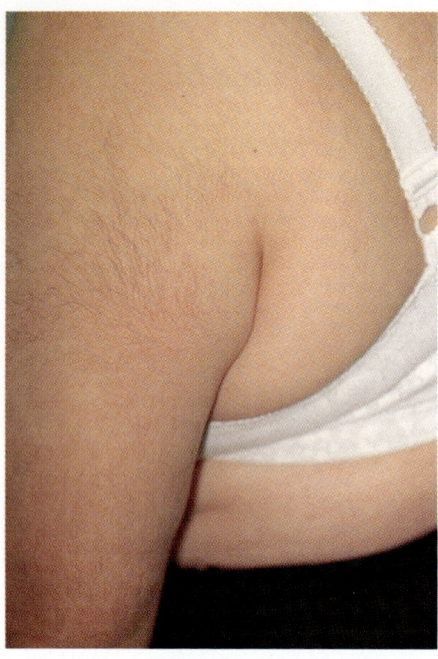

FIGURE 28–14 • Waxing is an excellent method of removing dark, unwanted hair, such as that found in a Becker's nevus.

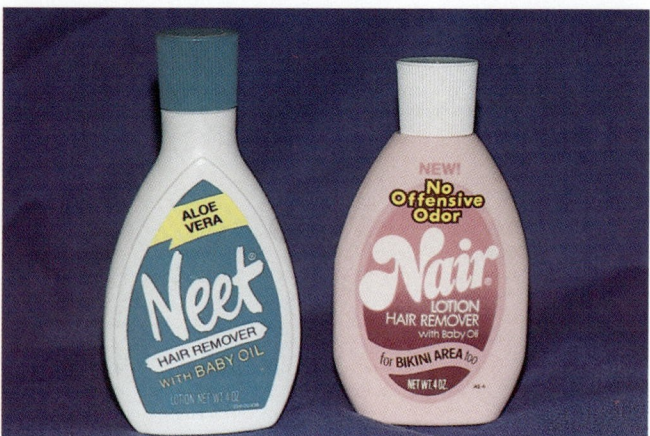

FIGURE 28–15 • Chemical depilatories can be used to remove hair on the legs and bikini line. Irritation is the major side effect.

the upper lip, chin, eyebrows, cheeks and groin of women where removal of all hair is desirable. Men generally do not find waxing of facial hair acceptable as the hair must grow to at least 1/16 of an inch before it can be reliably removed by waxing. Excess hair present in Becker's nevi, congenital hairy nevi, and benign hairy nevi can be removed in both males and females with this technique (Fig. 28–14).

5. Depilatories

Chemical depilatories function by softening the hair shaft above the skin surface to such a degree that it can gently be wiped away with a soft cloth. Hair removal is accomplished by softening the cysteine-rich hair disulfide bonds to the point of dissolution.

Chemical depilatories are designed to remain in contact with the skin for 5 to 10 minutes, with shorter contact periods for fine hair and longer contact times for coarse hair. The products are somewhat selective for hair shaft damage, as the hair shafts contain more cysteine than the surrounding skin, but are still irritating to skin, especially if contact is prolonged. The hairs are wiped away once they assume a corkscrew appearance (Fig. 28–15). Under no circumstances should chemical depilatories be applied to abraded or dermatitic skin.

Chemical depilatories are best used for removal of hair on the legs, including the upper thigh. Darkly pigmented hair seems somewhat more resistant to de-

pilatory removal than lighter hair, and coarse hair is more resistant than fine hair. This explains why these products are difficult to use on the male beard. However, a variety of powder depilatories containing barium sulfide are available for black men who have difficulty with pseudofolliculitis barbae.[9,10] These powdered products are mixed with water to form a paste and are then applied to the beard with a wooden applicator, remaining in place for 3 to 7 minutes (Fig. 28–16). The hair and depilatory are then removed with the same applicator and the skin is rinsed with cool water. This procedure should be performed no more frequently than every other day.

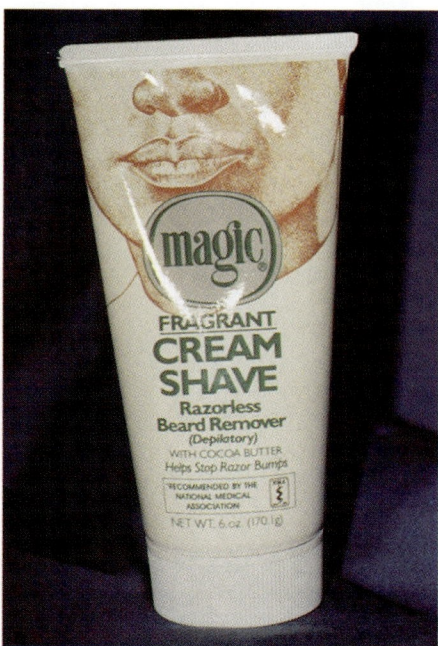

FIGURE 28–16 • Chemical depilatories are available to remove facial hair in men; however irritation is almost always present.

TABLE 28–2 Guidelines for Electrolysis

• • • • • •

1. Only telogen hairs, not anagen hairs, can be treated.
2. The electrolysis needle must be inserted into the depth of the hair follicle, as the water found in this location is necessary for transmitting electrical energy between the needle and dermal papillae.
3. The depth of needle insertion is determined by the hair shaft diameter. Large-diameter hairs require deep needle insertion for adequate destruction.
4. Coarse hairs require a longer treatment duration than fine hairs.[19]
5. Curly, wavy, or kinky hair is more difficult to treat owing to problems related to accurate needle placement in the hair follicle.

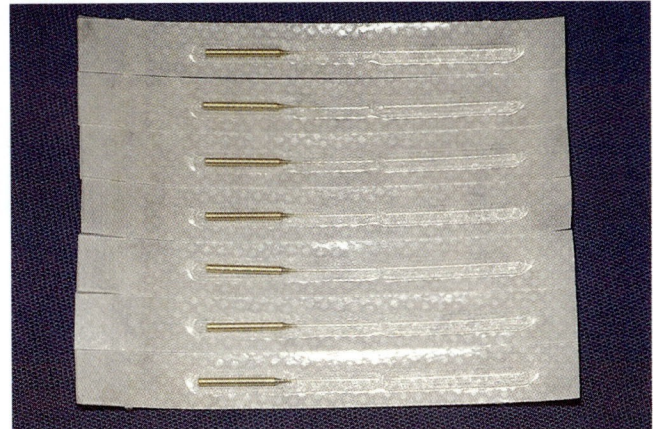

FIGURE 28–18 • Gold needles, sometimes called hypoallergenic needles, are preferred by some electrologists.

6. Electrolysis

Electrolysis is the only widely available permanent method of hair removal for patients. Physicians are well aware of the complications of electrolysis, which include scarring, failure to destroy the germinative follicular cells, and the transmission of viral and bacterial disease. Yet, electrolysis remains a tremendously popular hair removal technique among women with unwanted hairs on the face, chin, neck, and bikini areas.[11] There are three electrolysis techniques: galvanic electrolysis, thermolysis, and the blend. All electrolysis techniques involve the insertion of a needle into the follicular ostia down to the follicular germinative cells. The dermal papillae must be destroyed to prevent hair growth permanently. There are several important considerations in determining the effectiveness of electrolysis techniques, and these are summarized in Table 28–2.

Galvanic electrolysis utilizes direct current (DC), which is passed through a stainless steel or gold needle (Figs. 28–17 and 28–18) into sodium chloride and

water in the tissue surrounding the hair follicle. The current causes ionization of the salt (NaCl) and water (H_2O) into free sodium (Na^+), chloride (Cl^-), hydrogen (H^+), and hydroxide (OH^-) ions. These free ions then recombine into sodium hydroxide (NaOH), known as lye, and hydrogen gas (H_2). The caustic sodium hydroxide destroys the hair follicle while the hydrogen gas escapes into the atmosphere.[12] Galvanic electrolysis is the most effective method of producing permanent hair removal, but it is a tedious and slow process. Because of this, multiple-needle techniques have been developed (Fig. 28–19).

Thermolysis, also known as short-wave radio frequency diathermy, differs from galvanic electrolysis in

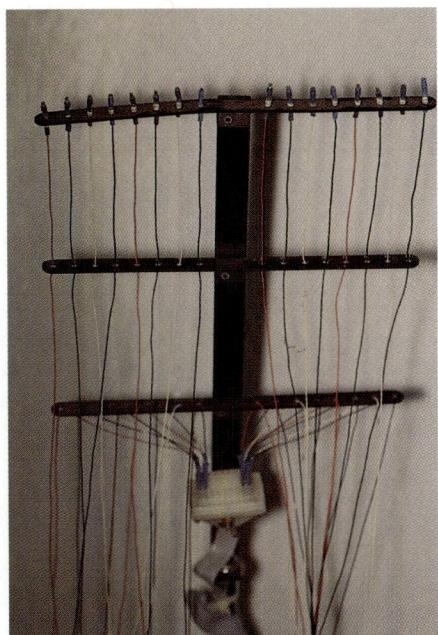

FIGURE 28–19 • Electrolysis needles are attached to each of these wires to allow multiple hairs to be treated simultaneously.

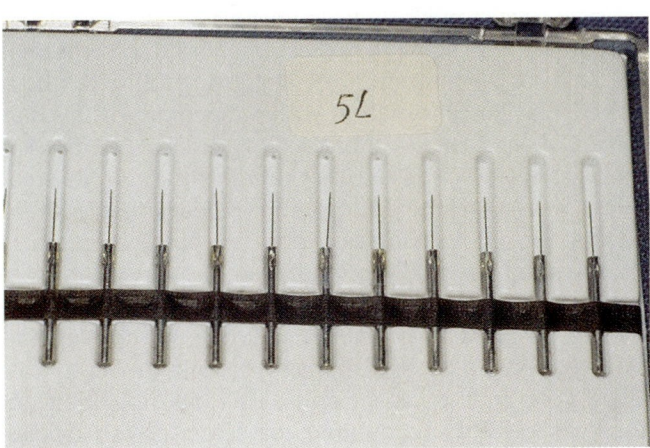

FIGURE 28–17 • These stainless steel needles are used for electrolysis.

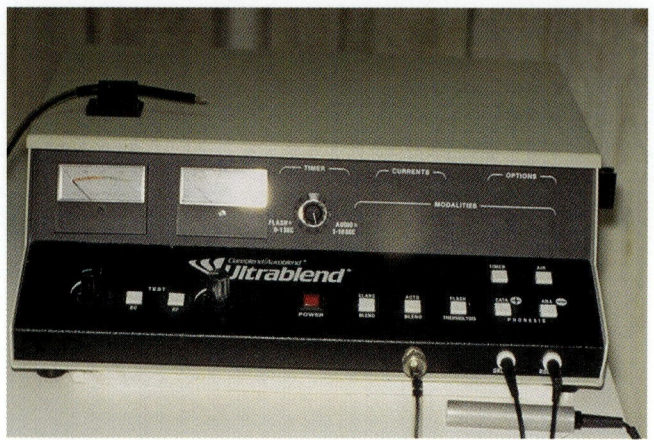

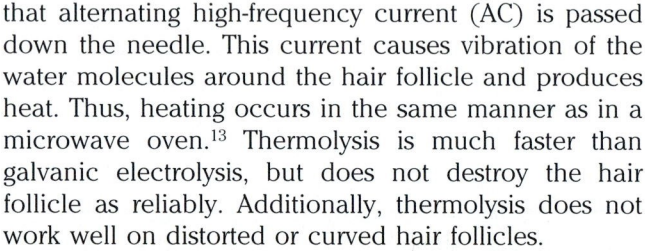

FIGURE 28–20 • This machine is used to perform electrolysis utilizing a technique known as the blend.

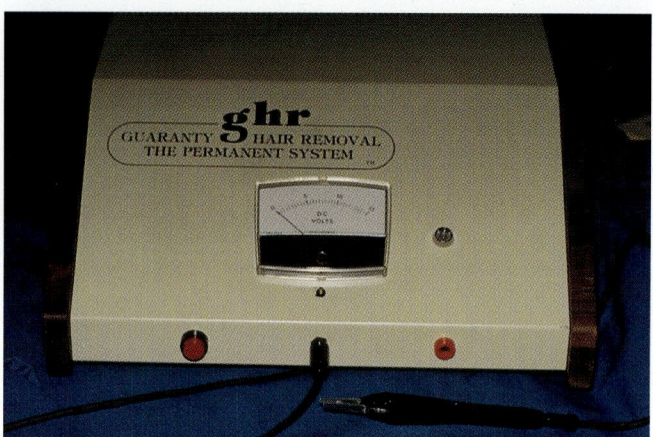

FIGURE 28–21 • Despite claims to the contrary electronic tweezers are not a permanent method of hair removal.

that alternating high-frequency current (AC) is passed down the needle. This current causes vibration of the water molecules around the hair follicle and produces heat. Thus, heating occurs in the same manner as in a microwave oven.[13] Thermolysis is much faster than galvanic electrolysis, but does not destroy the hair follicle as reliably. Additionally, thermolysis does not work well on distorted or curved hair follicles.

As its name suggests, the blend is a combination of both galvanic electrolysis and thermolysis (Fig. 28–20).[14] Both DC and high-frequency AC are passed down the needle at the same time to produce sodium hydroxide and heat. The hot lye is extremely effective in destroying the dermal papillae, allowing superior results with less regrowth. Furthermore, the tissue damage induced by the thermolysis allows the lye to spread through the hair follicle more rapidly. The blend requires only one-fourth the time of galvanic electrolysis alone.

Electrolysis must be performed properly to minimize scarring. Table 28–3 summarizes the guidelines

TABLE 28–3 Tips for Prevention of Scarring from Electrolysis

• • • • • •

1. The treated hair should be pulled effortlessly from the follicular ostia.
2. The needle size should be the same as the hair diameter.
3. The skin should be dry.
4. The skin should not blanch following treatment.
5. The current should only flow when the needle has been completely inserted in the follicular ostia to the level of the follicle.
6. The needle should only be removed when the current has stopped.
7. The same follicular ostia should not be reentered or treated more than once.

that must be followed for successful electrolysis.[15] Care must also be taken to perform the procedure under sanitary conditions to prevent the spread of bacterial and viral infection.[16] If a good operator with superior health standards can be found, electrolysis may be useful in the female with a few unwanted facial hairs on the upper lip or chin. This technique is not suitable for removal of large hairy areas, such as the male beard, as only 25 to 100 hairs can be removed per sitting.

Electronic tweezers, such as the machine shown in Figure 28–21, have not been shown to be effective in permanent hair removal.

7. Laser Treatment

The availability of lasers to permanently remove hair is the newest technique. Several different laser removal systems are presently available (Table 28–4).[17] The lasers function by producing light energy of a specific wavelength that is absorbed by a specific chromophore, such as melanin, inducing thermal damage or vaporization of the hair follicle.[18] It is hoped that the destruction will be specific for the hair follicle, based on the concept of selective photothermolysis. Selective thermolysis predicts that the thermal injury will be restricted to the intended target, if there is selective light absorption and the pulse duration is shorter than the cooling time, also known as the thermal relaxation time. For this reason, many laser companies have devised unique methods of cooling the skin to allow selective damage of hair melanin with sparing of cutaneous melanin. This has not been entirely successful, accounting for some of the dyspigmentation and scarring seen following laser hair removal treatments (Fig. 28–22).

TABLE 28–4 Hair Removal Lasers and Light Sources

Laser Name	Type	Wavelength (NM)	Target	Unique Features
Softlight	Neodymium: YAG	1064	Topical carbon	Hair epilation is followed by a topical carbon-in-mineral-oil application
LightSheer	Diode	800	Melanin	Cold sapphire tip
Epilight	Monochromatic, pulsed light source	590, 615, 645, 690 filters	Melanin	Not a laser; filters are used to tailor light spectrum to hair color
PhotoGenica LPIR	Alexandrite	755	Melanin	Cooling tip in handpiece
Apogee	Alexandrite	755	Melanin	None
EpiTouch 5100	Alexandrite	755	Melanin	Water-based gel to cool skin
GentleLase	Alexandrite	755	Melanin	Cryogen spray
Epilaser	Ruby	694	Melanin	Cold sapphire lens that produces a convergent beam
EpiTouch Silk Laser	Ruby	694	Melanin	Utilizes cooling gel
Chromos	Ruby	694	Melanin	None

YAG, yttrium aluminum garnet.

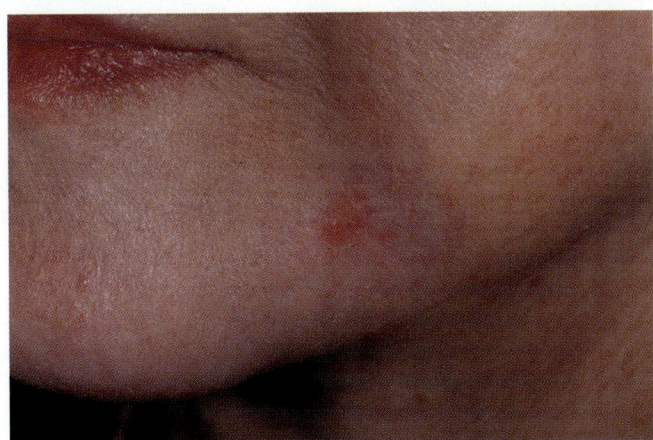

FIGURE 28–22 • Hypertrophic scarring may occur following laser hair removal on the face.

Even though laser has been touted as a permanent hair removal method, it should be remembered that the U.S. Food and Drug Administration (FDA) requires that hair removal devices, including lasers, produce a sustained reduction in hair growth for 3 months. Most patients would hardly consider this short-lived reduction permanent.

REFERENCES

1. Bhaktaviziam C, Mescon H, Matolsky AG. Shaving. Arch Dermatol 88:242–247, 1963.
2. Lynfield YL, MacWilliams P. Shaving and hair growth. J Invest Dermatol 55:170–172, 1970.
3. Bogaty H. Shaving with razor and blade. Cutis 21:609–611, 1978.
4. Brooks GJ, Burmeister F. Preshave and aftershave products. Cosmet Toiletr 105:67–69, 1990.
5. Richards RN, Uy M, Meharg G. Temporary hair removal in patients with hirsutism: A clinical study. Cutis 45:199–202, 1990.
6. Scott JJ, Scott MJ, Scott AM. Epilation. Cutis 46:216–217, 1990.
7. Wright RC. Traumatic folliculitis of the legs: A persistent case associated with use of a home epilating device. J Am Acad Dermatol 27:771–772, 1992.
8. Dilaimy M. Pseduofolliculitis of the legs. Arch Dermatol 112:507–508, 1976.
9. de la Guardia M. Facial depilatories on black skin. Cosmet Toiletr 91:37–38, 1976.
10. Halder RM. Pseudofolliculitis barbae and related disorders. Dermatol Clinics 6:407–412, 1988.
11. Goldberg HC, Hanfling SL. Hirsutism and electrolysis. J Med Soc NJ 62:9–14, 1965.
12. Cipollaro AD. Electrolysis: Discussion of equipment, method of operation, indications, contraindications, and warnings concerning its use. JAMA 110:2488–2491, 1938.
13. Wagner RF, Tomich JM, Grande DJ. Electrolysis and thermolysis for permanent hair removal. J Am Acad Dermatol 12:441–449, 1985.
14. Hinkel AR, Lind RW. Electrolysis, Thermolysis and the Blend. CA: Arroway Publishers, 1968, pp. 199–223.
15. Richards RN, Meharg GE. Cosmetic and Medical Electrolysis and Temporary Hair Removal. Ontario, Canada: Medric, Ltd., 1991, pp. 85–86.
16. Petrozzi JW. Verrucae planae spread by electrolysis. Cutis 26:85, 1980.
17. Olsen EA. Methods of hair removal. J Am Acad Dermatol 40:143–155, 1999.
18. Dover JS, Arndt KS. Illustrated cutaneous laser surgery: A practitioner's guide. Norwalk, CT: Appleton & Lange, 1990.
19. Hinkel AR, Lind RW. Electrolysis, Thermolysis and the Blend. CA: Arroway Publishers, 1968, pp. 181–187.

29

Hair Dyeing Techniques

Hair dyes represent a major hair cosmetic used by both men and women. The dyes may be used to blend gray tones, cover gray hair, add colored highlights, produce unnatural temporary colors, and lighten or darken the original hair color, depending on the interaction between the dye and the hair fiber (Table 29–1 and Fig. 29–1).

1. Gradual Hair Coloring

Gradual hair dyes, also known as metallic or progressive hair dyes, require repeated application to result in gradual darkening of the hair shaft. This product will change the hair color from gray to yellow-brown to black over a period of weeks (Fig. 29–2).[1] There is no control over the final color of the hair, only the depth of color. Lightening is not possible. They employ

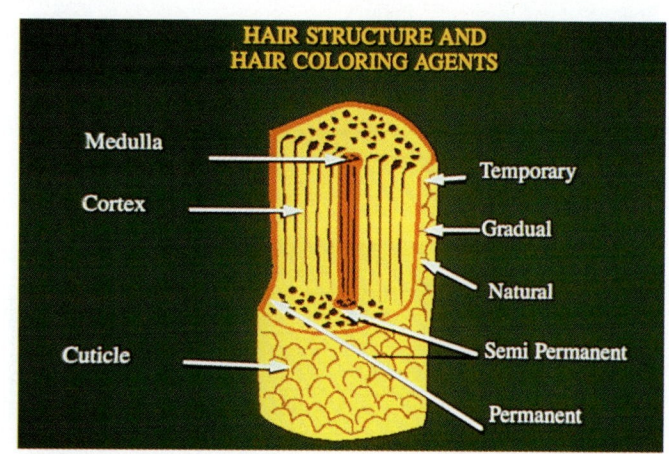

FIGURE 29–1 • Hair dyes vary in terms of their penetration into the hair shaft. Temporary hair dyes, removed with one shampooing, actually coat, rather than penetrate, the hair shaft, whereas permanent dyes, which are resistant to shampoo removal, penetrate to the level of the cortex. (Photo courtesy of Cosmetic, Toiletry, and Fragrance Association, Washington, DC.)

TABLE 29–1 Comparison of Hair Dyeing Techniques

Type	Main Ingredient	Duration of Effect	Effect on Hair	Advantages/Disadvantages
Gradual	Aqueous solution of lead or silver oxides, suboxides, and sulfides	Color persists with continued use	Darkens gradually by "plating" hair shaft	Cannot be combined with permanent dye or permanent wave
Temporary	High-molecular-weight, textile dyes	Removal with one shampooing	Large color molecules are deposited on hair shaft	Can blend or tone undesirable hair color
Semipermanent	Low-molecular-weight, natural or synthetic, textile-type dye	Removal with four to six shampooings	Small color molecules penetrate hair cortex	Provides tone-on-tone coloring; will cover less than 30% gray; may be allergenic
Permanent	Oxidation coloring employing primary intermediates, couplers, and an oxidant	Permanent	New color molecules are formed within hair shaft	Can lighten (two-step processing) or darken (one-step processing) hair; will cover gray 100%; need to cover new growth with monthly dyeing; may be allergenic

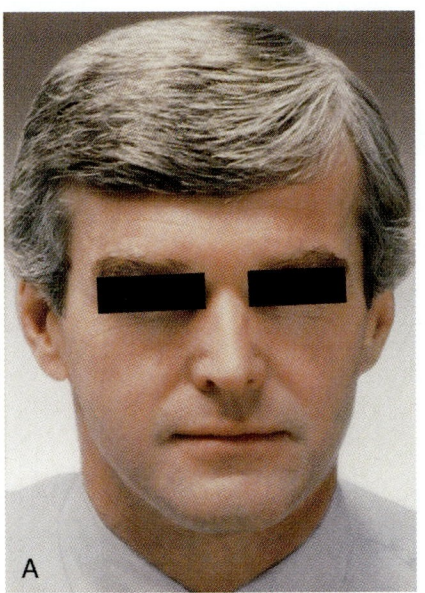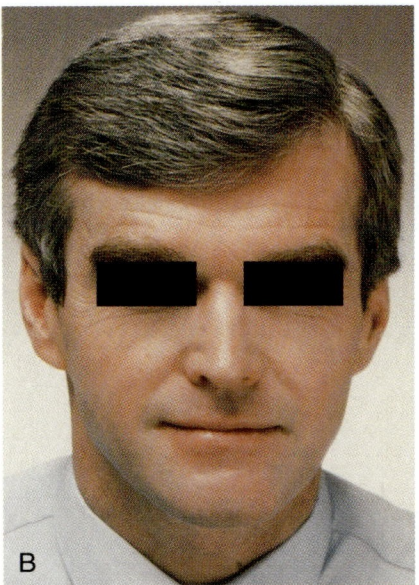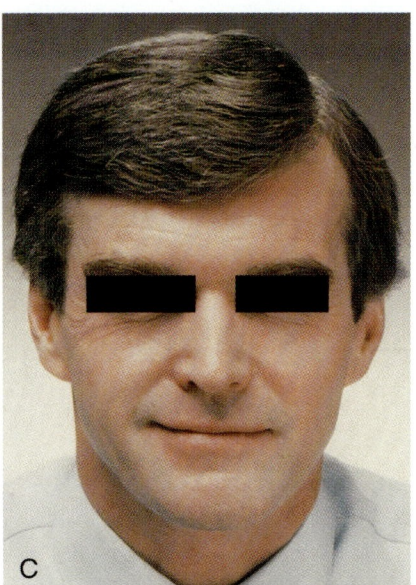

FIGURE 29–2 • Gradual hair dyes are popular among men for their ability to induce a gradual darkening of the hair color from gray to brown.

water-soluble metal salts which are deposited on the hair shaft in the form of oxides, suboxides, and sulfides (Fig. 29–3).[2]

2. Temporary Hair Coloring

Temporary hair coloring agents are designed to be removed in one shampooing.[3] They are used to add a slight tint, brighten a natural shade, or improve an existing dyed shade (Fig. 29–4). Their particle size is too large to penetrate through the cuticle, accounting for their temporary nature (see Fig. 29–1).[4] Temporary dyes can easily be rubbed off the hair shaft, however, and will run onto clothing if the hair gets wet from rain or perspiration. They can be formulated as a liquid, mousse, gel, or spray. The liquid rinse formulation is most popular, especially among mature patients

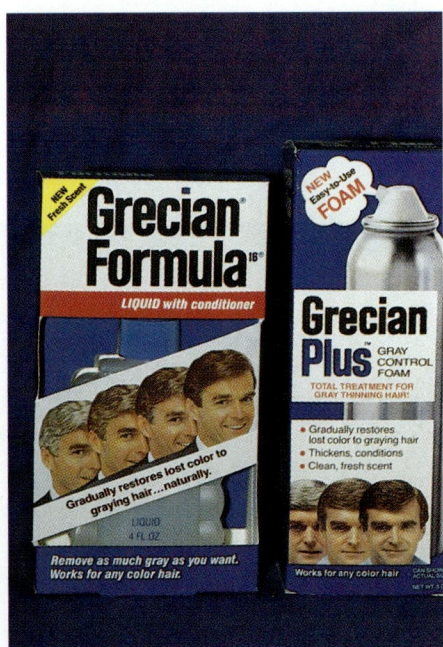

FIGURE 29–3 • Gradual hair dyes, also known as metallic or progressive hair dyes, deposit metal salts on the hair shaft.

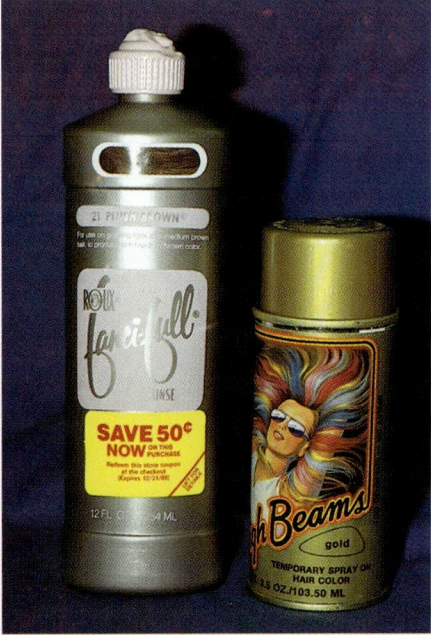

FIGURE 29–4 • Temporary hair dyes are rinses or sprays designed to brighten gray hair (*left*) or add colorful highlights (*right*).

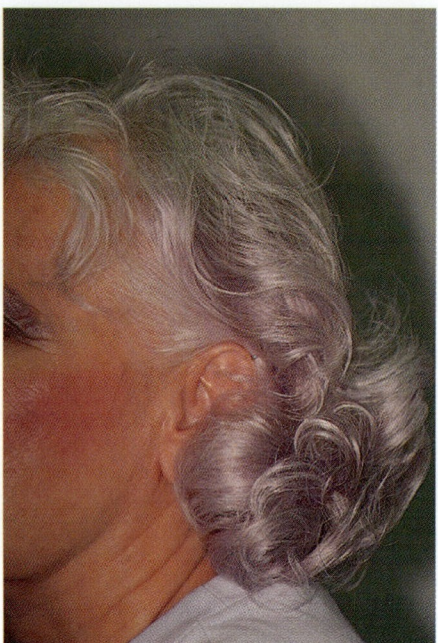

FIGURE 29–5 • Gray hair can be optically whitened with a purple temporary rinse. Unfortunately, the rinse adheres better to the damaged protein at the end of the hair shaft, which imparts a purple hue to the hair.

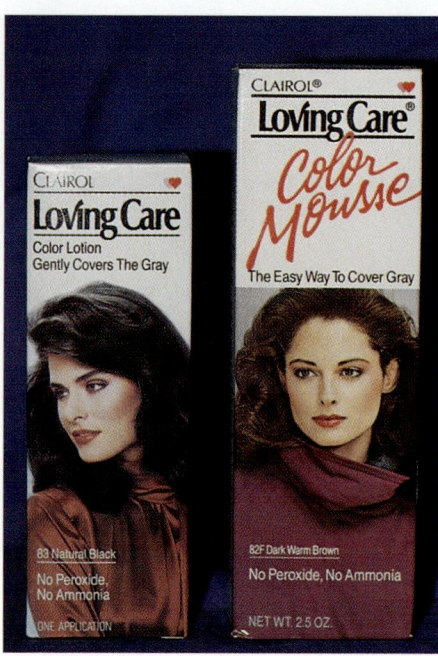

FIGURE 29–7 • Semipermanent hair dyes are removed in four to six shampooings.

with gray hair who wish to remove undesirable yellow tones and achieve a purer platinum color (Figs. 29–5 and 29–6).

3. Semipermanent Hair Coloring

Semipermanent hair coloring is popular with both men and women. Formulated for use on natural, unbleached hair, it can cover gray, add highlights, or rid

hair of unwanted tones (Fig. 29–7). Semipermanent hair dyes are removed in four to six shampooings due to their intermediate-sized particles, which can both enter and exit the hair shaft.[5] Recently, longer lasting products incorporating hydrogen peroxide have become available.[6] The dye is applied to wet, freshly shampooed hair and rinsed out within 20 to 40 minutes. Semipermanent dyes are best suited for patients with less than 30% gray hair who want to restore their natural color.[7]

Henna, a vegetable dye, also falls into the category of semipermanent hair coloring (Fig. 29–8). Today, natural henna dyes have been replaced by synthetic henna-type products with dye shades ranging from au-

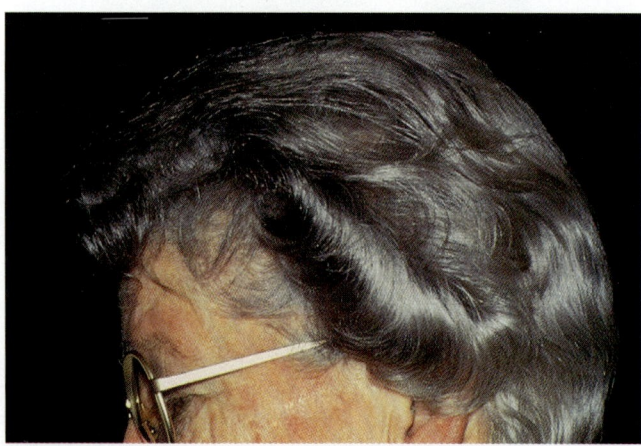

FIGURE 29–6 • Blue temporary dye can be used to remove the yellow tones from gray hair, yielding a platinum color.

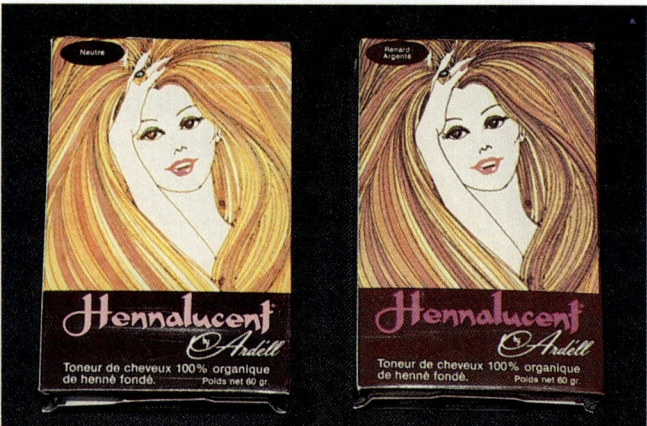

FIGURE 29–8 • Henna is another type of semipermanent hair dye used to produce red tones on brown hair.

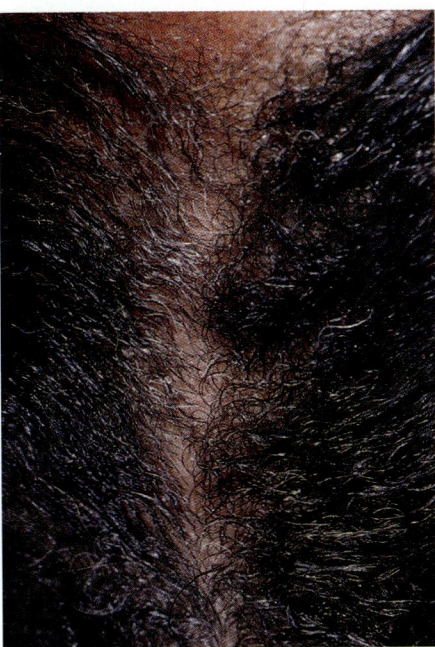

FIGURE 29–9 • Gray roots can be seen at the scalp of this patient with kinky hair who has permanently dyed her hair black.

TABLE 29–2 **Permanent Hair Dyeing Technique**

• • • • • •

1. Do not wash hair prior to dyeing unless it is heavily coated with styling products (e.g., hair spray, styling gel, mousse).
2. Remove two bottle containing dyestuffs from the packaging and mix immediately prior to application.
3. Immediately apply the mixture to the hair, beginning at the scalp, by parting hair into ¼-inch sections and thoroughly saturating. New hair growth at the scalp is more resistant to dyeing.
4. If this is the first time dye has been applied to the hair, work the dye through the entire scalp and allow to process for 30 minutes. If the hair is being redyed, allow the dye to remain on the scalp 25 to 30 minutes, and then work the remaining dye through the hair for an additional 15 minutes.
5. Rinse the dye from the hair with warm water until the water runs clear.
6. Apply an acid pH shampoo, usually supplied with the hair dye, and leave the product on 5 minutes to reverse hair shaft swelling induced by the dye exposure.
7. Rinse shampoo.
8. Allow hair to air dry to avoid heat damage.

burn to blonde to gray. These synthetic henna products combine a conditioning agent with the dye, but they are still powders mixed with water to form a paste that remains in contact with the hair for 40 minutes. Hennas can be used for darkening, but not lightening, of the original hair color.

4. Permanent Hair Coloring

Permanent hair coloring is so named because the dyestuff penetrates the hair shaft to the cortex and forms large color molecules that cannot be removed by shampooing (see Fig. 29–1).[8] It can be used to cover gray or produce a completely new hair color. Redyeing is necessary every 4 to 6 weeks, as new growth

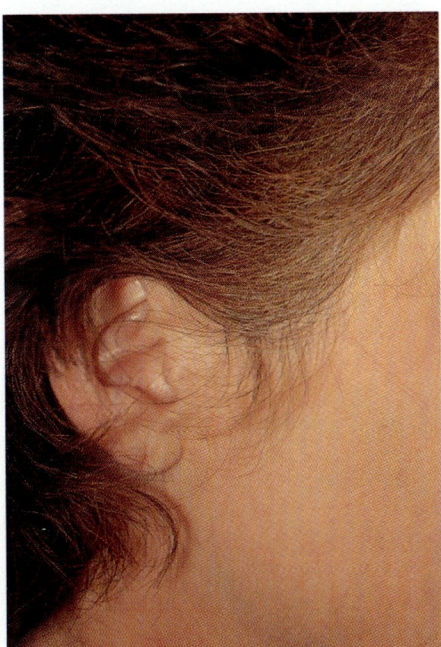

FIGURE 29–10 • Semipermanent hair dyes do not produce as dramatic a color change between the underlying gray hair and the dyed hair, as the dye rinses away slowly with time.

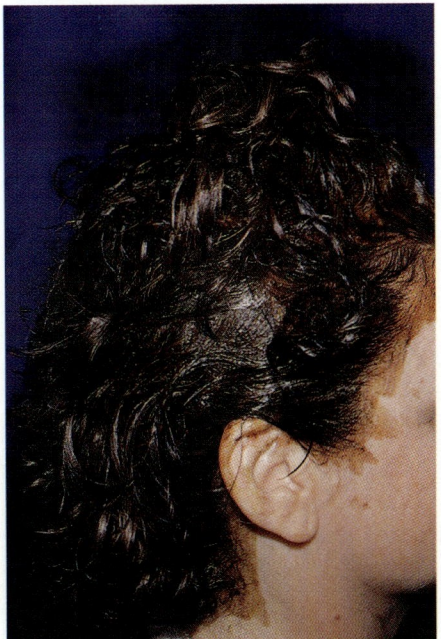

FIGURE 29–11 • Permanent hair dye changes color when the oxidative reaction has proceeded to completion. It should be applied evenly throughout the length of the hair shafts.

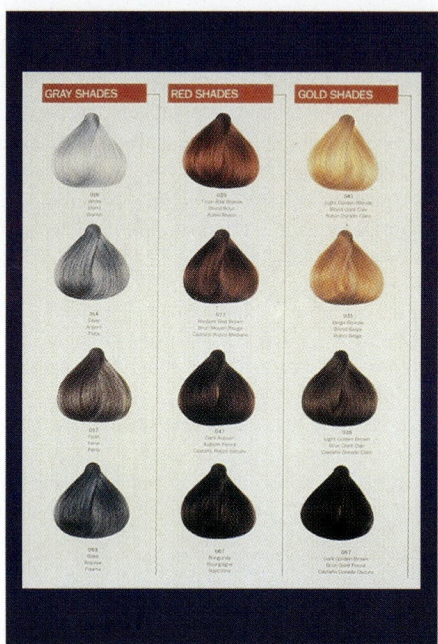

FIGURE 29–12 • Tremendous color possibilities are available with permanent hair dyes, allowing patients to either lighten or darken their existing hair color.

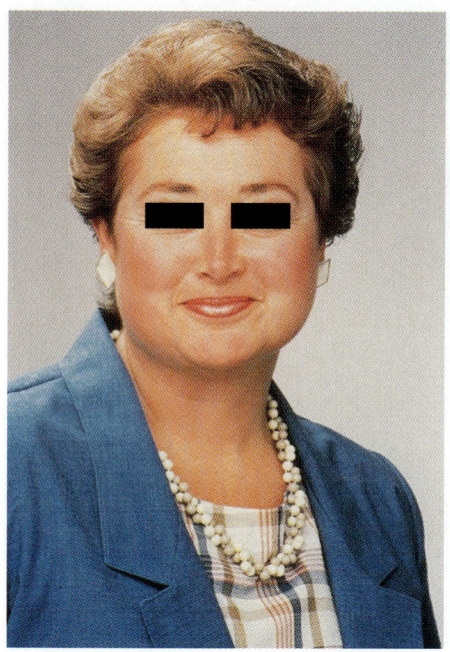

FIGURE 29–14 • A brown permanent oxidative dye has been used to achieve this color result on the same patient seen in Figure 29–13.

(known in the cosmetic industry as "roots") appears at the scalp (Figs. 29–9 and 29–10). This type of hair coloring does not contain dyes, but rather colorless dye precursors that chemically react with hydrogen peroxide inside the hair shaft to produce colored molecules (Table 29–2 and Fig. 29–11).[9] The process

entails the use of primary intermediates (p-phenylenediamines, p-toluenediamine, p-aminophenols), which undergo oxidation with hydrogen peroxide. These reactive intermediates are then exposed to couplers (e.g., resorcinol, l-naphthol, m-aminophenol), resulting in a wide variety of indo dyes. These indo dyes can

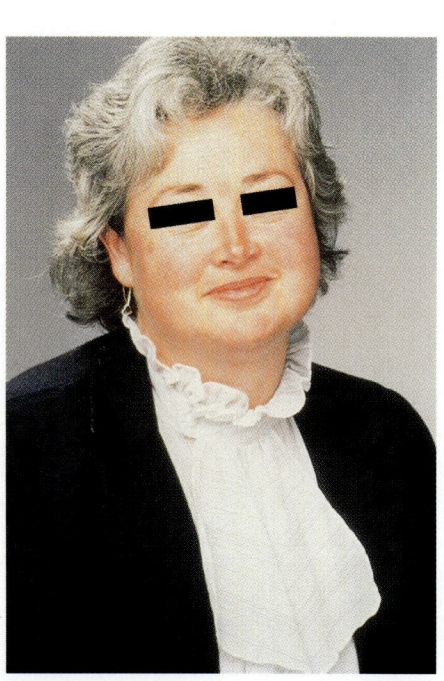

FIGURE 29–13 • This patient with 90% gray hair requires a permanent hair dye to darken her hair to its youthful color.

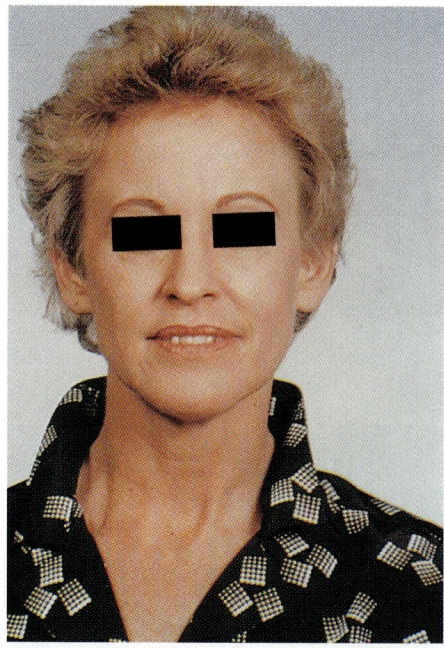

FIGURE 29–15 • Dull hair color, such as demonstrated here, can be brightened with a permanent hair dye.

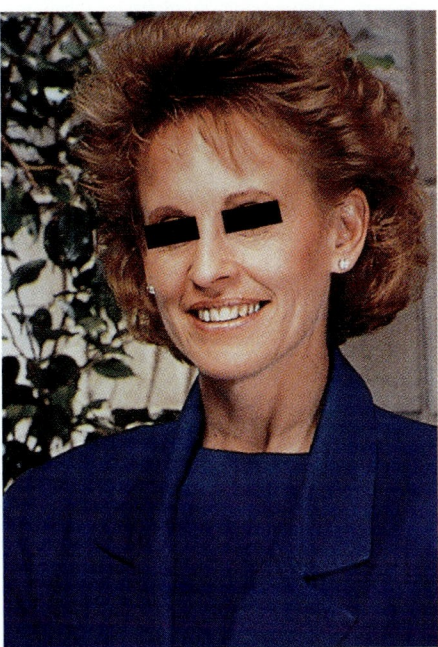

FIGURE 29–16 • An auburn permanent oxidative dye has restored vitality to the appearance this patient, the same one pictured in Figure 29–15.

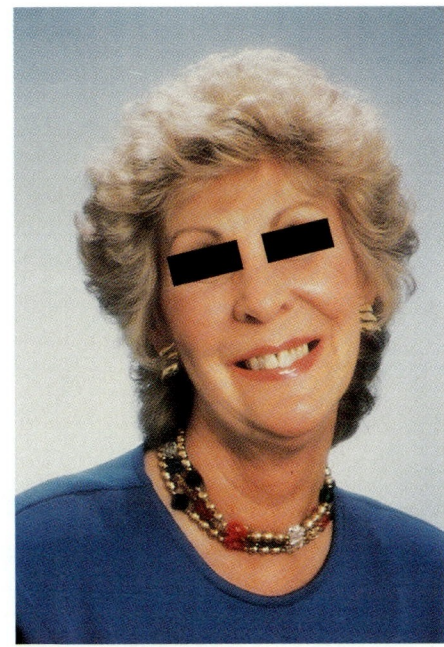

FIGURE 29–18 • Two-step processing was used to change the hair color of this patient, first pictured in Figure 29–17. The patient's brown hair was first bleached and then a toner was used to dye the hair the desired blonde color.

produce shades from blonde to brown to black with highlights of gold to red to orange (Fig. 29–12).[10]

Permanent dyeing allows shades either lighter and darker than the patient's original hair color to be obtained (Figs. 29–13 through 29–16). Higher concentra-

tions of hydrogen peroxide can bleach melanin; thus the oxidizing step functions both in color production and bleaching (Figs. 29–17 and 29–18). Most home products are designed to achieve a 35% coverage of gray hair. More dramatic color changes require professional products (Fig. 29–19).

Permanent hair dyes are also available for men (Fig. 29–20). Their formulation is identical to the products that are used by women, but the packaging

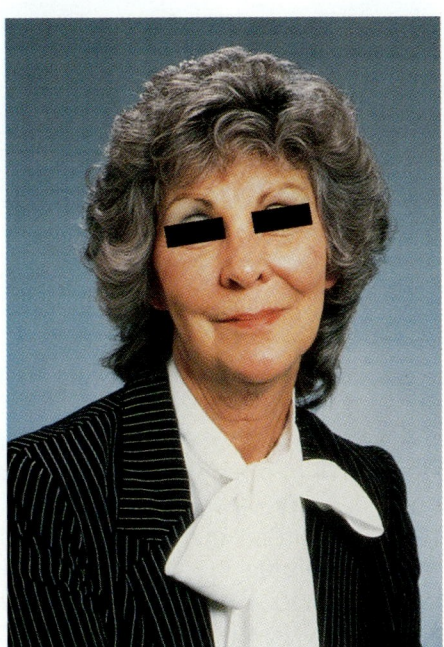

FIGURE 29–17 • This patient with 75% gray hair wished to lighten her hair outside of her color group rather than return to her natural brunette color. Hair color lightening can only be accomplished with oxidative permanent dyes.

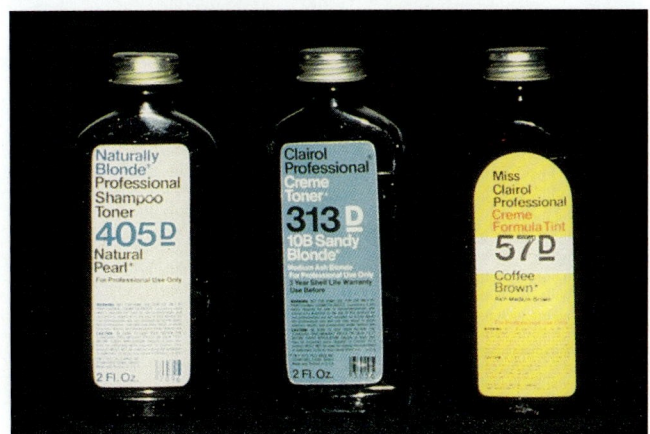

FIGURE 29–19 • These are examples of professional permanent hair dyes. Tints are used to darken hair color, whereas toners are used to replace the color in bleached hair.

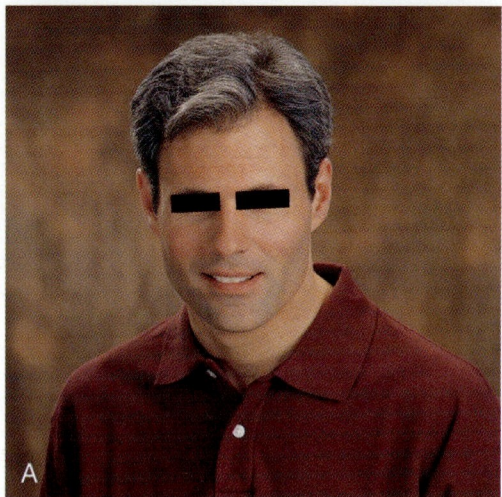

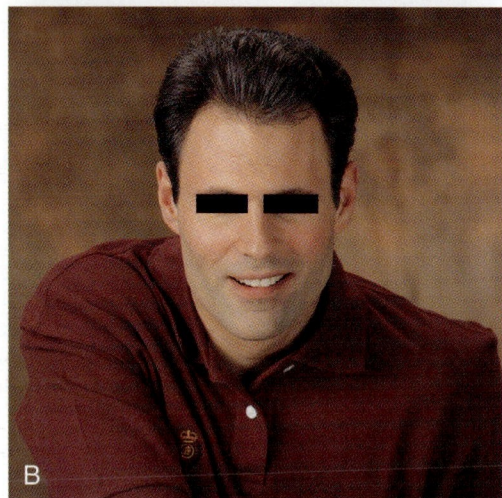

FIGURE 29–20 • *A* and *B,* Hair dyeing among men is becoming increasingly popular. This patient used a permanent hair dye to achieve this color result.

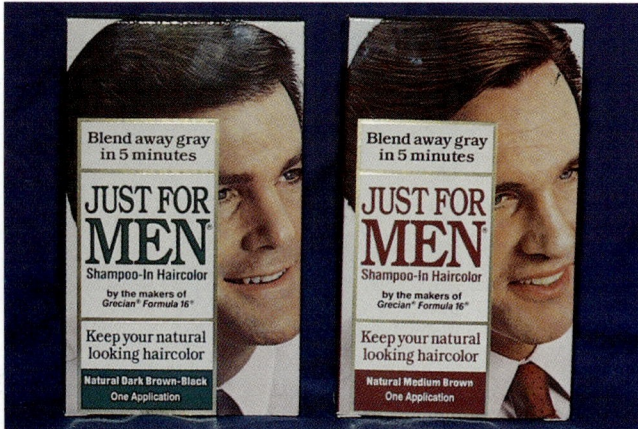

FIGURE 29–21 • Permanent hair colorings, such as this, are packaged for male consumers, but contain the same dyestuffs as products marketed to women.

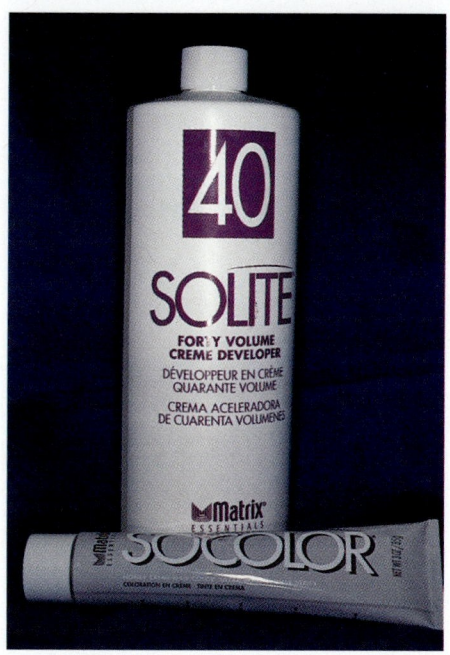

FIGURE 29–22 • This is an example of salon packaging for one color of permanent hair dye.

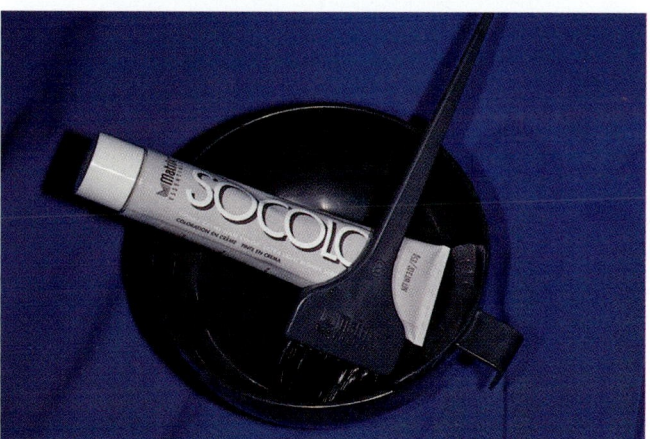

FIGURE 29–23 • The standard dyestuffs are mixed in a bowl to achieve the exact hair color the client desires.

and store location are more appealing to the male consumer (Fig. 29–21).

Some patients do not wish to lighten the hair on the entire scalp. For example, if only selected hairs are lightened in color (a technique known as "highlighting"), the dyestuff is applied to selected hairs and covered with foil during the processing period (Figs. 29–22 through 29–29). Fashion trends dictate the proportion of bleached to unbleached hairs in the scalp (Fig. 29–30). Melanin pigment is very resistant to reducing agents, but is easily degraded by oxidizing agents, such as hydrogen peroxide, causing oxygen to

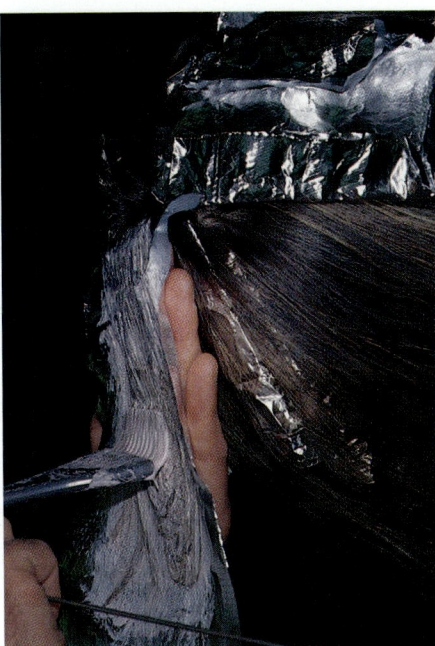

FIGURE 29–24 • This client wished to have a certain percentage of her brunette hairs bleached to a lighter blonde color. In this case, the permanent hair color is painted on the hair shafts.

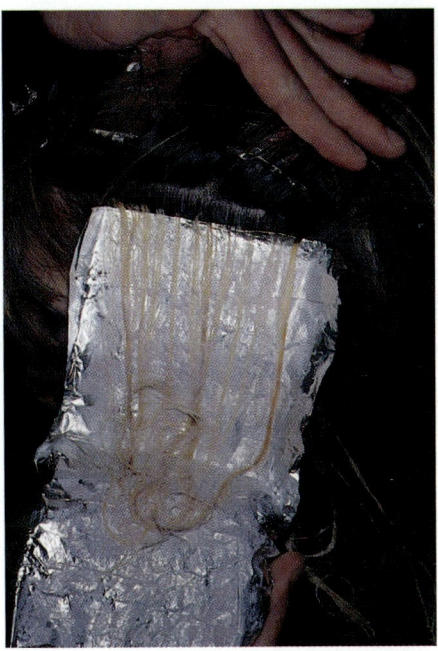

FIGURE 29–26 • After a predetermined period of time, usually 20 to 30 minutes, the foil is removed from the bleached hair shafts.

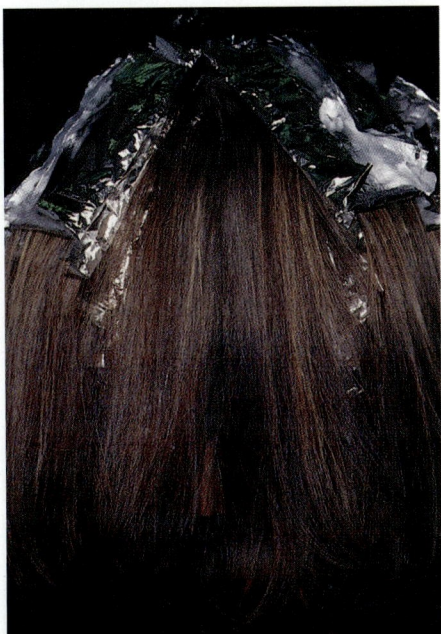

FIGURE 29–25 • Aluminum foil is used to wrap the dyed locks and protect the undyed hair. For this reason, this technique of selective hair bleaching is known as "foiling."

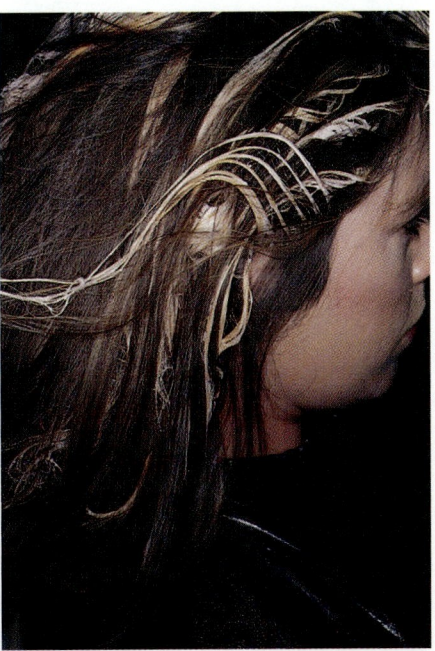

FIGURE 29–27 • The dyed hair shafts are now lighter than the client's original hair color.

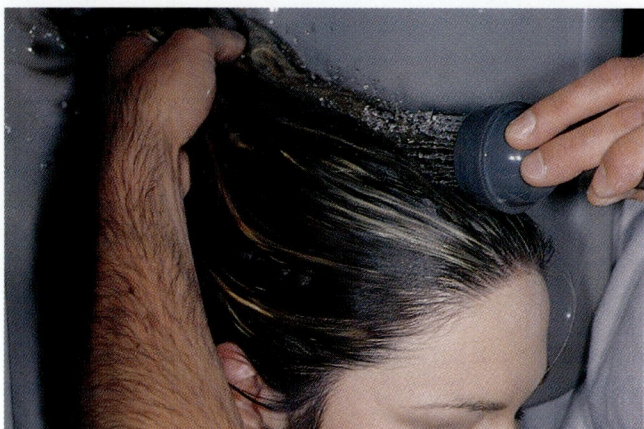

FIGURE 29–28 • Water is used to rinse the excess dyestuff from the hair shaft quickly, both to prevent excess lightening of the treated hairs and to prevent bleach contact with the hairs where no bleaching was desired.

be released from the hair keratin. The amount of hair lightening obtained is related to the amount of oxygen released, a quantity expressed as volumes by the cosmetic industry. The volume of a hydrogen peroxide solution is the number of liters of oxygen released by a liter of the bleaching solution (Fig. 29–31).

Problems associated with hair dyeing include dull, brittle, unmanageable, cosmetically unacceptable hair secondary to irreversible damage to the protein structure. This is especially prevalent when brown hair is

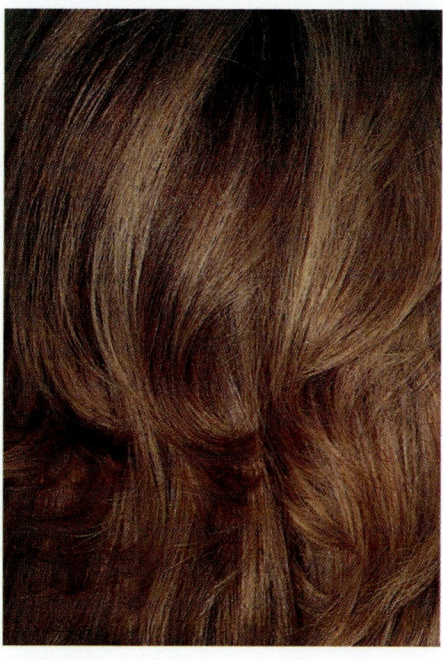

FIGURE 29–30 • This patient has elected to have some of her hair dyed auburn and some of her hair dyed blonde. Mixing of hair colors is thought to be cosmetically desirable, as natural hair possesses some color variation.

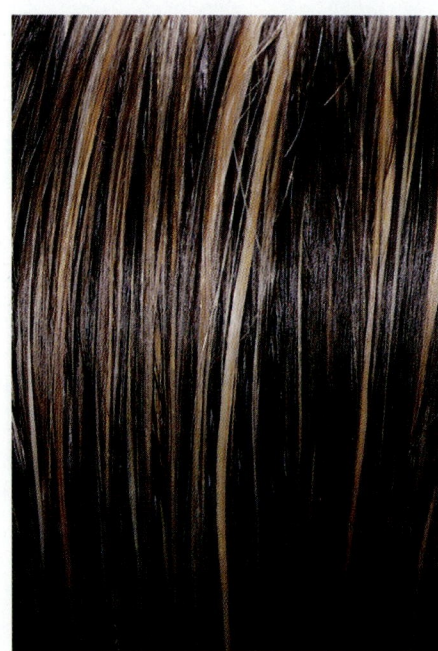

FIGURE 29–29 • This is the final appearance of the foiling technique.

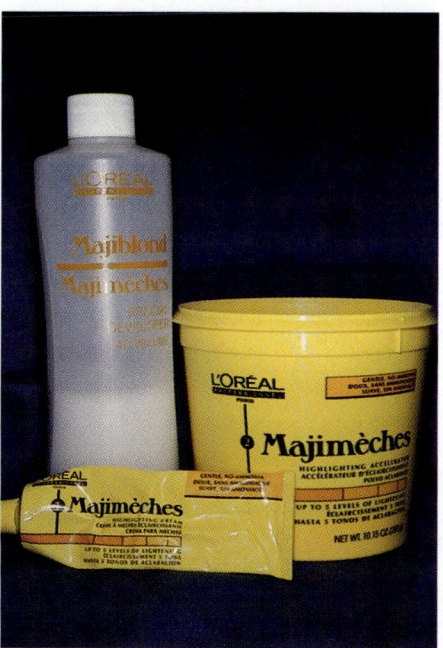

FIGURE 29–31 • This professional 40-volume salon hair lightening product is capable of producing blonde hair; however, hair shaft damage and subsequent hair breakage is an expected side effect.

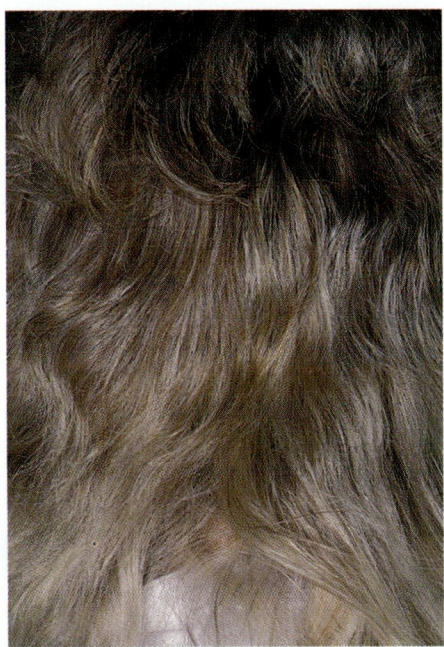

FIGURE 29–32 • This naturally brunette patient has bleached her hair extensively and frequently, resulting in weak hair shafts that have fractured, giving the appearance of thinning hair.

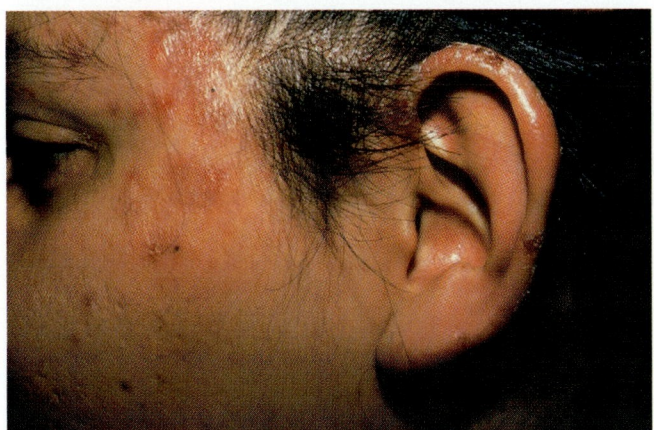

FIGURE 29–33 • Allergic contact dermatitis is most commonly seen with permanent hair dyes due to *p*-phenycenediamine.

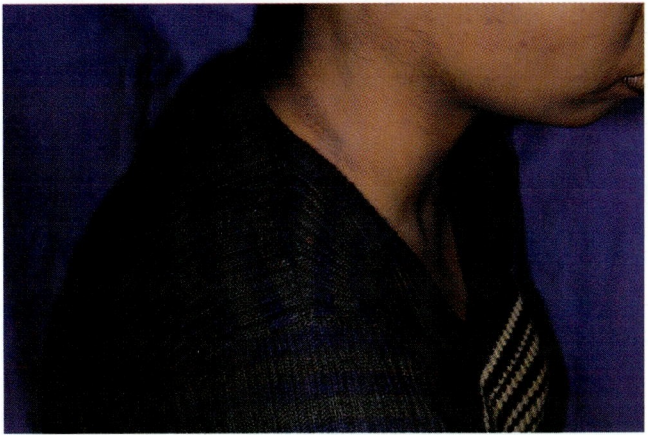

FIGURE 29–34 • Irritant contact dermatitis and subsequent postinflammatory hyperpigmentation has resulted from permanent hair dye contacting the skin in this patient.

bleached repeatedly to a light color (Fig. 29–32). Hair dyes can also cause an allergic contact dermatitis (Fig. 29–33) or, more frequently, an irritant contact dermatitis (Fig. 29–34).

REFERENCES

1. Pohl S. The chemistry of hair dyes. Cosmet Toiletr 103:57–66, 1988.
2. Spoor HJ. Part II: Metals. Cutis 19:37–40, 1977.
3. Spoor HJ. Hair Dyes: Temporary colorings. Cutis 18:341–344, 1976.
4. Corbett JF. Hair coloring. Clin Dermatol 6:93–101, 1988.
5. Spoor HJ. Semi-permanent hair color. Cutis 18:506–508, 1976.
6. Robbin CR. Chemical and Physical Behavior of Human Hair, 2nd ed. New York: Springer-Verlag, 1988, pp. 185–188.
7. Zviak C. Hair coloring, nonoxidation coloring. In Zviak C (ed.). The Science of Hair Care. New York: Marcel Dekker, 1986, pp. 235–261.
8. Tucker HH. Formulation of oxidation hair dyes. Am J Perfum Cosmet 83:69, 1968.
9. Corbett JF, Menkart J. Hair coloring. Cutis 12:190, 1973.
10. Zviak C. Oxidation coloring. In Zviak C (ed.). The Science of Hair Care. New York: Marcel Dekker, 1986, pp. 263–286.

30

Hair Curling Techniques

Hair that has a natural curl is irregular in cross section, accounting for the inability of the hair to hang straight (Figs. 30–1 and 30–2). However, an artificial curl can be created in naturally straight hair, either on a temporary or permanent basis, owing to the physical characteristics of the hair shaft. Temporary changes in hair shape involve the use of water, rollers, and possibly, heat. Wet hair is more elastic than dry hair, allowing partial transformation of the normal alpha-keratin structure to a beta-keratin structure when the hair is tightly wrapped around a roller (Figs. 30–3 through 30–5). This transformation shifts the relative position of the polypeptide chains and brings about a disruption of ionic and hydrogen bonds. During the drying process, new ionic and hydrogen bonds are formed, blocking return to the natural alpha-keratin configuration and allowing the hair to remain in its newly curled position. Wetting the hair, however, returns hair bonds immediately to the natural alpha configuration, accounting for the temporary nature of this type of hair curling.[1]

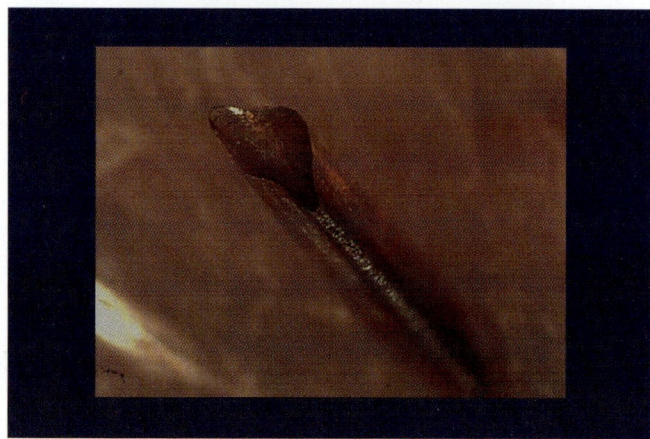

FIGURE 30–2 • This flattened elliptical hair shaft also will exhibit a natural curl (video microscope, X400).

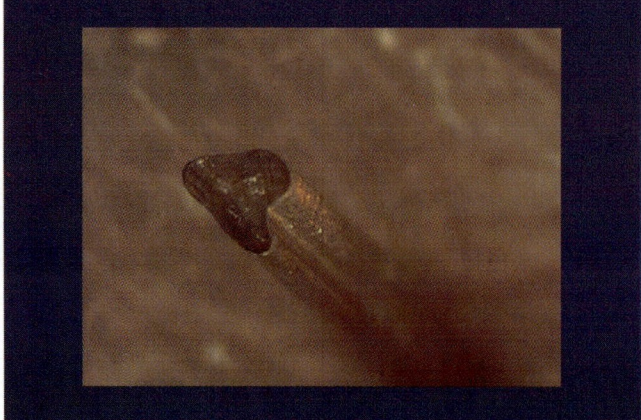

FIGURE 30–1 • A hair that is triangular in cross section will exhibit a natural curl (video microscope, X400).

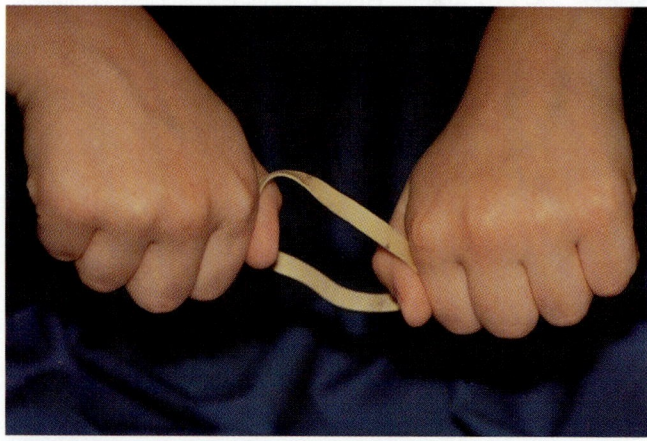

FIGURE 30–3 • This rubber band represents an unstretched hair shaft in an alpha-keratin configuration.

142

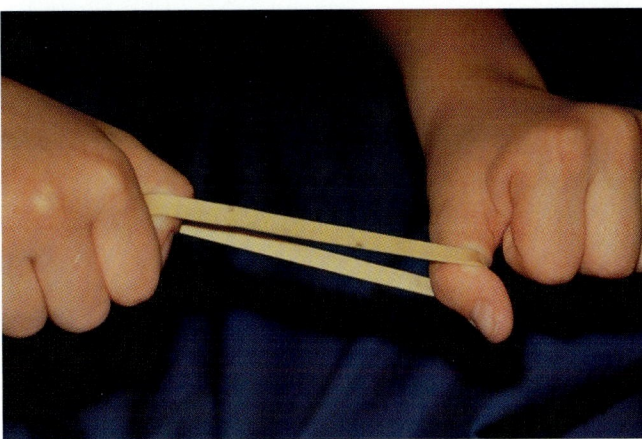

FIGURE 30–4 • As the hair is stretched, much like this rubber band, the hair shaft assumes a beta-keratin configuration. Hair can shift between alpha and beta configurations without irreversible trauma and maintain its elastic qualities with complete recoil.

Permanent waving utilizes three processes: chemical softening, rearranging, and fixing.[2] The basic chemistry involves the reduction of the disulfide hair shaft bonds with mercaptans,[3] as illustrated in Table 30–1.[4] The standard salon application procedure involves a waving lotion (Table 30–2) and a neutralizer (Table 30–3). The individual steps are presented in Table 30–4 (Figs. 30–6 and 30–7).[5] It usually takes about 90 minutes to complete the entire process, depending on the length of the hair. Careful factors to consider in the cold waving process are listed in Table 30–5.[6] Tips for troubleshooting patient problems related to permanent waving procedures are listed in Table 30–6. The hair changes that occur are listed in Table 30–7.

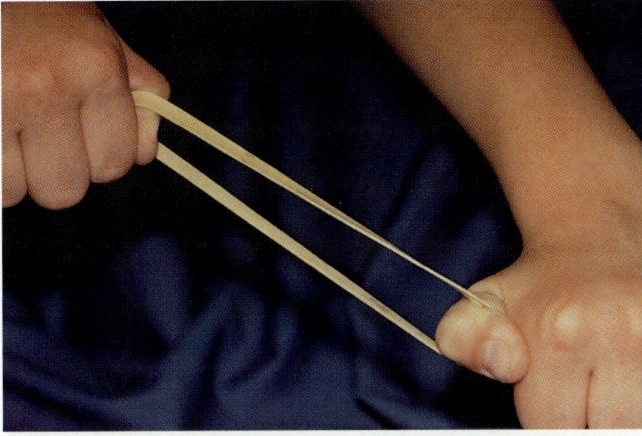

FIGURE 30–5 • Hair that is stretched beyond the elastic range, however, will become brittle and easily fracture, much like a tightly stretched rubber band that is no longer able to assume its original shape.

TABLE 30–1   Chemistry of Permanent Hair Waving

1. Penetration of the thiol compound into the hair shaft
2. Cleavage of the hair keratin disulfide bond (kSSk) to produce a cysteine residue (kSH) and the mixed disulfide of the thiol compound with the hair keratin (kSSR)

$$kSSk + RSH \rightleftharpoons kSH + kSSR$$

3. Reaction with another thiol molecule to produce a second cysteine residue and the symmetrical disulfide of the thiol waving agent (RSSR)

$$kSSR + RSH \rightleftharpoons kSH + RSSR$$

4. Rearrangement of the hair protein structure to relieve internal stress determined by curler size and hair wrapping tension
5. Application of an oxidizing agent to reform the disulfide cross-links

$$kSH + HSk \xrightarrow{\text{oxidizing agent}} kSSk + water$$

Several types of permanent waves are available, based on the composition of the waving solution. An evaluation of the various types of permanent waves is presented in Table 30–8.[3,7]

Adverse reactions associated with permanent wave procedures vary from irritant contact dermatitis to allergic contact dermatitis. Irritation is clearly most common owing to the nature of the chemical required to break the disulfide bonds in the hair shafts (Figs. 30–8 and 30–9).

TABLE 30–2   Permanent Waving Lotion Ingredients

Ingredient	Chemical Examples	Function
Reducing agent	Thioglycolates, sulfites	Breaks disulfide bonds
Alkaline agent	Ammonium hydroxide, triethanolamine	Adjusts pH
Chelating agent	Tetrasodium EDTA	Removes trace metals
Wetting agent	Fatty alcohols	Improves hair saturation with waving lotion
Conditioner	Proteins, humectants, quaternium compounds	Protects hair during waving process
Opacifier	Polyacrylates, polystyrene latex	Opacifies waving lotion

Adapted from Lee AE, Bozza JB, Huff S, de la Mettrie R. Permanent waves: An overview. Cosmet Toiletr 103:37–56, 1988.

TABLE 30–3 Function of Neutralizer Ingredients

Ingredient	Chemical Examples	Function
Oxidizing agent	Hydrogen peroxide, sodium bromate	Reforms broken disulfide bonds
Acid buffer	Citric acid, acetic acid, lactic acid	Maintains acidic pH
Stabilizer	Sodium stannate	Prevents hydrogen peroxide breakdown
Wetting agent	Fatty alcohols	Improves hair saturation with neutralizer
Conditioner	Proteins, humectants, quaternium compounds	Improves hair feel
Opacifier	Polyacrylates, polystyrene latex	Makes neutralizer opaque

Adapted from Lee AE, Bozza JB, Huff S, de la Mettrie R. Permanent waves: An overview. Cosmet Toiletr 103: 37–56, 1988.

TABLE 30–4 Permanent Hair Waving Technique

1. Wet hair thoroughly to increase flexibility in hair hydrogen bonds.
2. Section hair into 30 to 50 areas, depending on hair length and thickness.
3. Wind hair on rods with minimal tension to prevent excessive stretching of hair fibers. Select small rods for small curls and large rods for large curls.
4. Apply tissue paper squares to the ends of the hair shafts to prevent uneven wrapping and frizzy hair.
5. Apply a cotton wick to the scalp margins over a layer of petroleum jelly to prevent waving lotion contact with the facial and neck skin.
6. Saturate rods evenly with waving lotion and allow chemical reaction to process for 5 to 20 minutes, depending on the condition of the hair.
7. Perform a test curl to determine if the desired amount of curl has been obtained to prevent overprocessing.
8. Saturate the rods with ⅔ of the neutralizer and allow to set for 5 minutes.
9. Remove the rods from the hair and apply the remaining neutralizer.
10. Rinse hair carefully and thoroughly.
11. Dry and style hair as desired.
12. Avoid shampooing or manipulating the hair for 2 days to prolong curl retention.

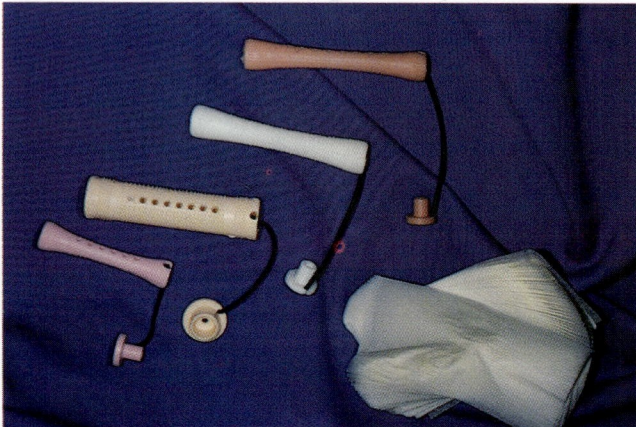

FIGURE 30–6 • Wet hair is tightly wound around these mandrels to initiate the permanent waving process. Small mandrels produce tight curls, whereas large mandrels produce loose curls. The white papers in the lower right hand corner are end papers that are wrapped around the distal hair shaft ends to prevent frizziness.

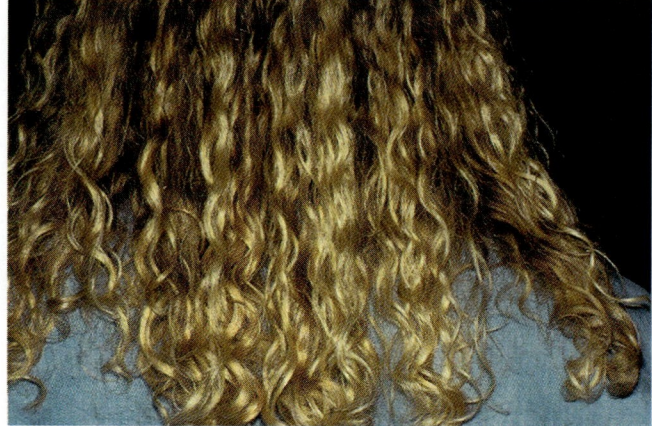

FIGURE 30–7 • This patient, who presented with straight hair, now has tightly curled hair owing to the use of small mandrels and strong permanent waving solution. Tighter curls produced with a permanent wave induce greater hair damage than looser curls because of the dramatic protein rearrangement of the hair shaft.

TABLE 30–5 Factors Influencing Cold Waving

• • • • • •

1. The hair must not be wound with excessive tension around the rods, or increased breakage may occur.[8]
2. Smaller rods will produce smaller curls, which are more damaging to the hair shaft.
3. The hair must fit around the rod at least once for complete curl formation in patients with short hair.
4. A stronger waving lotion will not produce a tighter curl. The curl diameter is determined by the rod diameter.
5. Weak waving lotions with shorter processing times should be used for damaged hair.
6. It may be necessary to use different strengths of waving lotions on new proximal growth and previously waved distal growth, especially in patients with bleached hair.
7. A test curl should be performed to avoid overprocessing the hair. Long processing times can excessively damage hair, increasing breakage.
8. Discoloration of the hair may occur in patients who have used para-phenylenediamine-based permanent dyes that have been oxidized incompletely.

TABLE 30–6 Troubleshooting Problems Related to Permanent Waving Procedures

• • • • • •

Problem	Cause	Solution
Foul odor	Incomplete reformation of the disulfide bonds[9]	Reneutralize hair professionally
Hair breakage	Waving solution left in contact with hair too long; hair stretched too tightly on rods	Apply protein-containing conditioner to increase strength; decrease processing time; select acid instead of alkaline permanent wave solutions
Hair breakage around face	Overprocessing of weathered hair around face	Place test curl at anterior, instead of posterior, hairline
Curl too loose	Select smaller rods	None
Curl too tight	Select larger rods	Curl will relax naturally with shampooing
Frizzy hair shaft	Excessive damage to cuticle	Apply deep and instant conditioners
Frizzy hair ends	Failure to smooth distal hair shafts on end papers	Pull hair shafts straight and carefully wrap in end papers
Hair color change	Permanent hair dye incompletely oxidized	Permanent wave hair at least 10 days prior to dyeing
Poor curl retention	Shampooing to soon after permanent wave procedure; inadequate processing time	Wait 2 days or longer prior to shampooing after undergoing a permanent wave, lengthen processing time if hair is coarse or has never been chemically treated
No curl retention	Hair unable to complete one revolution around perming rod	Select smaller perming rods or allow hair to grow longer

TABLE 30–7 Cosmetic Hair Changes Associated with Permanent Waving

• • • • • •

1. Permanently waved hair is 17% weaker than natural hair, accounting for increased hair breakage with grooming.[10]
2. Increased hair friction is present, creating more tangles and necessitating increased combing force.[11]
3. Disruption of the cuticle following permanent waving causes increased static electricity and decreased manageability.
4. Cortical damage following permanent waving predisposes to hair shaft swelling, allowing deeper penetration of subsequent permanent waving and dyeing procedures.[12]

TABLE 30–8   Types of Permanent Waves

Type	Chemical Composition	pH	Disadvantages	Advantages	Special Considerations
Acid	Glycerol monothioglycolate	6.5–7	Produces looser curl; may cause allergic contact dermatitis	Minimizes hair damage	Preferred for previously chemically treated hair
Exothermic	Hydrogen peroxide mixed with thioglycolate		Professional product only	Produces heat for client comfort	Must be mixed properly to prevent hair damage
Self-regulated	Dithioglycolic acid added to thioglycolate			Unlikely to overprocess	Prevents problems for the busy beautician
Alkaline	Ammonium thioglycolate	9–10	Harsh on hair	Tight curl	Reduces waving lotion concentration on bleached hair
Buffered alkaline	Ammonium bicarbonate	7–8.5	Harsh on hair	Less harsh than alkaline, but tight curl	None
Sulfite	Sulfite or bisulfite	6–8	Long processing time; harsh on hair; loose curl; home product only	Reduced odor	Must be combined with a conditioning agent

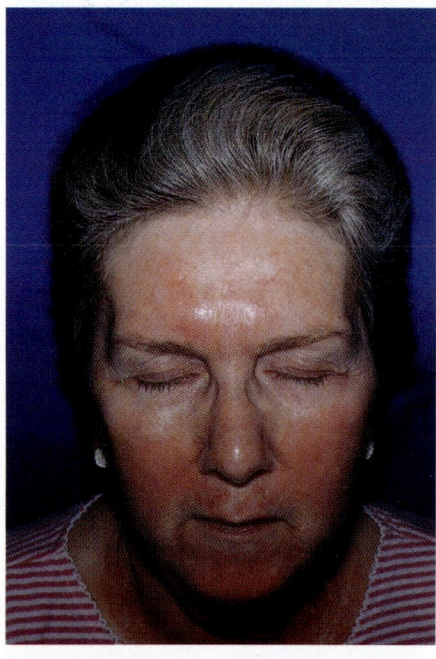

FIGURE 30–8 • Facial irritant contact dermatitis can occur if the permanent wave solution is mistakenly rinsed over the face.

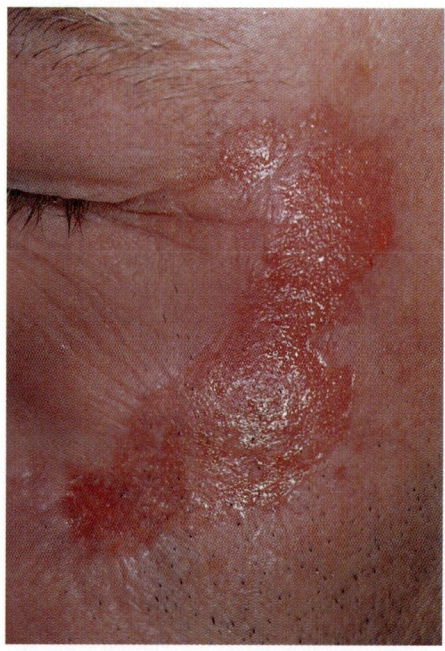

FIGURE 30–9 • A superficial second-degree burn can be induced if strong permanent waving solution contacts the skin for a prolonged time.

REFERENCES

1. Robbins CR. Chemical and Physical Behavior of Human Hair, 2nd ed. New York: Springer-Verlag, 1988, pp. 89–91.

2. Wickett RR. Permanent waving and straightening of hair. Cutis 39:496–497, 1987.

3. Zviak C. Permanent waving and hair straightening. In Zviak C (ed.). The Science of Hair Care. New York: Marcel Dekker, 1986, pp. 183–209.

4. Cannell DW. Permanent waving and hair straightening. Clin Dermatol 6:71–82, 1988.

5. Draelos ZK. Hair cosmetics. Dermatol Clin 9:19–27, 1991.

6. Heilingotter R. Permanent waving of hair. In de Navarre MG (ed.). The Chemistry and Manufacture of Cosmetics. Carol Stream, IL: Allured Publishing Co, 1988, pp. 1167–1227.

7. Gershon SD, Goldberg MA, Rieger MM. Permanent waving. In: Balsam MS, Sagarin E (eds.). Cosmetics Science and Technology, 2nd ed, Vol. 2. New York: Wiley-Interscience, John Wiley & Sons, 1972, pp. 167–250.

8. Wortman FJ, Souren I. Extensional properties of human hair and permanent waving. J Soc Cosmet Chem 38:125–140, 1987.

9. Brunner MJ. Medical aspects of home cold waving. Arch Dermatol 65:316–326, 1952.

10. Feughelman M. A note on the permanent setting of human hair. J Soc Cosmet Chem 41:209–212, 1990.

11. Robbins CR. Chemical and Physical Behavior of Human Hair. New York: Springler-Verlag, 1988, pp. 94–98.

12. Shansky A. The osmotic behavior of hair during the permanent waving process as explained by swelling measurements. J Soc Cosmet Chem 14:427–432, 1963.

31

Hair Styling Products

Hair styling products are intended to enhance and sustain an orderly arrangement of the hair. Styling aids also provide conditioning, shine, body, and increased manageability. These products are applied following shampooing and are intended to be completely removed with subsequent shampooing. The categories of modern styling products are listed in Table 31–1.

1. Hair Sprays

Hair sprays are applied either prior to hair styling to act as a setting lotion, or following hair styling to hold the finished hairstyle (Fig. 31–1). Copolymers, such as polyvinylpyrrolidone, vinyl acetate, vinylmethylether, and polyvinylpyrrolidone dimethylaminoethylmethacrylate, are the main ingredients in hair sprays, now widely available as aerosol pumps.[1-3] Conditioning agents, such as hydrolyzed animal proteins, quaternium-19, are also incorporated to enhance the cosmetic appearance of the hair.[4] Newer hair spray formulations provide a flexible hold (Fig. 31–2), which is desirable in patients with thinning hair so as to minimize hair shaft damage.

2. Hair Gels

Hair gels contain the same copolymers as hair sprays except that they are formulated into a gel and packaged in soft plastic squeeze tubes (Fig. 31–3). These products contain glossening and conditioning agents (e.g., hydrolyzed animal proteins, panthenol, keratin polypeptides, amino acids) that coat the hair shaft and restore shine (Fig. 31–4). Two formulations are available: styling gels and sculpturing gels. As the names suggest, sculpturing gels afford more hold than styling gels.

Hair gels may contain synthetic color, usually in unnatural shades, such as blue, red, or purple (Fig. 31–5). The colored gel coats the hair shaft, imparting tones of the color selected. The color molecules are too large to penetrate the undamaged hair shaft, though, so the colored coating can be removed with one shampooing. However, persons with chemically dyed or waved hair have a porous shaft that may absorb color molecules semipermanently, requiring four to six shampooings for removal. Glitter may also be added to hair gels for effect.

Hair gels are applied to towel-dried, damp hair and distributed on the hair shafts by combing to form a

TABLE 31–1 Hair Styling Products

Type	Formulation	Indication
Spray	Aerosol or pump	Hold finished style
Styling fix	Aerosol or pump	Provide strong hold to finished style
Styling gel	Gel	Applied to towel-dried hair to add body and increase hold
Sculpturing gel	Gel	Applied to towel-dried hair to add body and greatly increase hold
Mousse	Foam	Applied to towel-dried hair during styling to add body minimally and increase hold
Pomade	Cream	Applied during styling to moisturize kinky hair, add shine, decrease breakage, and/or aid in straightening hair
Glycerin curl activator	Gel	Applied during styling to condition kinky hair and add shine
Brilliantine	Liquid	Applied during styling to condition kinky hair and add shine

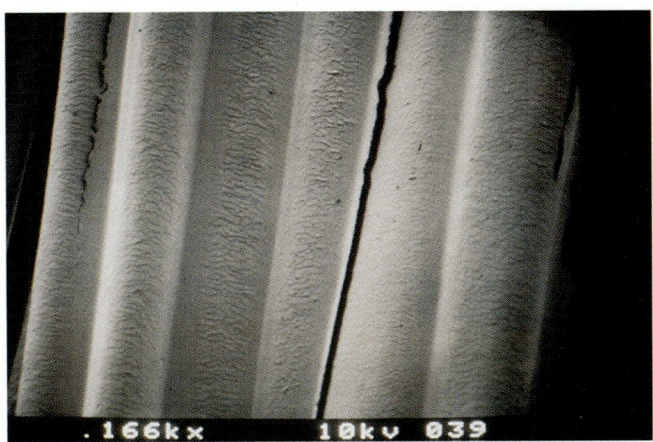

FIGURE 31–1 • Hair spray coats, stiffens, and bonds the hairs together.

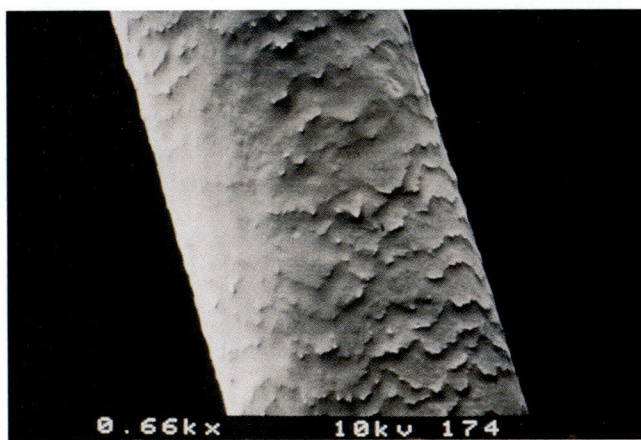

FIGURE 31–3 • Styling gels coat the surface of the hair shaft, providing stiffness and maintaining the desired hairstyle.

thin film. If a small amount of gel is applied, the hair will have a natural look and feel. If a large amount is applied, the hair will have a wet look and a stiff feel (Fig. 31–6). A small amount of hair gel can be useful in patients with thinning hair to hold the hair away from the scalp and create the illusion of fullness.[5,6]

3. Hair Mousses

Hair mousses contain copolymers in an aerosolized foam released under pressure from a can (Fig. 31–7).

Hair styling mousses may also contain glossening and conditioning agents and can be colored to provide either natural or unnatural highlights (Fig. 31–8). The color is temporary and can be removed with one shampooing unless applied to chemically treated hair.

The mousse is applied in the same manner as a hair gel to towel-dried hair, except that it provides less hold. Owing to their lower moisture content, hair styling mousses can more easily create natural-appearing fullness than hair gels. A half-dollar-sized mound of mousse is placed in the palm. Small amounts are then dabbed onto the fingers and massaged into the proximal hair shaft. Drying occurs al-

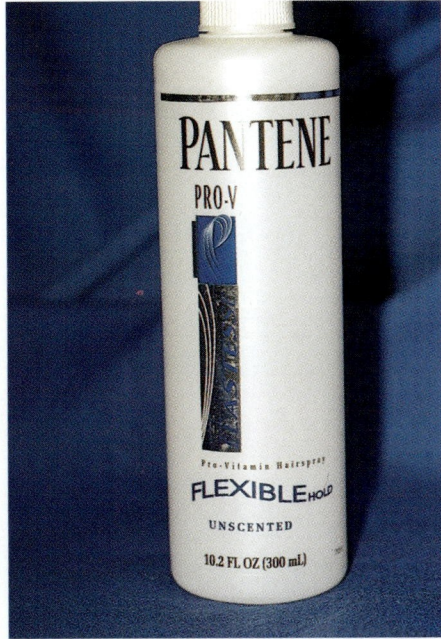

FIGURE 31–2 • Flexible hair sprays are recommended for patients with hair loss, since these products provide excellent hold, creating the illusion of fullness, while allowing movement of the hair and preventing hair shaft fracture.

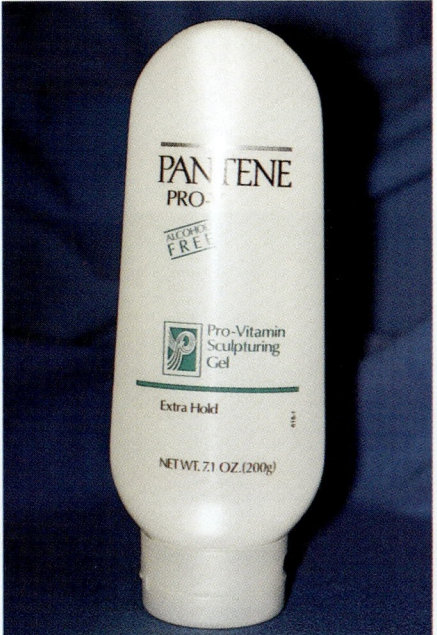

FIGURE 31–4 • Alcohol-free styling gels are recommended in the hair loss patient to minimize hair shaft dryness.

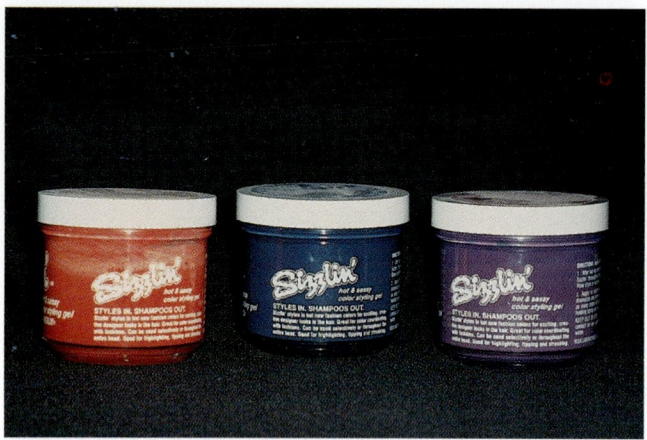

FIGURE 31–5 • Styling gels are available in party colors to create a temporary cosmetic hair effect.

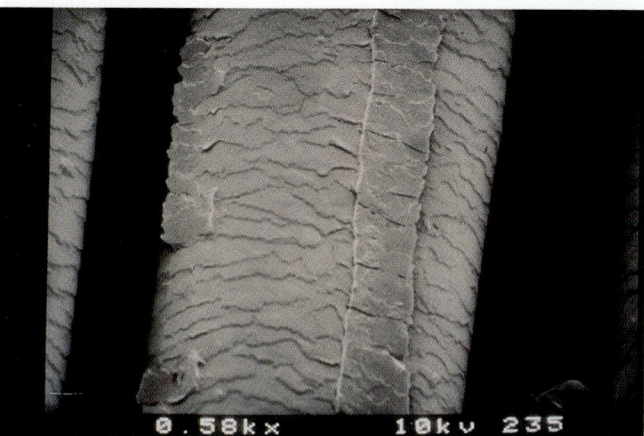

FIGURE 31–8 • Styling mousses leave an even film over the hair shaft, smoothing and protecting the damaged cuticular scales while increasing hair shine.

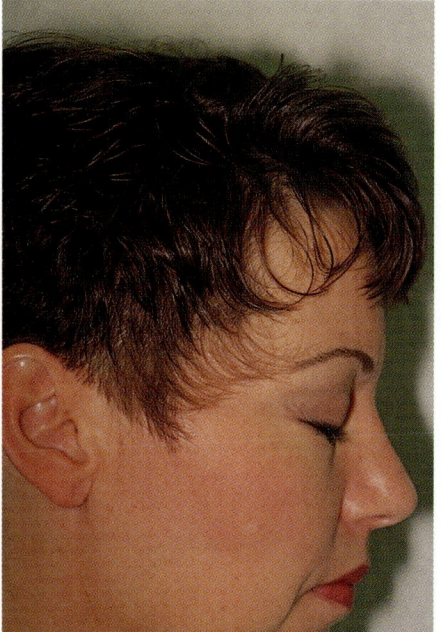

FIGURE 31–6 • Styling gel is used to maintain the hairs in this carefully arranged hairstyle.

most immediately. The mousse adds stiffness to the hair shaft, creating the illusion of fullness. This technique can be used by both men and women with thinning hair.

4. Pomades

Pomades, also known as cream brilliantines, are anhydrous products containing petrolatum, waxes, lanolin, and vegetable or mineral oils (Fig. 31–9).[7] They combine conditioning and styling properties, but can

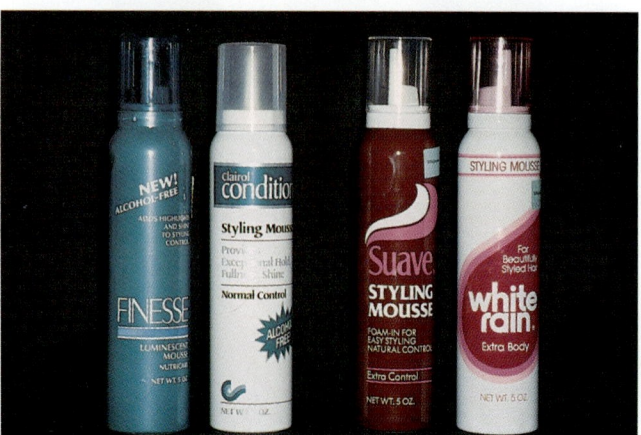

FIGURE 31–7 • Styling mousses are sprayed from a can onto the hands and dabbed into the hair to add shine and hold to the hair shafts.

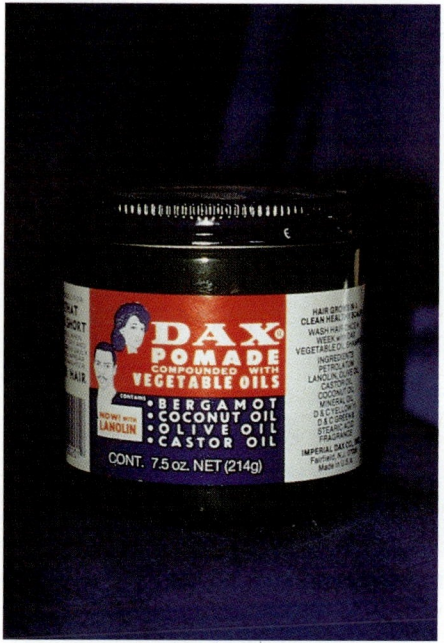

FIGURE 31–9 • Pomade is a heavy, petrolatum-based product designed to moisturize and style kinky hair.

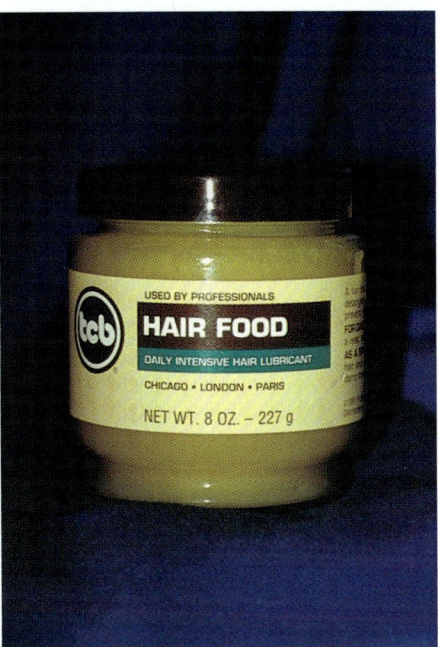

FIGURE 31–10 • Specialty additives can be incorporated into pomades.

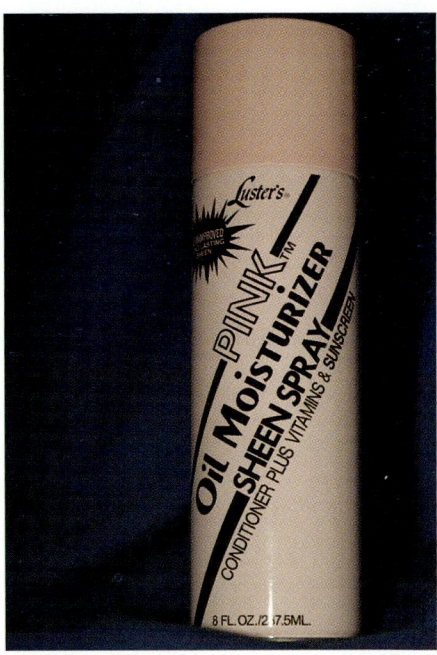

FIGURE 31–12 • Aerosolized oil sheen sprays are popular aids for adding shine to a finished hairstyle.

also contain sulfur or tar derivatives to aid in the treatment of seborrheic dermatitis (Fig. 31–10). The pomade adds shine, lubrication, and hold to allow the hair to remain close to the scalp with some curl reduction. These products are preferred by Black men who have close-cropped haircuts. Some of the newer glycerin-based products can be substituted for a petrolatum or olive oil pomade without producing acne.[8] These are known as gel curl activators, but they do not repel moisture or moisturize the hair quite as well as the traditional pomades (Fig. 31–11).

5. Brilliantines

Liquid brilliantines are popular for maintaining natural, kinky hairstyles. These products allow ease of styling, provide shine, and contain mineral and vegetable oils.[9] Newer formulations contain silicone to add lubricity, castor oil to aid in manageability, and soluble

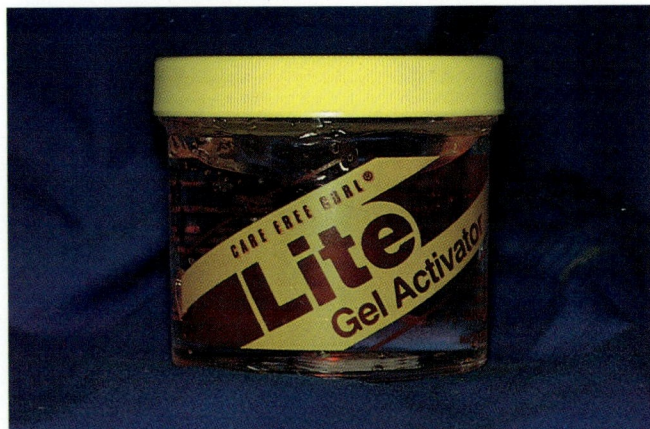

FIGURE 31–11 • Glycerin-based gel activator products are recommended for hair styling in the patient with pomade acne. However, these products provide less moisturization to the hair shafts.

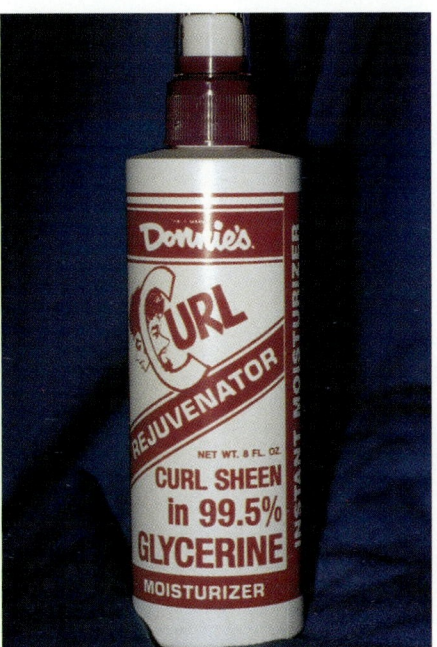

FIGURE 31–13 • Glycerin curl sheen products are preferred in patients with hairline comedonal acne.

glycoprotein to moisturize the hair shafts.[10] If the product is sprayed on to the hair, it is known as an oil sheen spray (Fig. 31–12). Products based on glycerin are also available for patients exhibiting comedones along the hairline, but the conditioning ability of these products is decreased (Fig. 31–13).

REFERENCES

1. Zviak C. The Science of Hair Care. New York: Marcel Dekker, 1986, pp. 153–165.
2. Stutsman MJ. Analysis of hair fixatives. In Senzel AJ (ed.). Newburger's Manual of Cosmetic Analysis, 2nd ed. Washington, DC: Association of Official Analytical Chemists, 1977, p 72.
3. Wells FV, Lubowe II. Hair grooming aids, Part III. Cutis 22:407–425, 1978.
4. Lochhead RY, Hemker WJ, Castaneda JY. Hair care gels. Cosmet Toiletr 102:89–100, 1987.
5. Clarke J, Robbins CR, Reich C. Influence of hair volume and texture on hair body of tresses. J Soc Cosmet Chem 42:341–352, 1991.
6. Rushton DH, Kingsley P, Berry NL, Black S. Treating reduced hair volume in women. Cosmet Toiletr 108:59–62, 1993.
7. Goode ST. Hair pomades. Cosmet Toiletr 94:71–74, 1979.
8. Plewig G, Fulton JE, Kligman AM. Pomade acne. Arch Dermatol 101:580–584, 1970.
9. Balsam MS, Sagarin E. Hair grooming preparations. In Cosmetics: Science and Technology, 2nd ed., Vol. 2. New York: Wiley-Interscience, 1972, pp. 119–123.
10. Wells FV, Lubowe II. Hair grooming aids, Part II. Cutis 22:270–301, 1978.

32

Hair Shampoos

The purpose of shampoo is to cleanse hair. Although this may sound like a simple task, the average woman has 4 to 8 m^2 of hair surface area to clean.[1] Shampoos are intended to remove sebum, sweat components, desquamated stratum corneum, styling products, and environmental dirt that is deposited on the hair.[2] It is very easy to formulate a shampoo that will remove dirt, but studies have shown that consumers do not favor a shampoo that only cleans efficiently. Hair that has had all the sebum removed is dull in appearance, coarse to the touch, subject to static electricity, and difficult to style (Fig. 32-1). Therefore, consumers want a shampoo that will not only clean, but also beautify.

The basic composition of shampoos is listed in Table 32-1. Basically, shampoos function by employing detergents, also known as surfactants, that are both lipophilic (oil-loving) and hydrophilic (water-loving). The lipophilic component adheres to sebum, whereas the hydrophilic component allows water to rinse away the sebum.[3] Most shampoos employ a variety of detergents

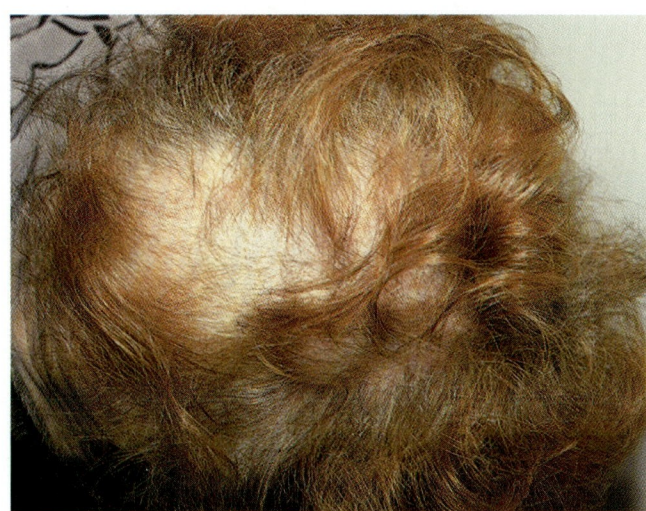

FIGURE 32-1 • Patients with female pattern hair loss require a shampoo that cleanses the hair to remove sebum, thereby reducing hair body, yet also conditions the hair to restore hair shine and eliminate static electricity.

TABLE 32-1 Shampoo Composition

Shampoo Component	Function
Detergents	Anionics, cationics, amphoterics, nonionics and natural surfactants are used to cleanse the hair (see Table 32-2)
Foaming agents	Introduce air bubbles in the shampoo to improve consumer acceptance
Thickeners	Increase the viscosity of the shampoo to improve consumer acceptance
Conditioners	Added to impart manageability, gloss, and antistatic properties to the hair
Sequestering agents	Chelate magnesium and calcium ions to prevent soap scum from forming on the hair shafts
pH adjuster	Acids added adjust the pH from alkaline to neutral to prevent hair shaft swelling
Opacifiers	Create the visual characteristics of the formulation by making it opaque
Fragrance	Mask the undesirable chemical smell of the formulation and leave a pleasant fragrance on the freshly washed hair
Specialty additives	Vitamins, plant extracts, proteins, and the like create consumer interest and support marketing claims

TABLE 32–2 **Shampoo Detergents**

Surfactant Type	Chemical Class	Characteristics
Anionics	Lauryl sulfates, laureth sulfates, sarcosines, sulfosuccinates	Deep cleansing; may leave hair looking harsh
Cationics	Long-chain amino esters, ammonioesters	Poor cleansing; poor lather; impart softness and manageability
Nonionics	Polyoxyethylene fatty alcohols, polyoxyethylene sorbitol esters, alkanolamides	Afford mildest cleansing; impart manageability
Amphoterics	Betaines, sultaines, imidazolinium derivatives	Nonirritating to eyes; mild cleansing, impart manageability
Natural Surfactants	Sarsaparilla, soapwort, soap bark, ivy, agave	Poor cleansing, excellent lather

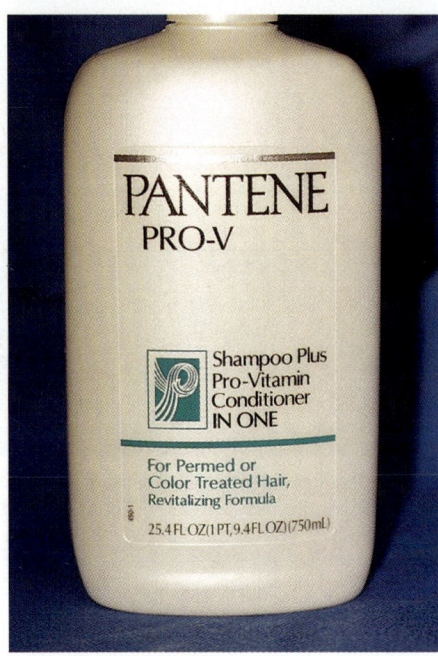

FIGURE 32–2 • Conditioning shampoos are recommended in patients with female pattern hair loss.

to combine both cleansing and conditioning properties (Table 32–2).

The biggest advance in shampoo development has resulted in so-called "2-in-1" shampoos that both cleanse and condition the hair in one step. This technology is made possible through development of silicones that are substantive to the hair shaft and not removed by rinsing. The silicones coat the hair shaft, reducing static electricity, minimizing combing friction, improving manageability, and adding shine (Fig. 32–2). These shampoos are useful in maximizing the appearance of damaged or thinning hair in dermatologic patients.

REFERENCES

1. Bouillon C. Shampoos and hair conditioners. Clin Dermatol 6:83–92, 1988.
2. Robbins CR. Interaction of shampoo and creme rinse ingredients with human hair. In Chemical and Physical Behavior of Human Hair, 2nd ed. New York: Springer-Verlag, 1988, pp. 122–167.
3. Zviak C, Vanlerberghe G. Scalp and hair hygiene. In Zviak C (ed.). The Science of Hair Care. New York: Marcel Dekker, 1986, pp. 49–86.

33

Hair Conditioners

The need for hair conditioners arose following the development of shampoos that so thoroughly removed sebum from the hair shaft that the hair became unmanageable, dull, and harsh to the touch (Figs. 33–1 through 33–3).[1] The role of a conditioner is to mimic sebum by making the hair manageable, glossy, and soft. Conditioners also attempt to recondition hair that has been damaged by chemical or mechanical trauma, such as brushing, blow-drying, shampooing, permanent waving, bleaching, and other procedures.[2] Clearly, because hair is nonliving tissue, any reconditioning that occurs is minimal and temporary until the next shampooing.

Healthy, undamaged hair is shiny, soft, resilient, and easy to disentangle owing to the presence of an intact cuticle (Fig. 33–4).[3] Unfortunately, the trauma

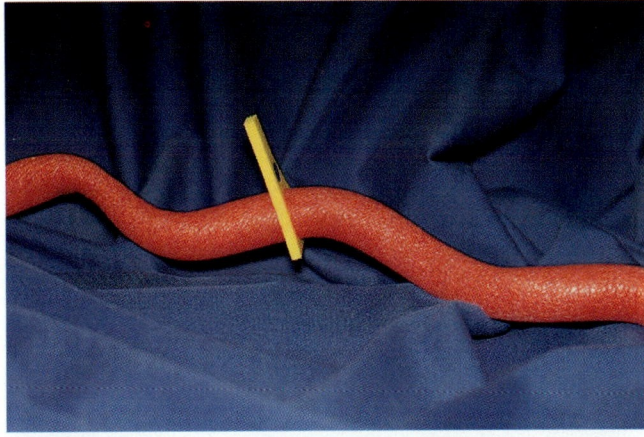

FIGURE 33–2 • Most Caucasians have slightly wavy hair, as illustrated by the red tube. The yellow sebum is not as easily wicked away from the scalp when the hair shaft is curly.

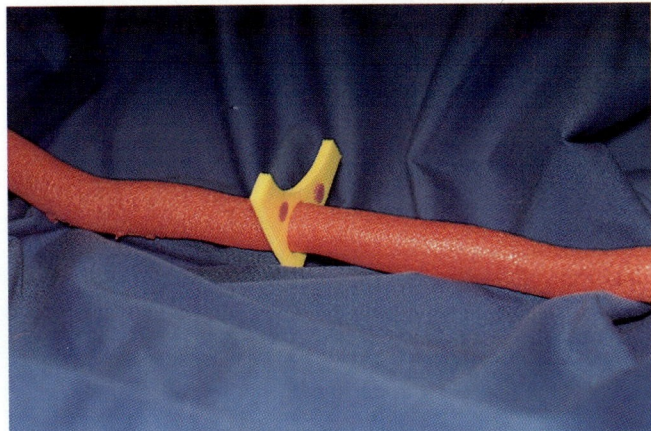

FIGURE 33–1 • The red tube represents the hair shaft, whereas the yellow triangle represents sebum. Straight hair needs less conditioning than curly or kinky hair because the sebum is easily wicked down the hair shaft away from the scalp. This explains the perceived need for frequent shampooing by Oriental individuals. Less conditioning is required with this hair configuration.

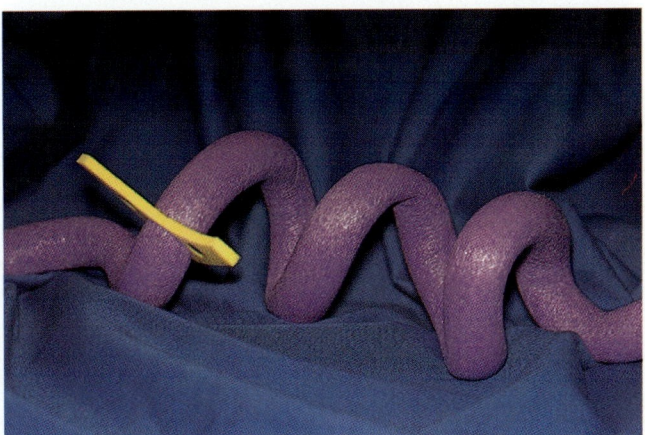

FIGURE 33–3 • Black individuals have tightly kinked hair, as demonstrated by the purple tube. Notice that the yellow triangle, representing sebum, is not as easily wicked from the scalp down the hair shaft. This means that the sebum does not moisturize the distal hair shaft well, thus frequent shampooing is not required. This type of hair shaft requires the use of a conditioner.

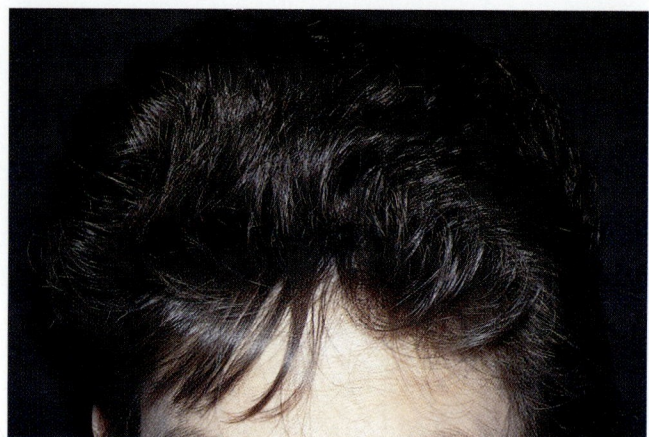

FIGURE 33–4 • Notice the high shine visible on healthy hair, representing an intact cuticle.

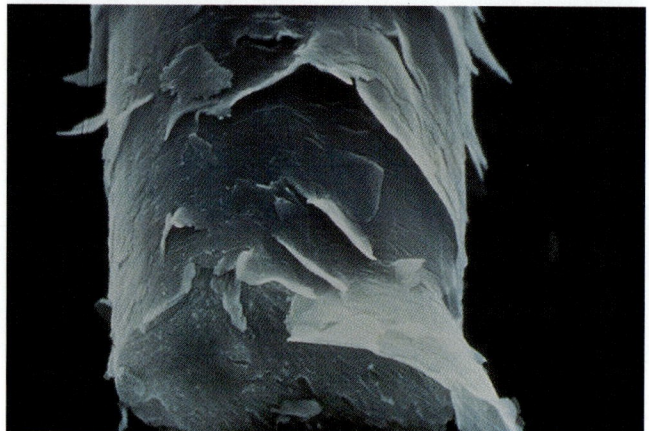

FIGURE 33–5 • A severely weathered cuticle, manifested by absent and lifted cuticular scales, requires the use of a conditioner to restore its cosmetic value.

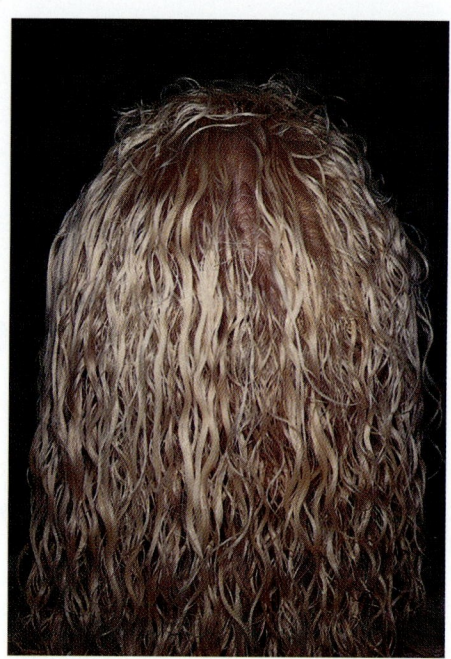

FIGURE 33–6 • Hair that has been bleached and permanently waved has extensive cuticular damage and a dull appearance.

caused by shampooing, drying, combing, brushing, styling, dyeing, and permanent waving damages the hair by disrupting the cuticular scales (Fig. 33–5). This leaves hair that is dull, harsh, brittle, and difficult to disentangle (Fig. 33–6).[4] Hair conditioners are designed to reverse this hair damage by improving sheen, decreasing brittleness, decreasing porosity, increasing strength, and restoring degradation in the polypeptide chain. Conditioners also attempt to mend

TABLE 33–1 Hair Conditioner Formulations

Type	Ingredient(s)	Advantage	Hair Type
Cationic detergent	Quaternary ammonium compounds	Smooths cuticle, decreases static electricity	Chemically processed hair
Film former	Polymers	Fills hair shaft defects, decreases static electricity, adds shine	Dry hair, not fine hair
Protein-containing	Hydrolyzed proteins	Penetrates hair shaft	Temporarily mends split ends

TABLE 33–2 Hair Conditioner Products

Type	Use	Indication
Instant	Applied following shampoo, then rinsed	Minimally damaged hair; aids wet combing
Deep	Applied and left in place for 20 to 30 minutes, then hair is shampooed and rinsed	Chemically damaged hair
Leave-in	Applied to towel-dried hair prior to styling	Prevents hair dryer damage; aids in combing and styling
Rinse	Applied following shampooing, then rinsed	Aids in disentangling hair if creamy rinse; removes soap residue if clear rinse

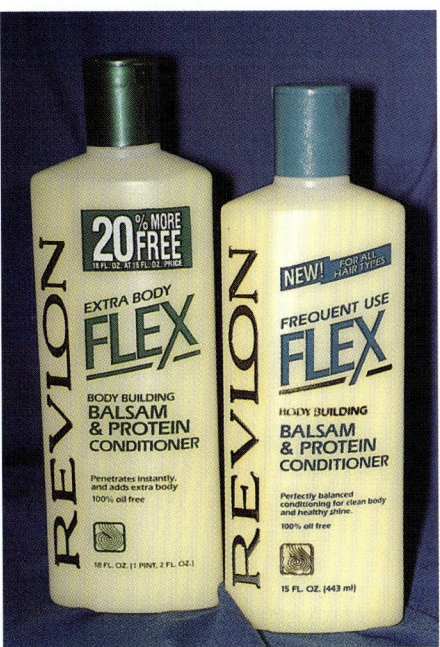

FIGURE 33–7 • Instant protein-containing conditioners that are left on the hair for 5 minutes and rinsed in the shower are excellent for minimally damaged straight hair.

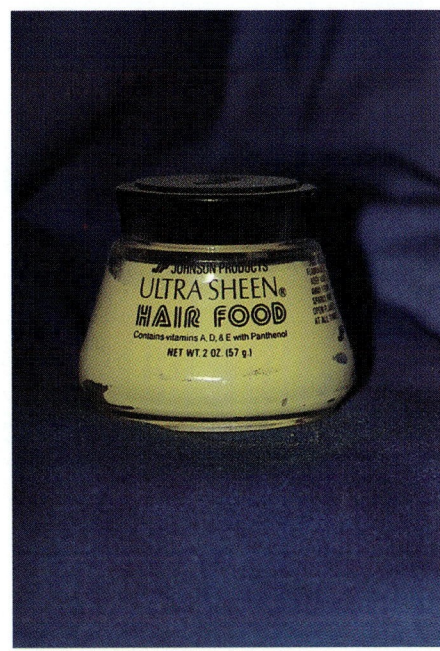

FIGURE 33–9 • Leave-in conditioners, such as pomades, can condition the hair shaft and assist in styling.

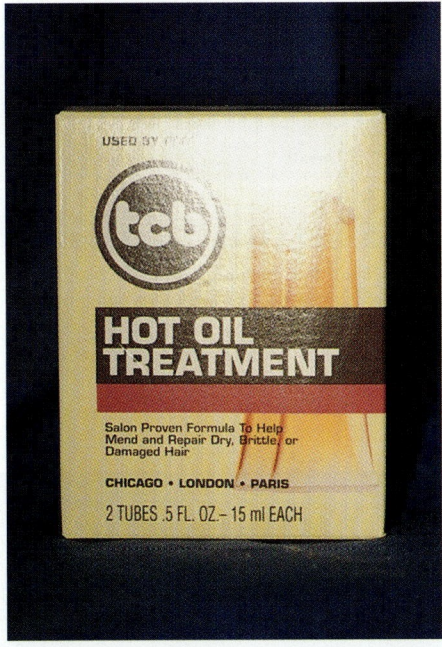

FIGURE 33–8 • Deep conditioners, such as hot oil treatments, are applied to the hair for 30 minutes and removed with shampooing. These products are used by individuals with chemically treated, kinky hair to provide necessary conditioning.

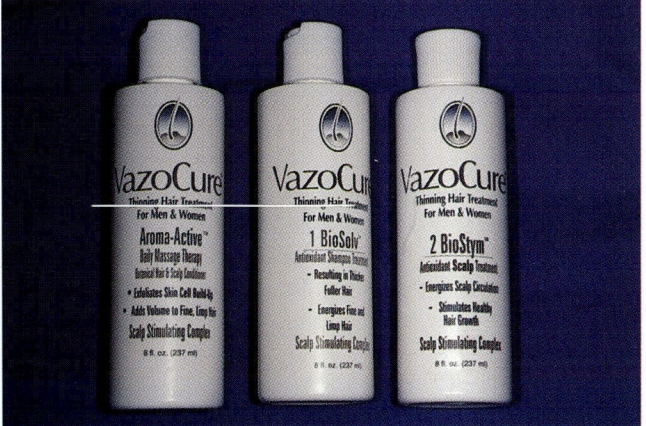

FIGURE 33–10 • Most cosmetic hair growth treatments include a leave-in conditioner, shampoo, and instant conditioner.

the split ends resulting from missing cortex, the structural component responsible for hair shaft strength, by temporarily reapproximating frayed remnants of the remaining medulla and cortex.

The basic conditioner formulations on the market today and their appropriateness for patient use are listed in Table 33–1. Table 33–2 lists the various categories of conditioning products (Figs. 33–7 through 33–10).

REFERENCES

1. Goldemberg RL. Hair conditioners: The rationale for modern formulations. In Frost P, Horwitz SN (eds.). Principles of Cosmetics for the Dermatologist. St. Louis: CV Mosby 1982, pp. 157–159.
2. Swift JA, Brown AC. The critical determination of fine change in the surface architecture of human hair due to cosmetic treatment. J Soc Cosmet Chem 23:675–702, 1972.
3. Garcia ML, Epps JA, Yare RS, Hunter LD. Normal cuticle-wear patterns in human hair. J Soc Cosmet Chem 29:155–175, 1978.
4. Corbett JF. Hair conditioning. Cutis 23:405–413, 1979.

34

Hair Care Techniques for Blacks

The hair of Blacks is identical to Caucasian hair in terms of its amino acid content, but it has a slightly larger diameter, lower water content, and, most importantly, a different cross-sectional shape.[1] Caucasian hair is symmetrical and elliptical on cross section, which allows the hair to be slighty wavy (Fig. 34–1). By contrast, the hair of Blacks is flattened, and elliptical on cross section (Fig. 34–2).[2] It is the asymmetry of this cross section that accounts for the irregular, kinky appearance of the hair. Hair that is straight, such as Oriental hair, appears perfectly round on cross section (Fig. 34–3).

However, the cross-sectional shape of the hair fiber accounts for more than the degree of curl, it also determines the amount of shine and the ability of sebum to coat the hair shaft. This topic is fully discussed in the previous chapter.[3]

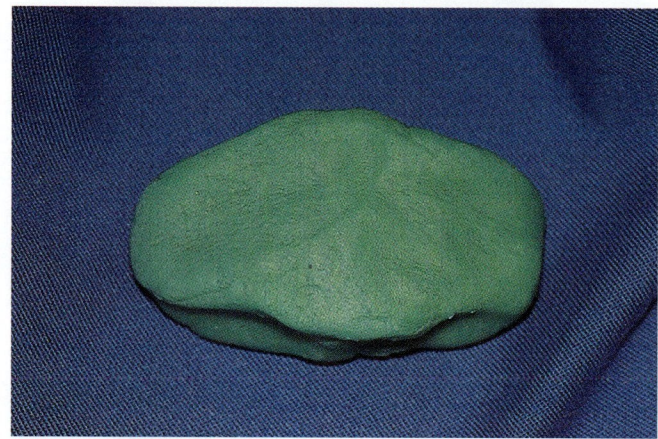

FIGURE 34–2 • Hair that is flattened and elliptical on cross section will be kinky owing to the dramatic assymmetry of the hair shaft.

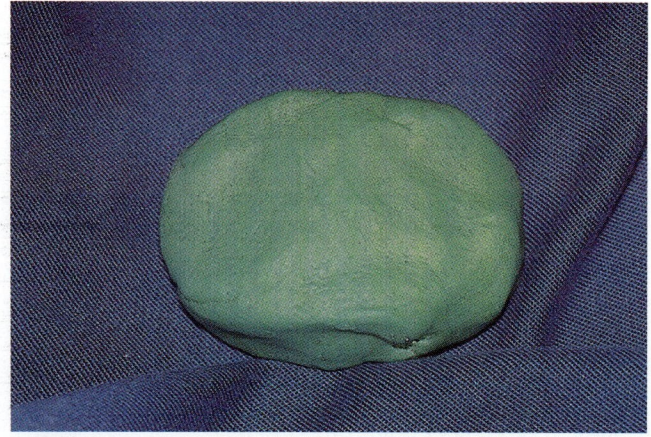

FIGURE 34–1 • Hair that is elliptical on cross section will have a mild curl owing to the slight assymmetry of the hair shaft.

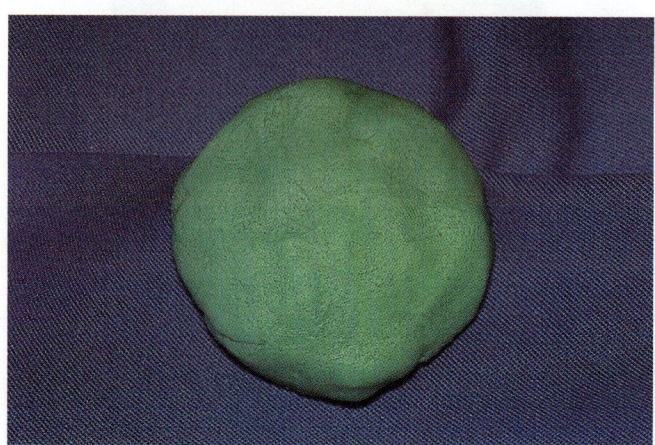

FIGURE 34–3 • Hair that is perfectly circular on cross section will hang straight owing to the symmetry of the hair shaft.

The shape of the hair shaft also determines grooming ease. Straight hair is the easiest to groom because combing friction is low and the hair is easy to arrange in a fashionable style. Kinky hair, on the other hand, demonstrates increased grooming friction, resulting in increased hair shaft breakage. Kinky hair also does not easily conform to a predetermined hairstyle, unless the shafts are short. This creates a predisposition to trichorrhexis nodosa, trichonodosis, and pseudofolliculitis barbae.[4] Therefore, Black hair requires special grooming tools to minimize friction and unique styling to increase manageability.

1. Hair Styling Techniques in Blacks

Several hair styling options available to the black patient are pictorially demonstrated in this chapter.[5] Fashion and personal style dictate the popularity of the techniques.

a. NATURAL STYLES

Black hair cutting techniques are designed to control the tightly kinked hair so it can be arranged into a fashionable hair style (Fig. 34–4).

b. BRAIDED STYLES

Another manner of organizing kinky hair is twisting or braiding. A popular hair style in young Black children

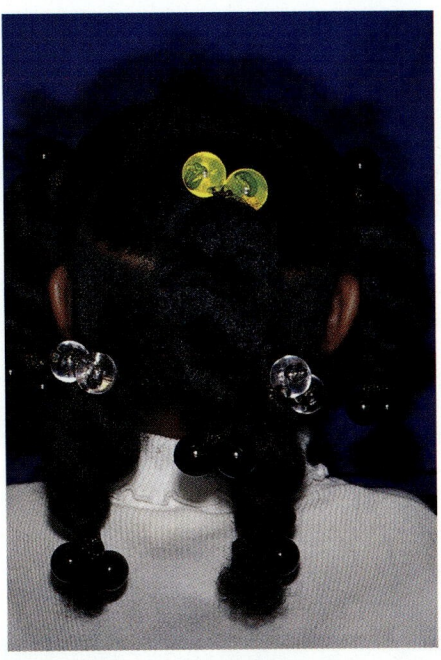

FIGURE 34–5 • This hairstyle is achieved by pulling the hair tightly and twisting the shafts into bundles, which are held together with elastic band clasps.

involves sectioning the hair into quadrants on the top, sides, and posterior scalp. The hair is then gathered in each quadrant and secured with a rubber band or clasp and twisted or braided (Fig. 34–5). This is an easy method of styling the hair that does not require chemical processing. Problems arise if the hair is repeatedly pulled too tightly, resulting in traction alopecia, or if the hair is sectioned in the same location for a prolonged period of time, resulting in increased localized hair breakage (Fig. 34–6).[6]

Braiding of scalp hairs may also be accomplished by a technique known as "cornrowing." The hair is

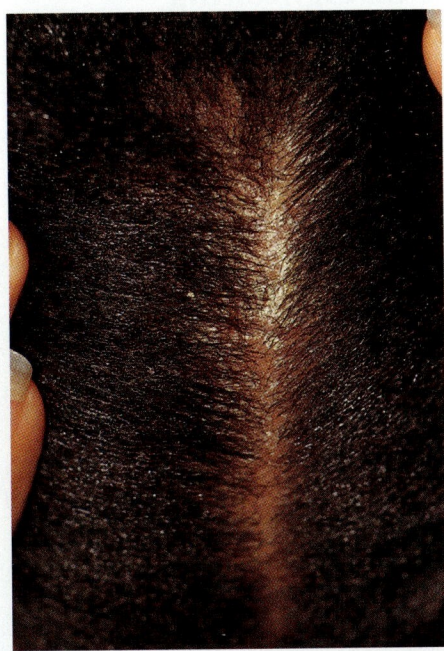

FIGURE 34–4 • An example of unprocessed kinky hair.

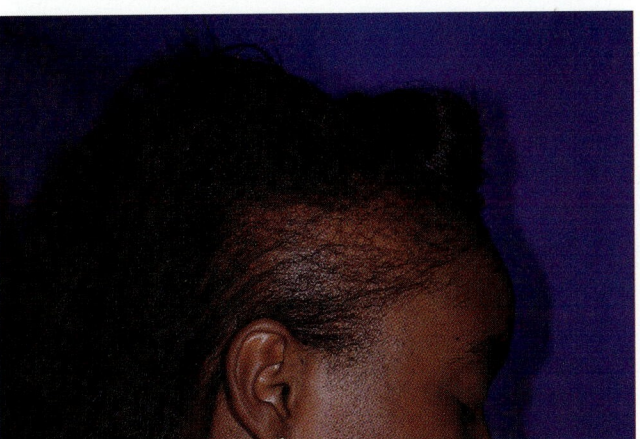

FIGURE 34–6 • Traction alopecia is a common side effect of hairstyles such as those demonstrated in Figure 34–5.

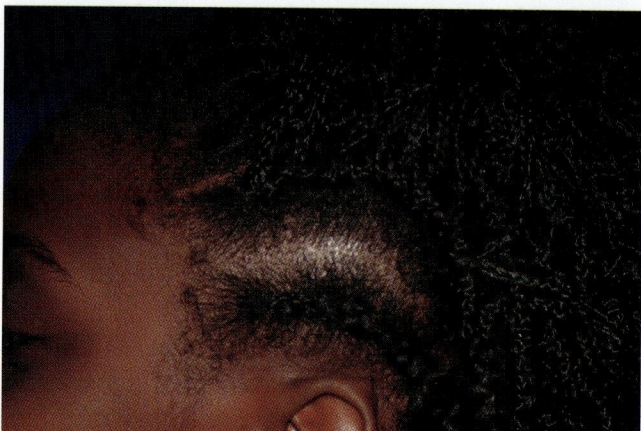

FIGURE 34–7 • Braiding on the scalp, also known as cornrowing, may contribute to traction alopecia if the hair is pulled too tightly.

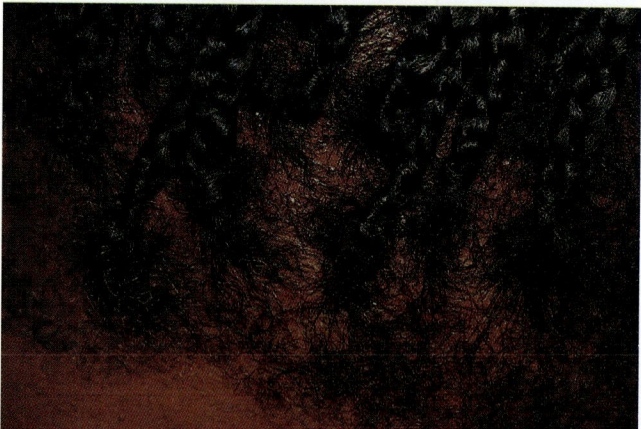

FIGURE 34–8 • Hair extensions are synthetic or natural hair fibers that are braided into cornrows on the scalp and are designed to create the illusion of long hair.

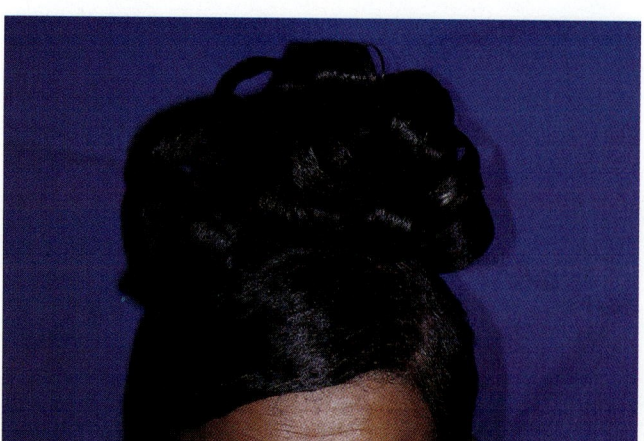

FIGURE 34–9 • Synthetic, precurled hair can be used to create the illusion of a large curled bun on top of the head in a woman with short hair.

pulled tightly to form continuous braids on the scalp in various patterns (Fig. 34–7). Beads or other jewels can be woven into the hairstyle if desired. Usually, the hairstyle is worn for 2 to 4 weeks and then undone and rebraided. This continuous tension on the hair shaft can result in traction alopecia, especially at the temples.[7–10] Even though the hair is shampooed with the braids in place, thorough cleansing of the scalp is not possible, and seborrheic dermatitis may occur.

c. HAIR ADDITIONS

The hair addition techniques most popular among Black patients are hair extensions and hair lacing. Hair extensions are natural or synthetic hair fibers braided along with the patient's natural hair, initially on the scalp and then off the scalp (Fig. 34–8). The extensions create the illusion of long, braided hair and can be woven in many patterns and adorned with beads or jewels (Fig. 34–9). The hairstyle remains in place for 2 to 8 weeks and is shampooed, but requires minimal grooming. Traction alopecia and seborrheic dermatitis may result.[11]

Another related technique is hair lacing. Hair lacing involves braiding the patient's natural hair with synthetic or natural hair fibers, except the braids are stopped 1 to 2 inches from the scalp and the added hair is allowed to flow freely (Fig. 34–10). The hair can then be styled as desired. Since it is difficult for the Black patient with tightly kinked hair to grow long hair owing to hair breakage, hair lacing is popular.

2. Hair Straightening Techniques

Kinky hair can be straightened and styled using heat or chemical techniques. Heat-induced straightening

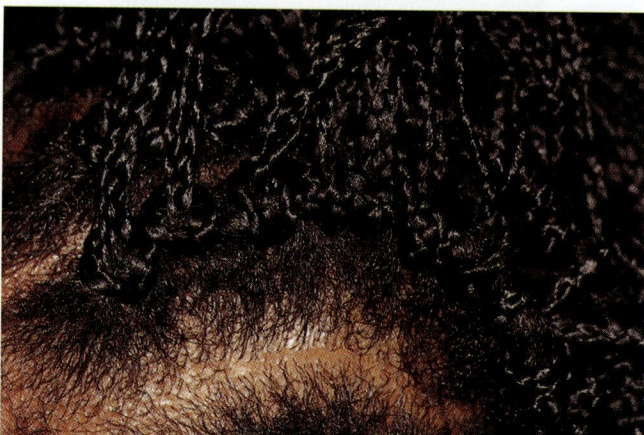

FIGURE 34–10 • Hair lacing, using synthetic hair, can create the appearance of hair fullnesss and length.

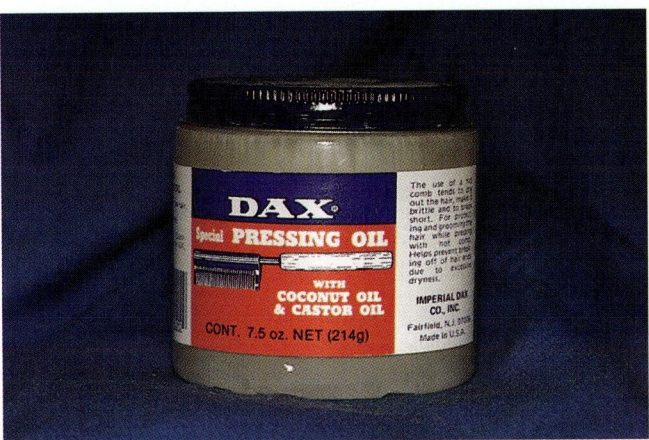

FIGURE 34–11 • Pressing oil is used to enhance heat transfer from the Marcel rod or hot hair iron to the hair.

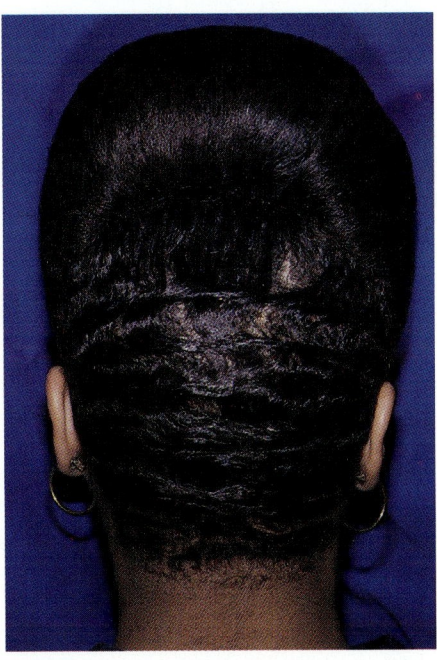

FIGURE 34–13 • This patient has a Marcel rod hairstyle on the back of the scalp, and has used hair extensions and a hair form to create the large bun on the top of the head.

techniques, including hot combing, hair pressing, and use of the Marcel rod,[12] employ metal combs, plates, or rods that are heated to a minimum of 300° F and placed in contact with the hair (Figs. 34–11 through 34–13). This breaks the water-reformable bonds and allows the hair to be rearranged structurally. The change is temporary, however, as moisture from perspiration, humidity, or shampooing allows the bonds to reform, and the hair returns to its natural kinky state.[13] A scarring alopecia, known as hot comb alopecia, is seen in some patients who use this hair styling technique (Fig. 34–14). There is some controversy as to whether the scarring is attributable to scalp heat damage or the idiopathic follicular degeneration syndrome.[14]

Chemical hair straightening, also known as hair relaxing or lanthionization, uses substances to break disulfide bonds in the hair shaft (Fig. 34–15). The technique is detailed in Table 34–1. The key to successful hair relaxing is an experienced beautician who can quickly apply and remove the chemicals and determine when the desired degree of disulfide bond

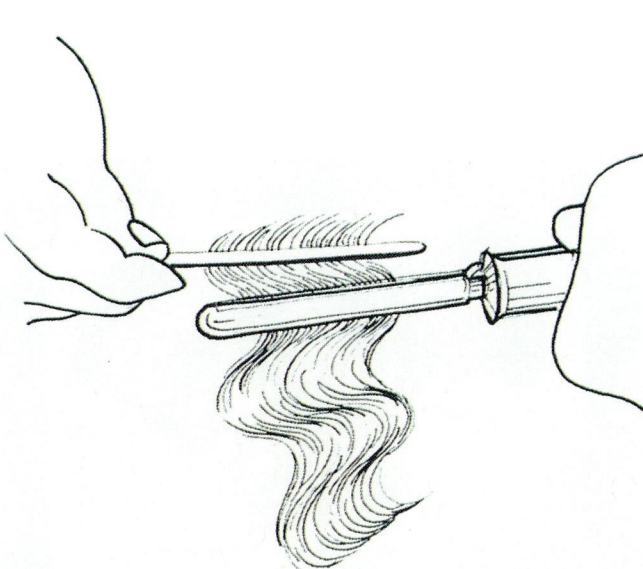

FIGURE 34–12 • "Marceling" involves waving the hair with a comb and a heated rod.

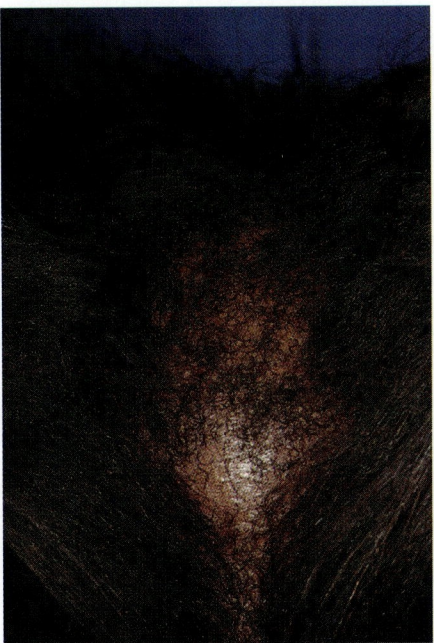

FIGURE 34–14 • Hot comb alopecia may be a follicular degenerative disease unrelated to the use of a hot comb for hairstyling.

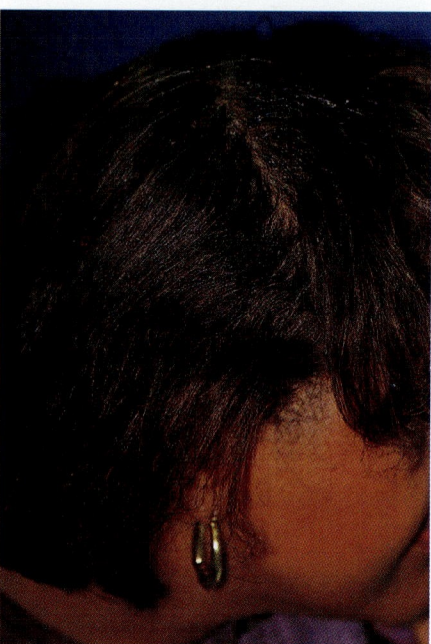

FIGURE 34–15 • Chemical hair straightening allows increased manageability and more styling options for kinky hair.

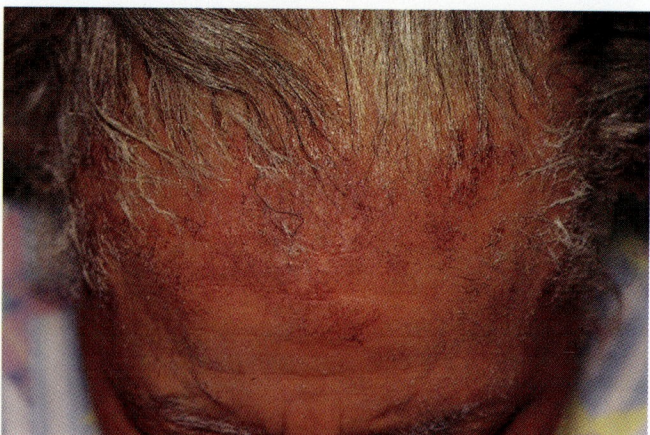

FIGURE 34–16 • Irritant contact dermatitis can occur if the chemical hair straightener is allowed to remain in contact with the scalp for a prolonged period of time.

breaking has occurred. It is estimated that virgin hair loses about 30% of its tensile strength following a properly performed chemical straightening procedure.

Chemical relaxing can be accomplished with lye-based, lye-free, ammonium thioglycolate, or bisulfite creams.[15] Lye-based (or up to 3.5% sodium hydroxide) straighteners are alkaline creams with a pH of 13. They convert one third of the hair cystine content to lanthionine, along with minor hydrolysis of the peptide bonds (Fig. 34–16).[16] Guanidine hydroxide and lithium hydroxide are known as "no-lye" chemical hair straighteners. These relaxing kits contain 4% to 7% cream calcium hydroxide and liquid guanidine car-

bonate. The guanidine carbonate activator is mixed into the calcium hydroxide cream to produce calcium carbonate and guanidine hydroxide (Fig. 34–17).

Kinky hair that has been overexposed to chemical straighteners can become brittle, and is likely to fracture with only minimal combing trauma, usually at the scalp. The dermatologist may encounter patients who report that they are losing their hair following an aggressive straightening procedure (Fig. 34–18). Hair breakage can be verified by noting that the lost hairs do not include the hair bulb. Unfortunately, if the hair has been appropriately neutralized, there is nothing that can be done to repair the damaged disulfide bonds. The brittle hair must be trimmed, and overprocessing of the new growth should be avoided. Hair breakage can be minimized by combing or styling the hair as little as possible, applying moisturizing conditioning agents, and avoiding any further chemical treatments, such as permanent hair dyeing or bleaching.[17]

TABLE 34–1 Chemical Hair Straightening Procedure

• • • • • •

1. Do not shampoo the hair for several days to allow sebum to coat the scalp.
2. Coat the scalp with petroleum jelly to minimize scalp irritation.
3. Section the hair into quadrants.
4. Apply the chemical from hair root to end, beginning at the nape of the neck and moving forward to the anterior hairline. For previously treated hair, apply the chemical to new growth only.
5. Allow the chemical to remain in contact with the hair for 10 to no more than 30 minutes while gently combing the hair straight.
6. Rinse hair with water.
7. Apply neutralizer while smoothing straight hair.
8. Shampoo straightened hair with a nonalkaline shampoo; then condition and style hair.

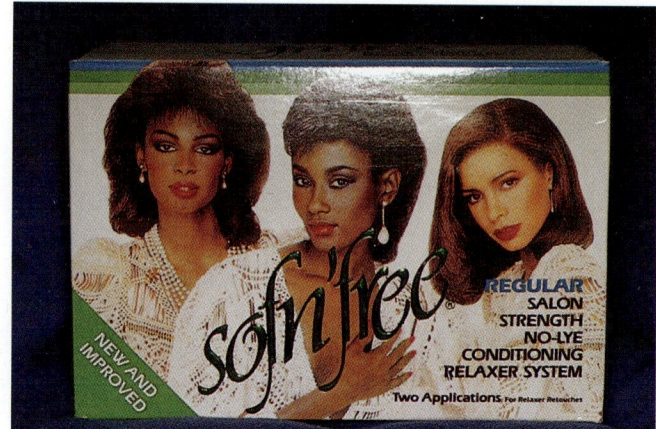

FIGURE 34–17 • No-lye hair straighteners are not necessarily less damaging to the hair than their lye-based counterparts.

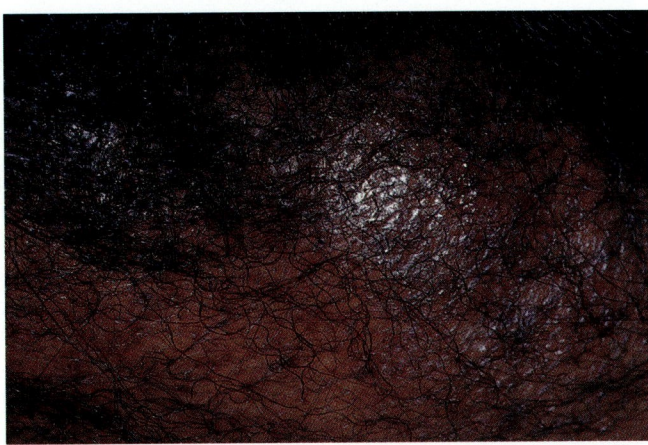

FIGURE 34–18 • Hair breakage is the most common side effect of chemical hair straightening owing to weakening of the hair shaft protein structure.

REFERENCES

1. Brooks G, Lewis A. Treatment regimens for styled black hair. Cosmet Toiletr 98:59–68, 1983.
2. Lindelof B, Forslind B, Hedblad M, et al. Human hair form: Morphology revealed by light and scanning electron microscopy and computer-aided three-dimensional reconstruction. Arch Dermatol 124:1359–1363, 1988.
3. Johnson BA. Requirements in cosmetics for black skin. Dermatol Clin 6:409–492, 1988.
4. Dawber RPR. Knotting of scalp hair. Br J Dermatol 91:169–173, 1974.
5. Vaughan-Richards A. Black and Beautiful. Published in association with Johnson Products Co., Collins Publishing, 1986, pp. 81–101.
6. Rollins TG. Traction folliculitis with hair casts and alopecia. Am J Dis Child 101:639–640, 1961.
7. Scott DA. Disorders of the hair and scalp in blacks. Dermatol Clin 6:387–395, 1988.
8. Rudolph RI, Klein AW, Decherd JW. Corn-row alopecia. Arch Dermatol 108:134, 1973.
9. Morgan HV. Traction alopecia. Br Med J 1:115–117, 1960.
10. Slepyan AH. Traction alopecia. Arch Dermatol 78:395–398, 1958.
11. Harman RRM. Traction alopecia due to hair extension. Br J Dermatol 87:79–80, 1972.
12. Syed AN. Ethnic hair care. Cosmet Toiletr 108:99–107, 1993.
13. Grimes PE, Davis LT. Cosmetics in blacks. Dermatol Clin 9:53–68, 1991.
14. Sperling LC, Sau P. The follicular degeneration syndrome in black patients. Arch Dermatol 128:68–74, 1992.
15. Cannell DW. Permanent waving and hair straightening. Clinics in Dermatol 6:71–82, 1988.
16. Hsuing DY. Hair straightening in The Chemistry and Manufacture of Cosmetics, MG deNavarre ed, 2nd ed.
17. Burmeister F, Bollatti D, Brooks G. Ethnic hair: Moisturizing after relaxer use. Cosmet Toiletr 106:49–51, July 1991.

PART

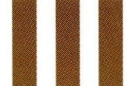

NAIL CARE

PART

III

35

Nail Manicuring Techniques

The main goal of a manicure should be proper trimming of the nails to maintain a strong, healthy nail plate. However, nail appearance seems to dominate current salon manicuring practices. The first step in a salon manicure is to soak the nails in a mild detergent solution (Fig. 35–1). This softens the cuticle and the nail plate and cleanses the nails. Following soaking, the nails are dried and the cuticle is pushed back from the nail plate and trimmed (Figs. 35–2 through 35–4). This is the most problematic part of salon grooming. It is the removal of the cuticle that creates an entry portal for water and other substances into the proximal nail fold, allowing the secondary growth of yeast, superficial fungi, and bacteria (Fig. 35–5). Aggressive removal of the cuticle also contributes to nail plate pitting and horizontal lines in the nail plate (Fig. 35–6). The patient may not correlate the nail dystro-

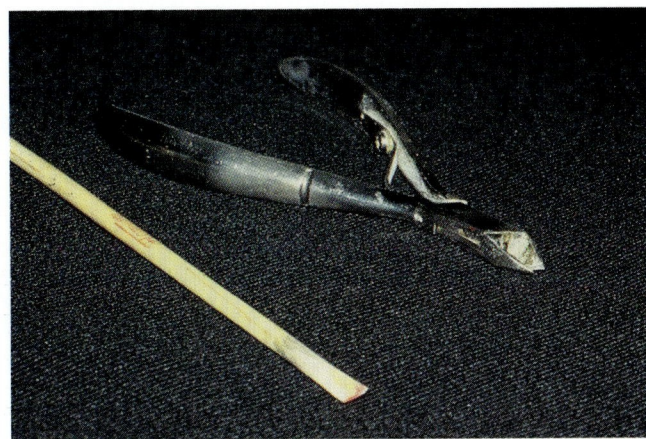

FIGURE 35–2 • Tools to groom the cuticle include a wooden stick to push back the cuticle to the proximal nail fold and cuticle scissors to remove any loose tissue.

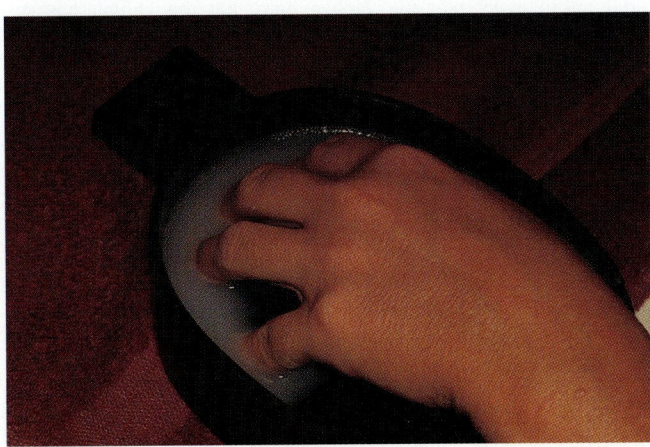

FIGURE 35–1 • The manicuring procedure is begun by soaking nails in a mild detergent for 10 to 15 minutes.

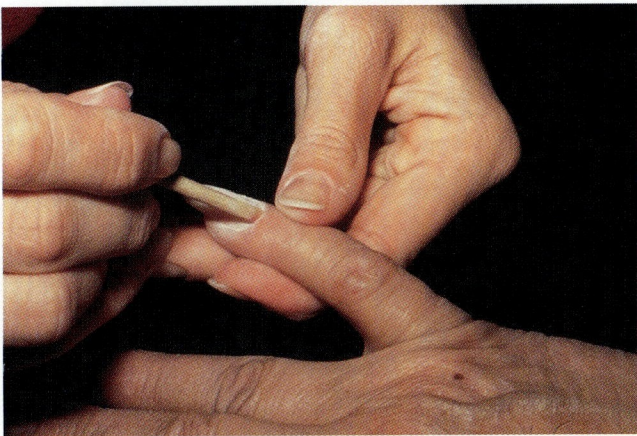

FIGURE 35–3 • Pushing back the cuticle forcefully with a wooden stick can easily damage the nail matrix, resulting in nail dystrophy. The latter becomes apparent about 1 to 3 months after the injury, depending on the rate of nail growth. This wooden instrument cannot be sterilized adequately between clients and, therefore, should be discarded.

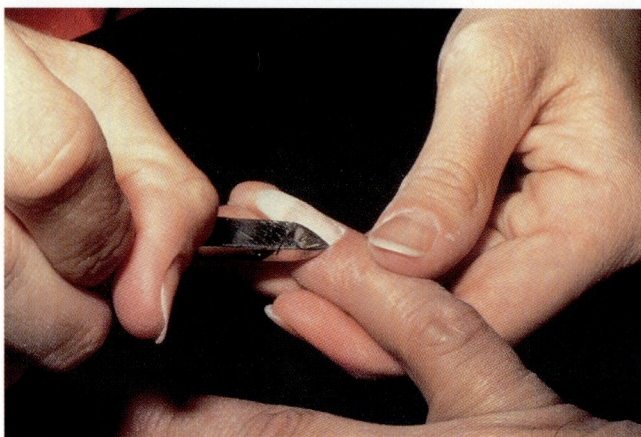

FIGURE 35–4 • Cuticle scissors remove any excess or loose cuticle, but can become easily contaminated with blood or other infectious agents.

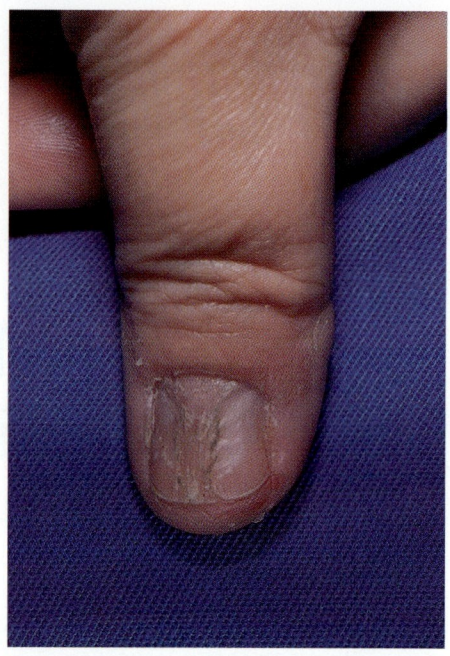

FIGURE 35–6 • Aggressive removal of the cuticle can cause severe, permanent nail trauma.

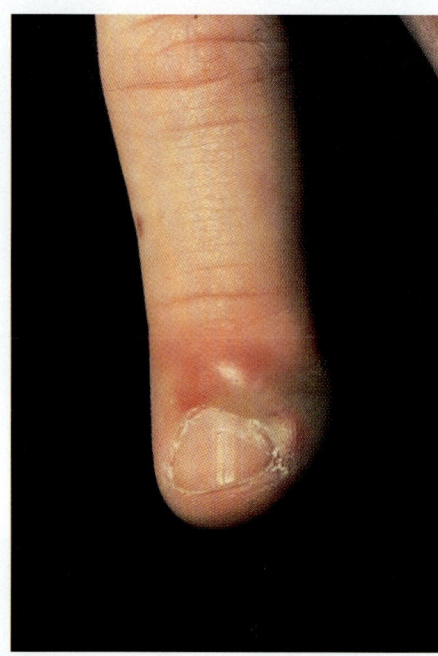

FIGURE 35–5 • Bacterial paronychia may be caused by contaminated cuticle scissors.

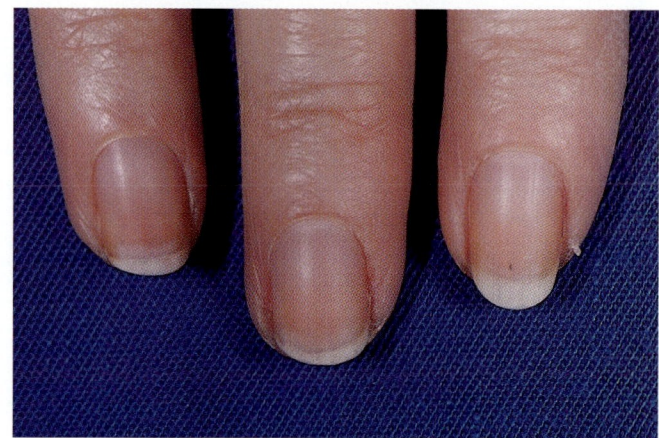

FIGURE 35–7 • A pleasant curve to the distal nail plate is considered aesthetically pleasing. Notice here that the patient has sustained splinter hemmorhages secondary to aggressive use of a pointed nail file to remove subungual debris.

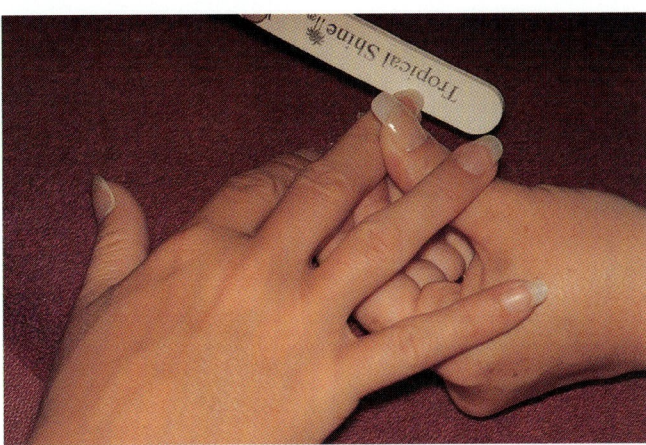

FIGURE 35–8 • Nail files may be used to groom the free edge of the nail plate, as well as to smooth contour irregularities on the nail surface.

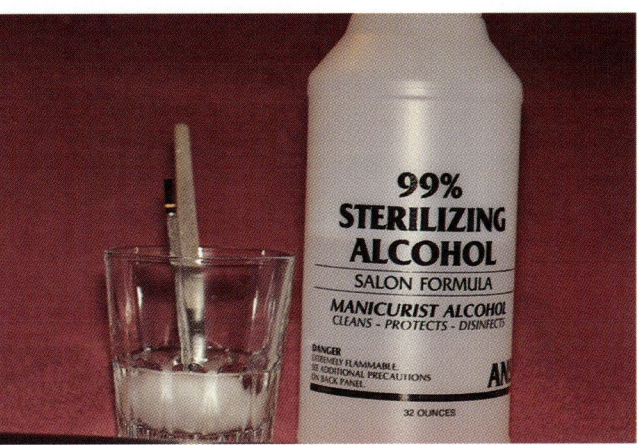

FIGURE 35–9 • The typical technique used by nail sculpture artists to sterilize manicuring instruments between clients is soaking in alcohol.

phy with the manicure procedure, since the nail damage may not be apparent for 3 to 4 weeks.

The next manicuring step is the shaping of the nail plate.[1] The nail should be rounded at the tip for aesthetics, but the corners should be left square to maximize strength (Fig. 35–7). Too sharp an arc extending from the lateral to medial nail margin will weaken the nail structurally. Most manicurists prefer to file the nail to shape, as cutting can fracture the nail plate.[1] The surface of the nail may also be filed to smooth imperfections (Fig. 35–8).

The instruments used by the nail manicure artist must be sterilized between customers to prevent the spread of viral, bacterial, yeast, and fungal infections. Most manicurists soak their instruments in 99% sterilizing alcohol between clients; however, if the salon is busy, insufficient time may have elapsed for complete sterilization (Fig. 35–9). A better solution is to autoclave the instruments, or have customers purchase and bring their own equipment to the nail salon.

REFERENCE

1. Engasser PG, Matsunaga J. Nail cosmetics. In Scher RK, Daniel CR (eds.). Nails: Therapy, Diagnosis, Surgery. Philadelphia: WB Saunders, 1990, pp. 214–215.

36

Nail Cosmetics

Nail cosmetics include nail polish, nail hardener, and nail polish remover (Table 36–1). Nail cosmetics can also be artistically applied to achieve nail camouflage, a technique known as a French manicure.

1. Nail Polish

The most popular nail cosmetic is nail polish. Nail polishes are available in a wide variety of colors (Fig. 36–1), but the basic formulation is as given in Table 36–2.[1]

A professional nail enamel application requires three layers of polish: a base coat, a pigmented nail enamel, and a top coat (Fig. 36–2). The base coat ensures good adhesion to the nail plate and prevents chipping of the polish. It contains no pigment, reduced primary film-former, and more secondary film-former resin, and is of a lower viscosity, as a thinner film is desirable. The second layer is the actual pigmented nail enamel. The top coat, or third layer, provides gloss and resistance to chipping. It contains increased amounts of primary film-former, more plasticizer, and less secondary film-forming resins. Some top coats may contain sunscreens but do not contain pigment. Sometimes, ultraviolet (UV) radiation is used to speed drying of nail polish, a possible source of photo-onycholysis (Fig. 36–3).

Generally, nail polishes are not the source of dermatologic problems; rarely, however, adverse reactions can occur. The first resin developed for nail polish was toluene-sulfonamide-formaldehyde. Some individuals are sensitive to this substance (Fig. 36–4), which is found on the standard dermatology patch test tray. The resin has been eliminated in some hypoallergenic nail enamels. A polyester resin or cellulose acetate butyrate is employed instead, but sensitivity is still possible and the enamel is less resistant to

TABLE 36–1 Nail Cosmetics

Nail Cosmetic	Main Ingredients	Function	Adverse Reactions
Nail polish	Nitrocellulose, toluene-sulfonamide resin, plasticizers, solvents, and colorants	Adds color and shine to nail plates	Allergic contact dermatitis to toluene-sulfonamide resin; nail plate staining
Nail hardener	Formaldehyde, acetates, acrylics, or other resins	Increases nail strength and prevents breakage	Allergic contact dermatitis to formaldehyde
Nail enamel remover	Acetone, alcohol, ethyl acetate, or butyl acetate	Removes nail polish	Irritant contact dermatitis
Cuticle remover	Sodium or potassium hydroxide	Destroys the keratin that forms excess cuticular tissue on the nail plate	Irritant contact dermatitis
Nail white	White pigments	Whitens free nail edge	Practically none
Nail bleach	Hydrogen peroxide	Removes nail plate stains	Irritant contact dermatitis
Nail polish drier	Vegetable oils, alcohols, or silicone derivatives	Speeds drying time of nail polish	Practically none
Nail buffing cream	Pumice, talc or kaolin	Smooths ridges in nails	Practically none
Nail moisturizer	Occlusives, humectants, lactic acid	Increases water content of nails	Practically none

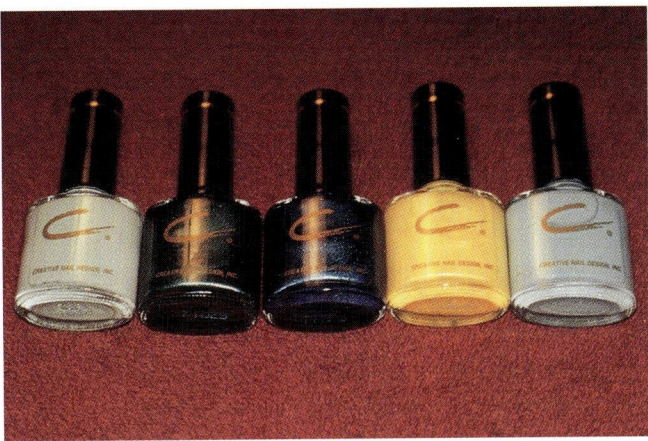

FIGURE 36–1 • Tremendous variety is available in nail polish color, although the basic formulation is the same.

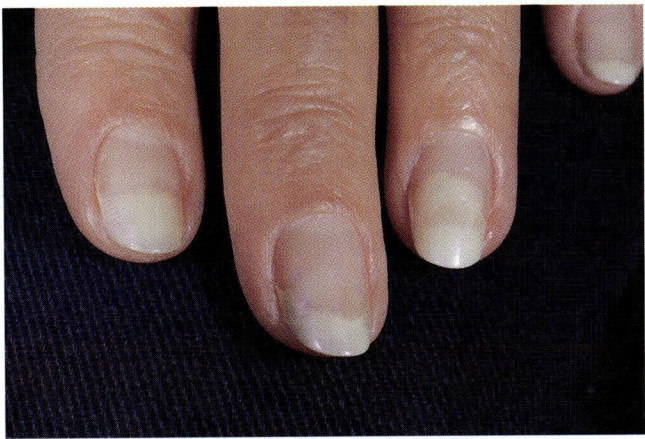

FIGURE 36–3 • Nail polish dryers using ultraviolet radiation are possible sources of photo-onycholysis in the patient with acne taking tetracycline.

TABLE 36–2   Nail Polish Formulation

Function in Nail Polish	Example Ingredients
Primary film-former	Nitrocellulose, methacrylate polymers, vinyl polymers
Secondary film-forming resin	Formaldehyde, p-toluene sulfonamide, polyamide, acrylate, alkyd and vinyl resins
Plasticizers	Dibutyl phthalate, dioctyl phthalate, tricresyl phosphate, camphor dibutyl phthalate, dioctyl phthalate, tricresyl phosphate, camphor
Solvents and diluents	Acetates, ketones, toluene, xylene, alcohols
Colorants	Organic D&C pigments, inorganic pigments
Specialty fillers	Quanine fish scale or titanium dioxide–coated mica flakes, or bismuth oxychloride for iridescence

wear.[2] The North American Contact Dermatitis Group determined that 4% of positive patch tests were attributable to toluene–sulfonamide–formaldehyde resin.[3] Even though the allergic reaction is most commonly due to wet nail enamel, Tosti et al. found that 11 of 59 patients who were test positive to wet polish by patch test, also reacted to the dried enamel.[4] The specifics of patch testing nail polishes is presented in Table 36–3.

Nail staining is another, more common, adverse reaction that can also occur with dissolved rather than suspended pigments. It is most common in deep red nail polishes containing D&C Reds No. 6, 7, 34, or 5 Lake (Fig. 36–5).[5] The nail plate will be stained yellow after 7 days of continuous wear (Fig. 36–6). The staining will fade without treatment in approximately 14 days, once the enamel has been removed. Scraping of the nail plate with a scalpel blade may help to confirm that only the nail surface has been stained, an important distinction in nail pigmentation abnormalities.[6]

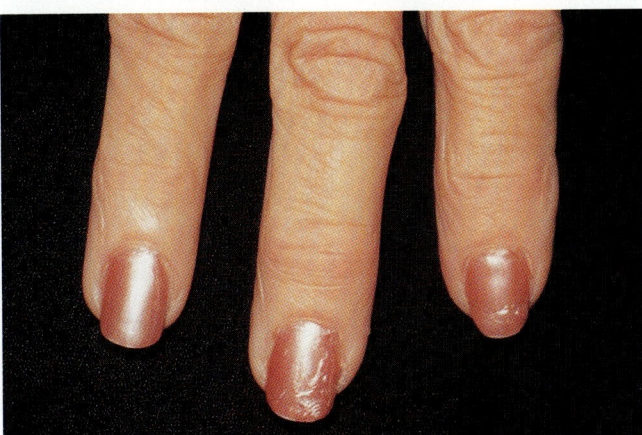

FIGURE 36–2 • Drying time is prolonged with application of several coats of nail polish. The polish can dent with pressure if the coat is not completely dry.

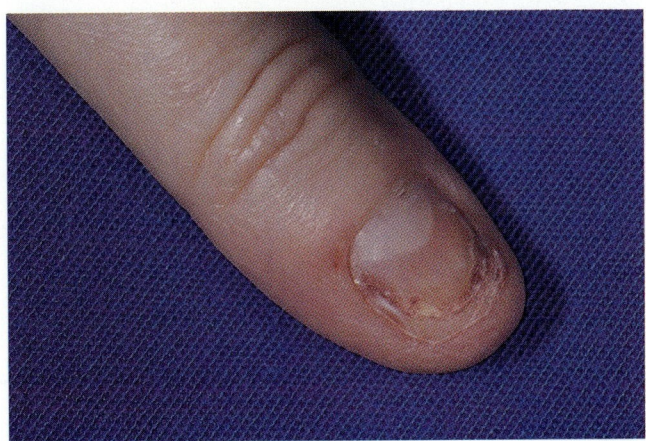

FIGURE 36–4 • An allergic reaction to nail polish can cause circumferential swelling and pain around the nail plate.

TABLE 36–3 Nail Cosmetic Patch Testing Guidelines

Nail Cosmetic	Allergen	Patch Testing Guidelines	Special Precautions
Nail polish	Toluene–sulfonamide–formaldehyde resin	Patch test as is, or in 10% petrolatum	Allow to dry thoroughly prior to closed patch testing
Hypoallergenic nail polish	Polyester resin or cellulose acetate butyrate	Patch test as is, or in 10% petrolatum	Allow to dry thoroughly prior to closed patch testing
Nail hardener	Formaldehyde and/or toluene–sulfonamide–formaldehyde resin	Patch test as is, or in 10% petrolatum	Allow to dry thoroughly prior to closed patch testing
Nail polish remover	Irritant reactions (primarily)	Patch test as 10% in olive oil	Open patch test only

There is some concern among manicurists that nail polish can contribute to nail dryness and brittleness. This actually is not the case. Nail polish prevents contact of detergents with the nail, thus acting as a protectant. Furthermore, it decreases nail water vapor loss from 1.6 to 0.4 mg/cm/hour[2].[7] This is important, as water is the plasticizer of the nail, providing for flexibility and preventing nail plate fracture and onychoschizia (Fig. 36–7).

2. Nail Hardener

Nail hardeners are sometimes used by manicurists to increase the strength of brittle nails, thus allowing the nails to reach longer lengths before traumatic breakage occurs (Fig. 36–8). The cause of brittle nails is thought to be dehydration of the nail plate, largely due to excessive contact with detergents and water. Some of the dehydration can be prevented by protecting the nail plate and applying lactic acid moisturizers designed to increase the water holding capacity of the nail plate.

Nail hardeners can be formulated with a variety of additives. Free formaldehyde in concentrations of 1% to 2% may be used, but acetates, toluene, nitrocellulose, acrylic, and polyamide resins are commonly incorporated to reinforce the nail plate structurally. Some products actually contain 1% nylon fibers and are known as "fibered nail hardeners." Other additives purported to strengthen the nail include hydrolyzed proteins, modified vegetable extracts, glycerin, propylene glycol, metal salts, and others.[8]

3. Nail Polish Remover

Following the application of numerous coats of nail hardener and nail enamels, it is necessary to remove the cosmetics from the nail plate. This is done with nail polish remover, which may contain solvents, such as acetone, alcohol, ethyl acetate, or butyl acetate. The solvents can be dehydrating to the nail plate, so conditioning agents, such as cetyl alcohol, cetyl palmi-

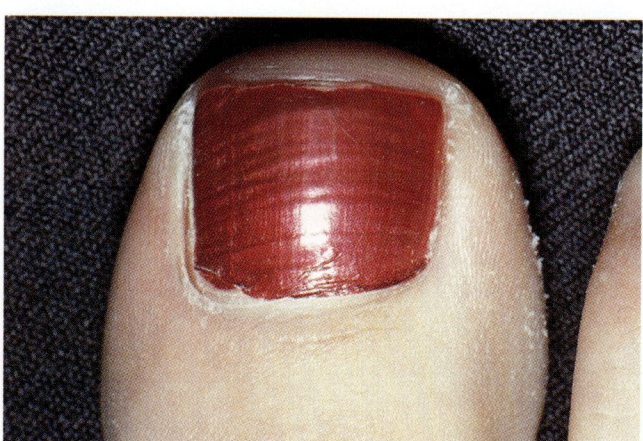

FIGURE 36–5 • Deep burgundy nail polish can cause temporary yellowish staining of the nail plate.

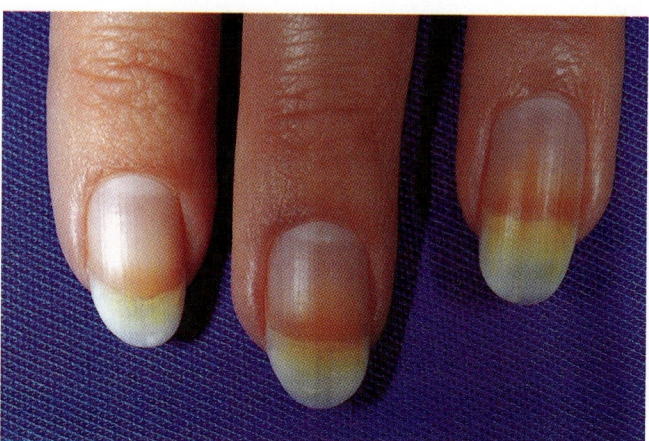

FIGURE 36–6 • Yellow staining can be separated from true nail disease by scraping off the surface of the nail plate with a No. 15 blade to reveal normal-colored nail beneath.

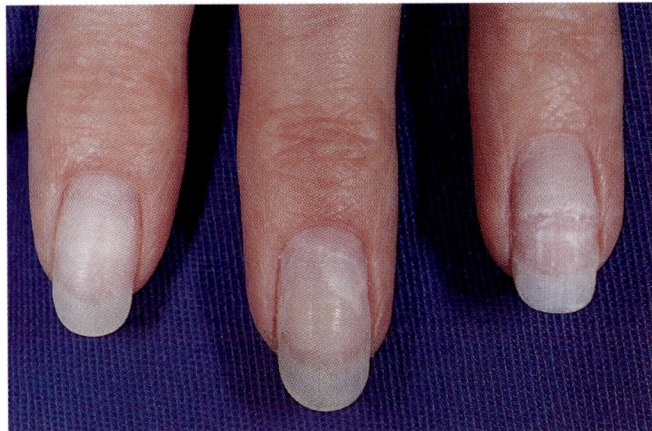

FIGURE 36–7 • Onychoschizia, or lamellar layering of the nail plate, results from nail dryness.

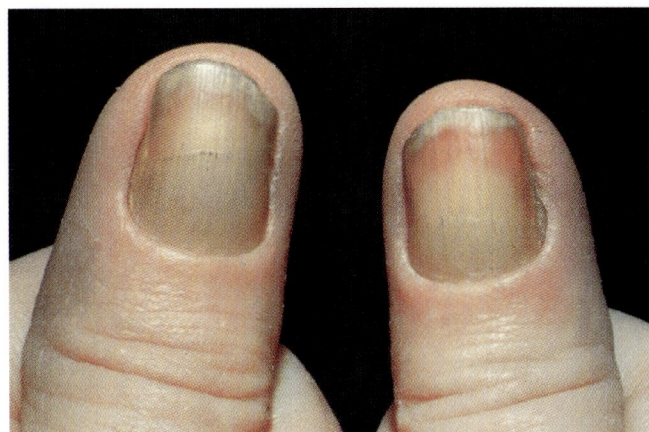

FIGURE 36–10 • Nail discoloration can easily be camouflaged with a French manicure.

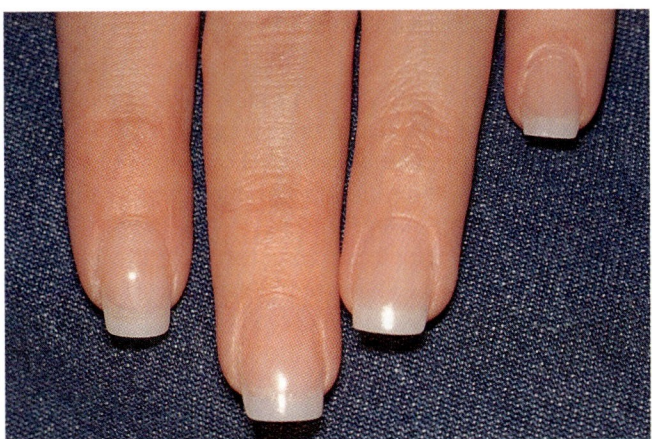

FIGURE 36–8 • Some patients believe that nail hardeners are helpful in achieving long nail plates, which are considered cosmetically desirable.

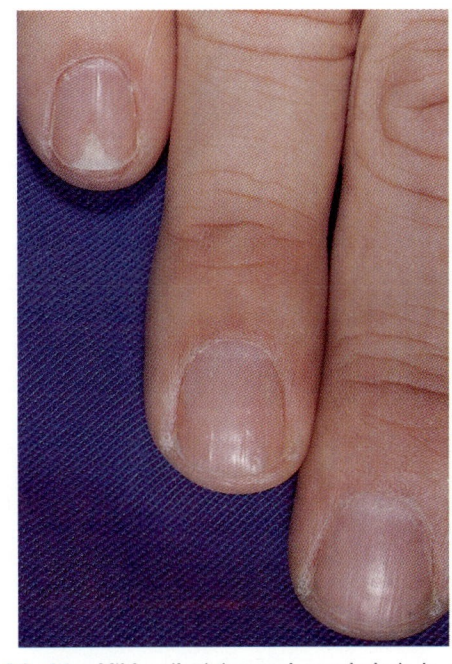

FIGURE 36–11 • Mild nail pitting and onycholysis in this patient with psoriasis can be camouflaged with a French manicure.

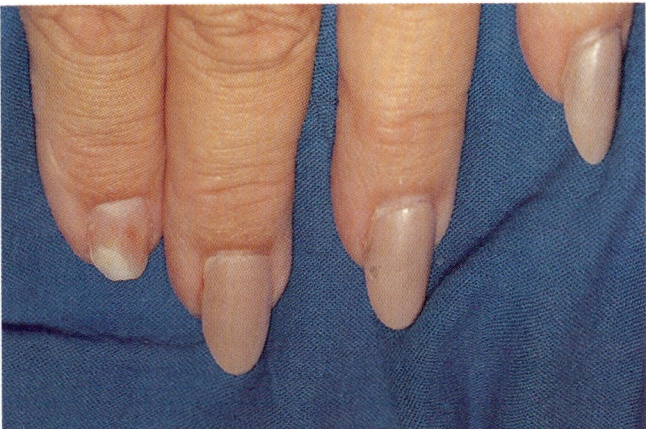

FIGURE 36–9 • Acetone is used to remove nail polish and artificial nails. This patient has soaked the artificial nail in acetone for an insufficient amount of time to break the methacrylate polymer bond. Onycholysis is evident from traumatic removal of the prosthesis.

tate, lanolin, castor oil, or other synthetic oils, are generally added. It is thought that these oily substances act as occlusive nail moisturizers, retarding water evaporation.

Nail enamel remover is applied to a tissue or cotton ball and wiped across the nail plate to remove old or unwanted nail polish or artificial nails (Fig. 36–9). Several applications and rubbing may be required to remove the polish, particularly if several coats have been applied. Nail polish remover can irritate and dry the nail plate and paronychial tissues.[9] It also can contribute to nail dryness and resulting brittleness. These problems can be minimized by using the product once a week or even less often.

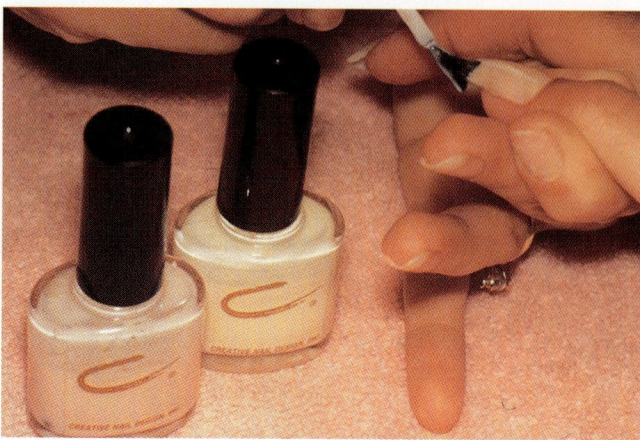

FIGURE 36–12 • An opaque coat of nail polish is applied to cover the entire underlying nail bed. A light pink coat is applied next, to simulate the natural nail bed.

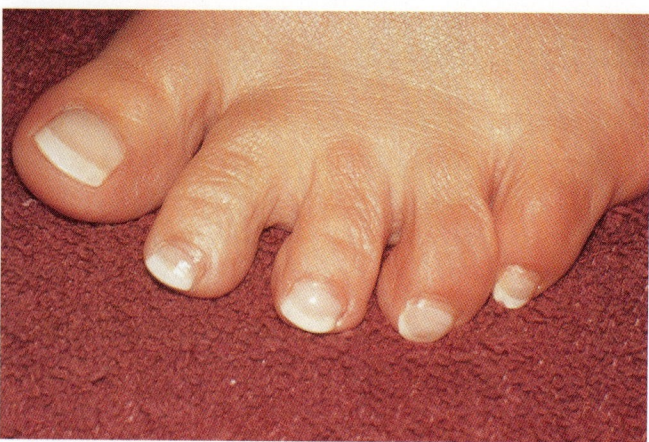

FIGURE 36–15 • The French manicure technique can also be applied to the toenails.

4. French Manicure

The cosmetic appearance of discolored nails in both men and women can be improved with a technique known as a French manicure (Figs. 36–10 and 36–11). A French manicure utilizes a number of colored nail enamels to simulate the natural appearance of unpainted nail. Initially, the nail is painted with an unpigmented opaque base coat to cover the discoloration (Fig. 36–12). A light pink enamel is then added to the entire nail plate, followed by white enamel to the tip, simulating the nail free edge (Fig. 36–13). Lastly, a clear top coat is applied to prevent enamel chipping. French manicures can be applied to both the fingernails and toenails (Figs. 36–14 and 36–15).

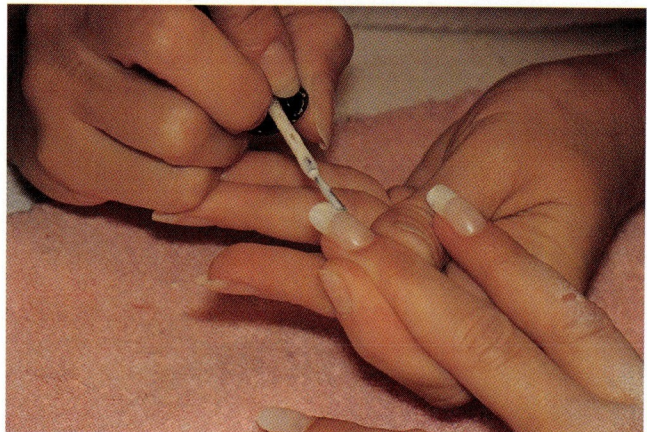

FIGURE 36–13 • A white nail polish is applied to simulate the distal free edge of the nail.

REFERENCES

1. Wing HJ. Nail preparations. In deNavarre MG (ed.). The Chemistry and Manufacture of Cosmetics. Carol Stream, IL: Allured Publishing Co., 1988, pp. 983–1005.
2. Schlossman ML. Nail-enamel resins. Cosmet Technol 1:53, 1979.
3. Adams RM, Maibach HI. A five-year study of cosmetic reactions. J Am Acad Dermatol 13:1062–1069, 1985.
4. Tosti A, Buerra L, Vincenzi C, et al. Contact sensitization caused by toluene sulfonamide-formaldehyde resin in women who use nail cosmetics. Am J Contact Dermatitis 4:150, 1993.
5. Samman PD. Nail disorders caused by external influences. J Soc Cosmet Chem 28:351, 1977.
6. Daniel DR, Osmet LS. Nail pigmentation abnormalities. Cutis 25:595–607, 1980.
7. Mast R. Nail products. In Whittam JH (ed.). Cosmetic Safety: A Primer for Cosmetic Scientists. New York: Marcel Dekker, 1987, pp. 265–313.
8. Wing HJ. Nail preparations. In deNavarre MG (ed.). The Chemistry and Manufacture of Cosmetics, 2nd ed. Carol Stream, IL: Allured Publishing Co., 1988, pp. 983–1005.
9. Wallis MS, Bowen WR, Guin JD. Pathogenesis of onychoschizia (lamellar dystrophy). J Am Acad Derm 24:44–48, 1991.

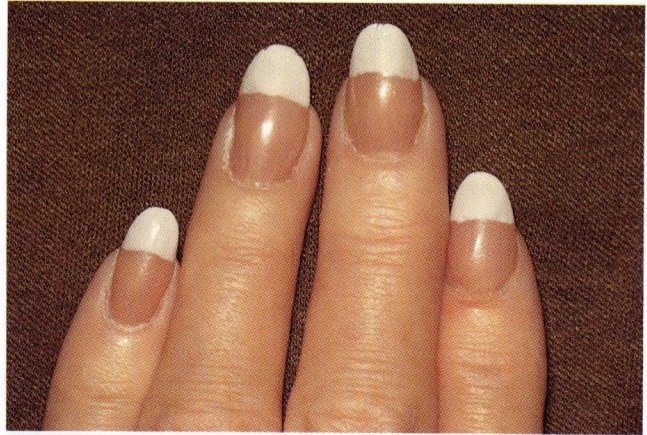

FIGURE 36–14 • The manicurist's artistic skill determines the final cosmetic appearance of a French manicure.

37

Nail Prostheses

Nail prostheses are considered separately from the nail cosmetics previously discussed, as they are nail attachments designed to elongate or beautify the nail plate, as opposed to nail grooming aids or nail coloring cosmetics. Nail prostheses can also function as effective camouflage for discolored, dystrophic, or malformed fingernails, but may be responsible for both irritant and allergic contact dermatitis, as well as nail damage (Table 37–1).

1. Preformed Artificial Nails

Preformed artificial nails are popular among those individuals who wish to elongate their nails at home with minimal expense, time, and skill. The prostheses are sold in several sizes designed to fit the most common sizes and shapes of fingernails. They are glued over the natural nail plate, usually with a methacrylate-based glue (Fig. 37–1). Preglued varieties are also available.[1] Even with the variety available, most patients do not find a suitable preformed nail, which fact accounts for the increasing popularity of custom-made sculptured nails.

Problems arise when preformed nails are traumatically removed, resulting in onychoschizia, nail pitting, and onycholysis (Fig. 37–2).[2] The tendency for onycholysis is increased as the artificial nail is advanced with growth of the natural nail plate (Fig. 37–3). Preformed nails cannot be used effectively by patients with nail dystrophy, congenital nail deformity, or nail plate irregularities, as a smooth nail surface is required for adhesion.

TABLE 37–1   Nail Prostheses

Nail Prostheses	Technique	Advantages	Disadvantages
Preformed	Preformed plastic pieces glued to natural nail plate	Inexpensive; quick; can be done at home	Possible ACD to methacrylate glue
Sculptures	Polymer formed on natural nail plate	Natural appearance; customized nail	Time consuming; onycholysis; paronychia; onychodystrophy; ACD
Photo-bonded sculptures	Light-cured polymer formed on natural nail plate	Natural appearance; customized nail	Photo-onycholysis, paronychia, onychodystrophy, ACD
Sculptures with tips	Preformed plastic piece glued to distal nail with sculpture placed over proximal nail plate	Less time consuming and less expensive than completely sculptured nails; natural appearance	Increased incidence of onycholysis, paronychia, onychodystrophy, and ACD
Sculptures with wraps	Linen or silk coth embedded in sculptured nail polymer	Adds strength to sculptured nail	Same as for sculptured nails

ACD, allergic contact dermatitis.

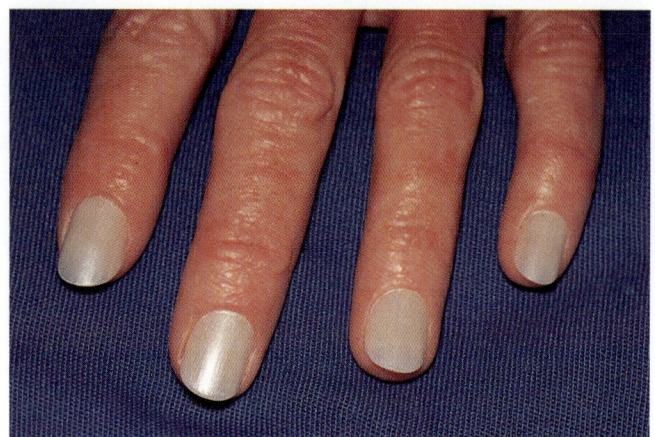

FIGURE 37–1 • Preformed, press-on nails are available already polished for quick nail adornment.

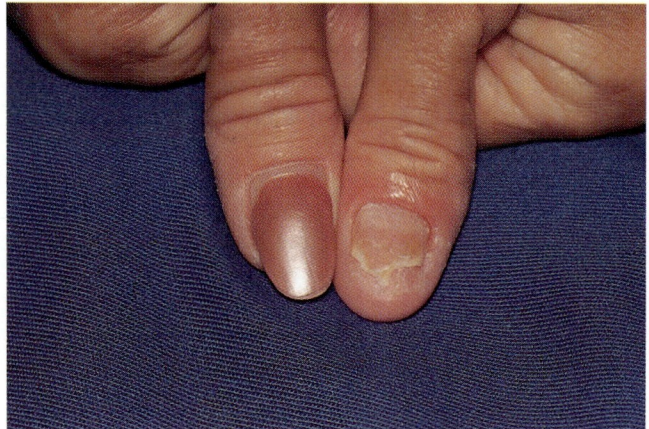

FIGURE 37–2 • Onycholysis is a common complication of press-on nails.

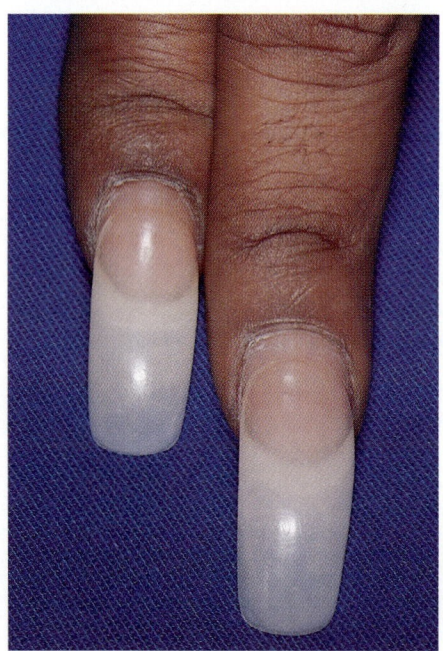

FIGURE 37–3 • Preformed nails move distally as the natural nail plate grows, requiring removal and reapplication.

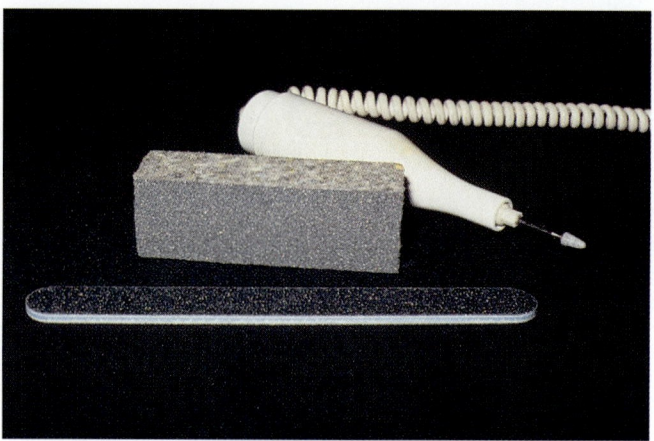

FIGURE 37–4 • A high-speed drill, pumice stone, and diamond file are used to apply nail sculptures.

2. Sculptured Nails

Sculptured nails are custom-made nail prostheses formed by polymerizing an acrylic on the natural nail plate. This procedure is generally performed in a salon as follows:

1. The nail is roughened with a coarse emery board, pumice stone, or grinding drill to create an optimal surface for sculpted nail adhesion (Figs. 37–4 and 37–5).
2. All nail polish and oils are removed from the nail with a primer (Figs. 37–6 and 37–7).
3. An antifungal, antibacterial liquid, such as decolorized iodine, is applied to the entire nail plate to minimize onychomycosis and paronychia (Fig. 37–8).
4. The loose edges of the cuticle are either trimmed, removed, or pushed back, depending on the operator (Fig. 37–9).

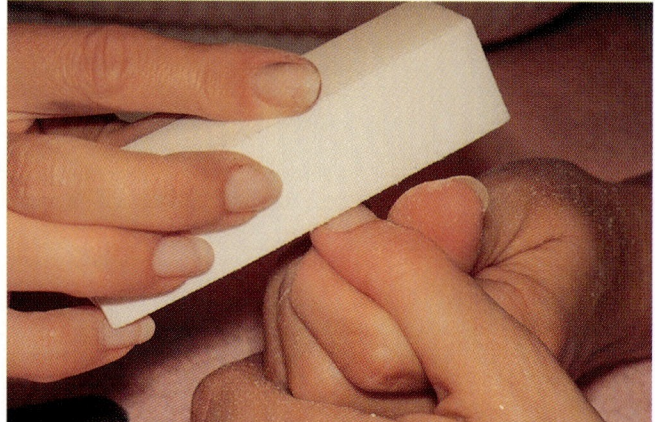

FIGURE 37–5 • The nail surface must be sanded to achieve a large surface area for attachment of the nail sculpture.

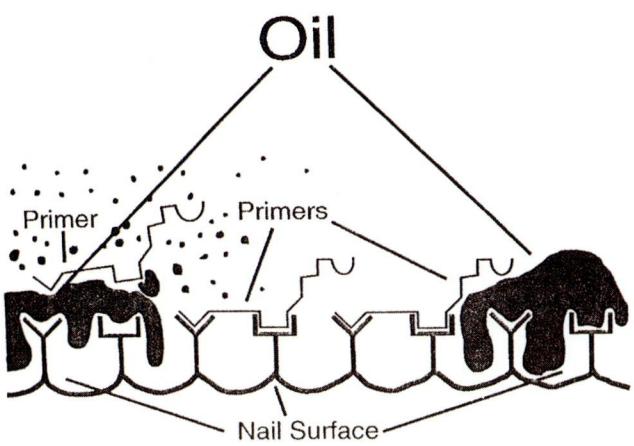

FIGURE 37–6 • A primer is applied to the sanded natural nail plate to remove oils and further etch the nail surface.

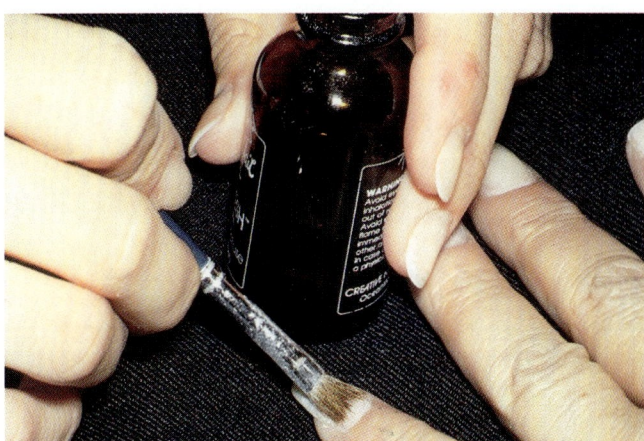

FIGURE 37–8 • Decolorized iodine is applied to decrease the chances of fungal and candidal growth between the natural nail plate and the prosthesis.

5. If the prosthesis is to be longer than the natural nail plate, a flexible template is fit beneath the natural nail plate upon which the elongated sculpted nail will be built (Fig. 37–10).

6. The acrylic is mixed and applied with a paint brush to cover the entire natural nail plate (Figs. 37–11 through 37–13). If nail elongation is desired, the acrylic is extended onto the template to the desired nail length (Fig. 37–14).

7. The final sculpture is sanded to a high shine (Fig. 37–15).

8. Nail polish, jewels, decals, and air-brushed designs may be added, depending on the fashion tastes of the patient (Figs. 37–16 through 37–21).

Sculptured nails utilize liquid ethyl or isobutyl methacrylate as the monomer, powdered polymethyl methacrylate as the polymer, and benzoyl peroxide as the accelerator. Usually, hydroquinone, the mono-

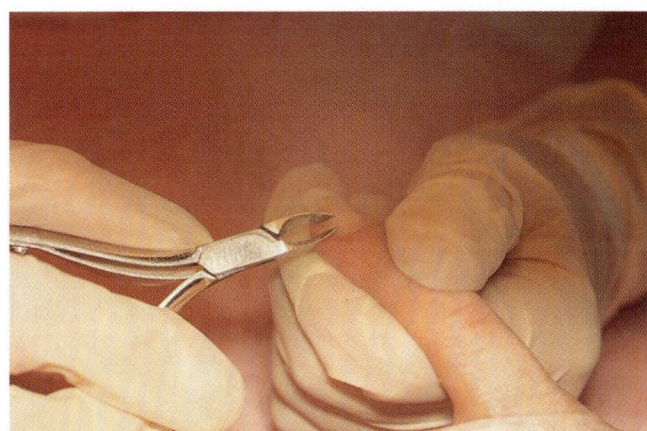

FIGURE 37–9 • Removal of the cuticle is the single most common cause of problems related to the use of nail sculptures.

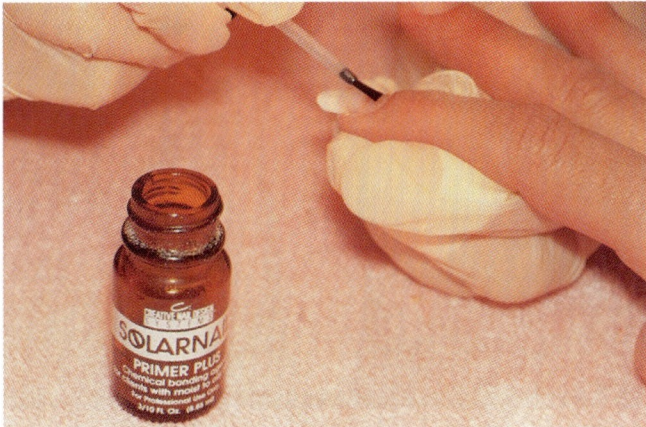

FIGURE 37–7 • The primer is necessary to insure good adhesion between the natural and artificial nail plates.

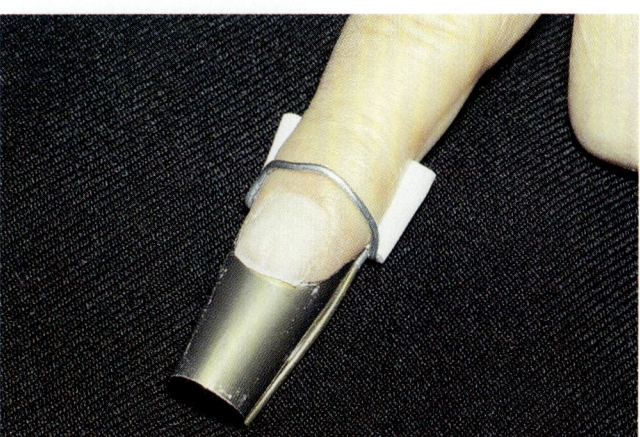

FIGURE 37–10 • A formable template provides a guide for application of the custom-made nail sculpture.

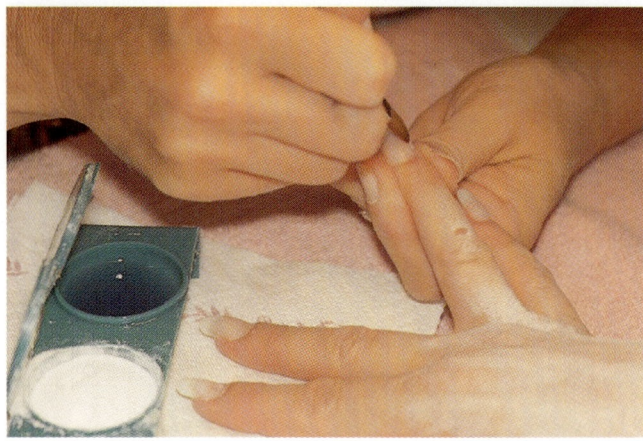

FIGURE 37–11 • The polymer is mixed immediately prior to application to the nail with a brush.

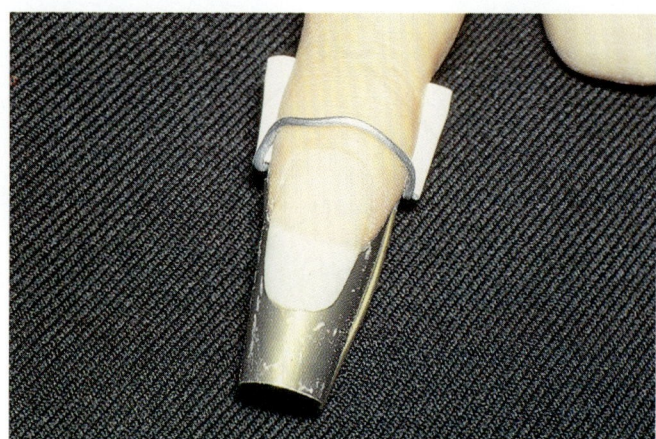

FIGURE 37–14 • If nail elongation is desired, the polymer is applied over the template until the final nail length is achieved.

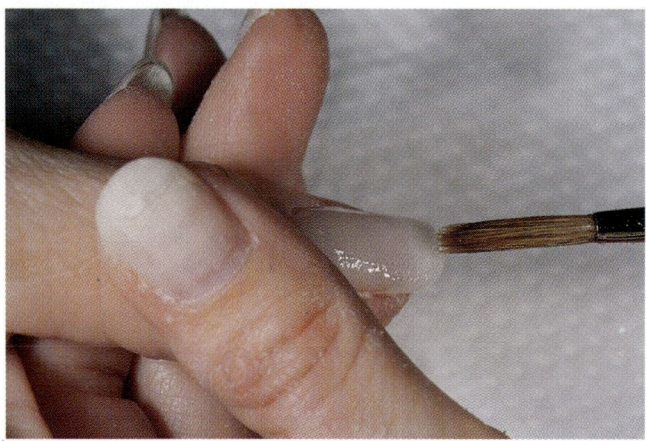

FIGURE 37–12 • The polymer is dabbed onto the nail in several coats.

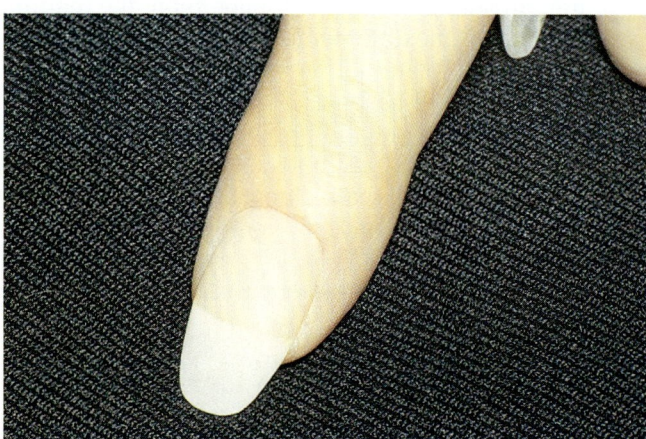

FIGURE 37–15 • To simulate the appearance of a natural nail, a clear polymer is used for the proximal nail plate prosthesis, whereas a white polymer is used for the distal nail prosthesis.

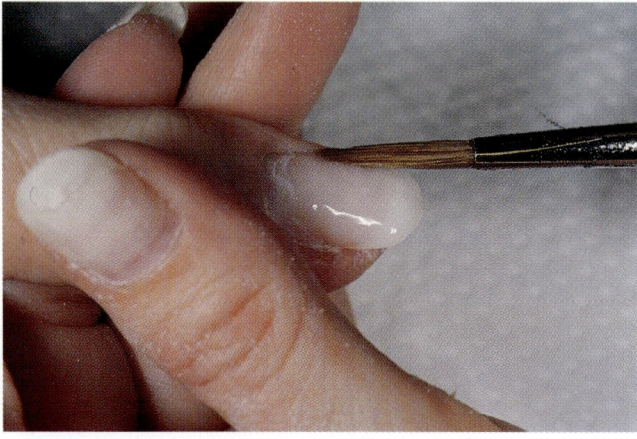

FIGURE 37–13 • The final polymer coat is brushed smooth and allowed to air dry.

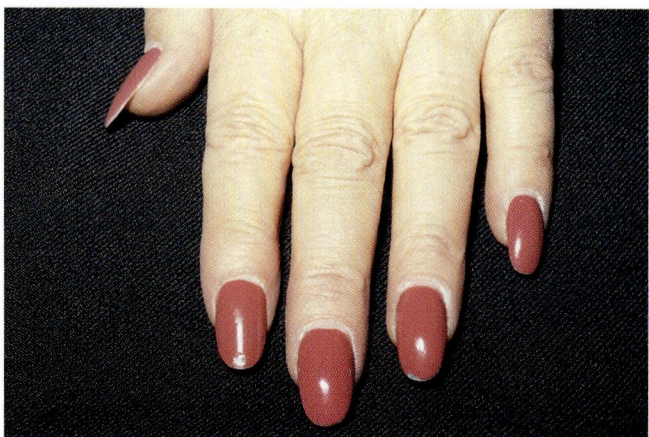

FIGURE 37–16 • Nail sculptures can be painted with nail polish to any color desired. Nail polish resists chipping better on a nail prosthesis than on a natural nail plate.

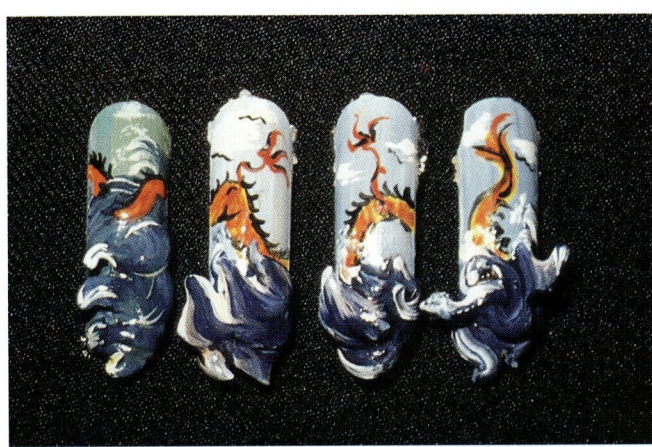

FIGURE 37–17 • Elaborate, artistic nail designs can be created by applying many layers of polymer.

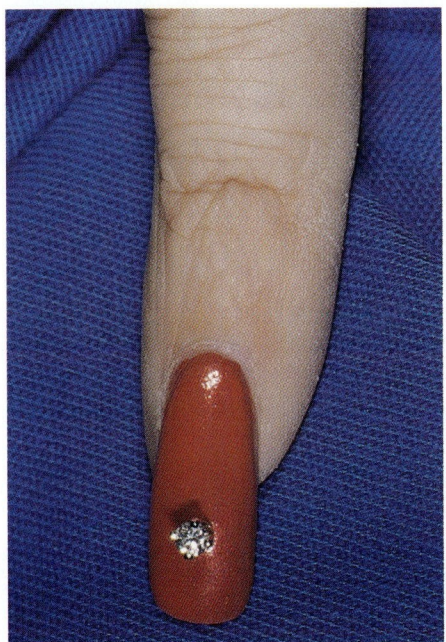

FIGURE 37–18 • Nail jewels are drilled through the distal sculptured nail plate.

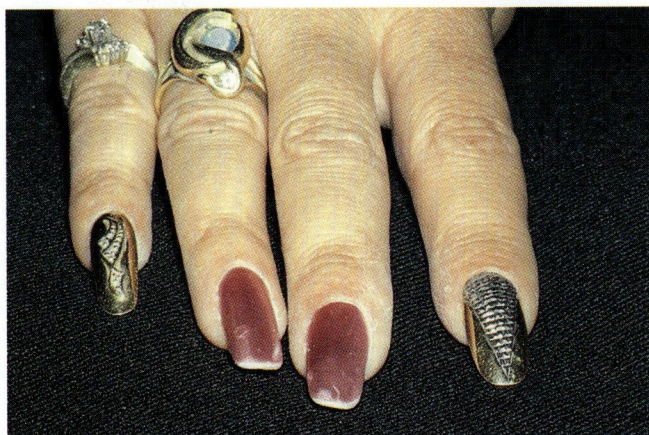

FIGURE 37–19 • Preformed gold nail plates can be attached to the natural nail plate with formable nail acrylic.

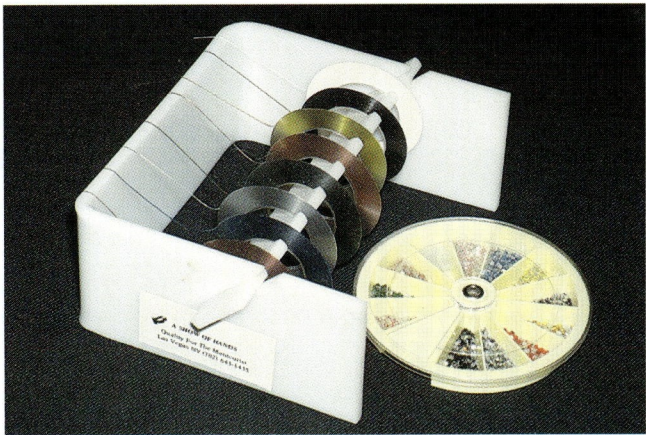

FIGURE 37–20 • Decals and metal strips may also be applied to sculptured nails by embedding the adornment in the polymer prior to application of the final layer.

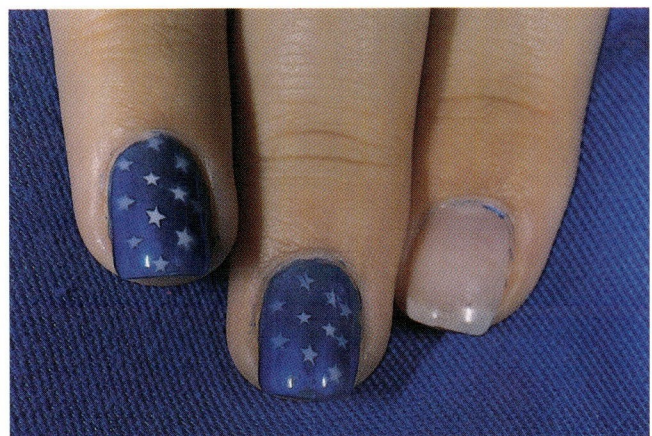

FIGURE 37–21 • Designs may be applied to the nail prostheses with air brush equipment.

methyl ether of hydroquinone or pyrogallol, is added to slow down polymerization.[3] Combining these ingredients results in a formable acrylic that hardens in 7 to 9 minutes.[4]

Nail sculptures require more care than natural fingernails. With continued wear, the acrylic loosens from the natural nail, especially around the edges. These loose edges must be clipped and new acrylic applied approximately every 3 weeks as the nail plate grows, a procedure known as "filling" (Fig. 37–22). Failure to undergo filling every 2 to 3 weeks will predispose the natural nail plate to traumatic onycholysis (Fig. 37–23). If necessary, the sculptured nails can be removed by soaking in acetone.

Damage to the natural nail plate may still occur with nail sculpture use, even if the patient is conscientious. After 2 to 4 months of wear, the natural nail plate becomes yellowed, dry, and thin. This is due to interference with the nail's normal vapor exchange, nail plate trauma during the removal process, and

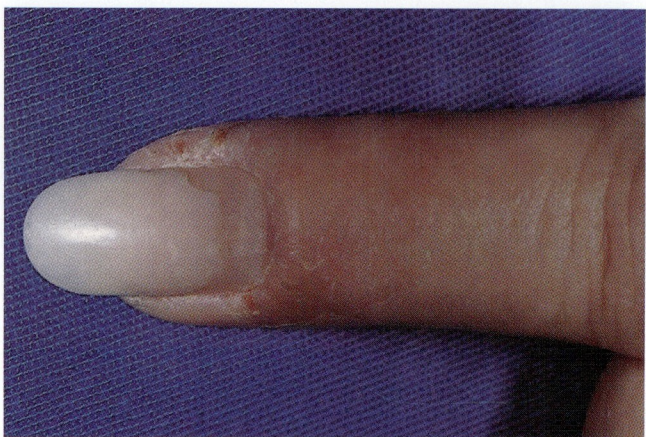

FIGURE 37–22 • The nail prosthesis requires regular maintenance. New polymer is required at the proximal nail fold as the sculpture moves with the growth of the natural nail plate.

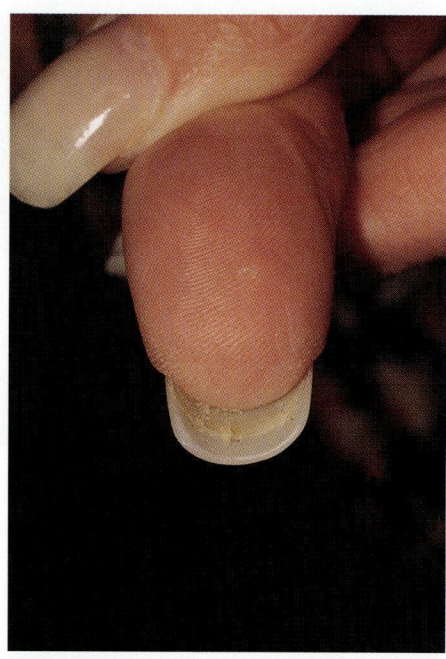

FIGURE 37–24 • The natural nail plate can be visualized beneath the nail prosthesis.

damage to the underlying nail bed.[5] Most operators prefer to allow the patient's natural nail to grow and act as a support for the sculpture; however, the nails become thin, bendable, and weak (Fig. 37–24). For this reason, it is not advisable to wear sculptured nails for more than 3 months consecutively, allowing 1 month's rest between applications.

Numerous problems are associated with the use of artificial nails. Poorly trained operators may allow liquid acrylic to enter the proximal nail fold, resulting in nail matrix damage (Fig. 37–25). Allergic contact dermatitis remains an issue even though methyl methacrylate is no longer used; isobutyl, ethyl, and tetrahydrofurfuryl methacrylate are still strong sensitizers.[6,7] Sensitivity to the acrylic can cause onycholysis[8,9] or, rarely, permanent loss of the fingernails.[10] It should be remembered that the polymerized cured acrylic is not sensitizing, only the liquid monomer.[11] Therefore, a careful operator who avoids skin contact with the uncured acrylic can avoid sensitizing the patient. Patch testing should be performed in individuals thought to be sensitized using methyl methacrylate monomer, 10% in olive oil, and methacrylate acid esters, 1% and 5% in olive oil and petrolatum.[12]

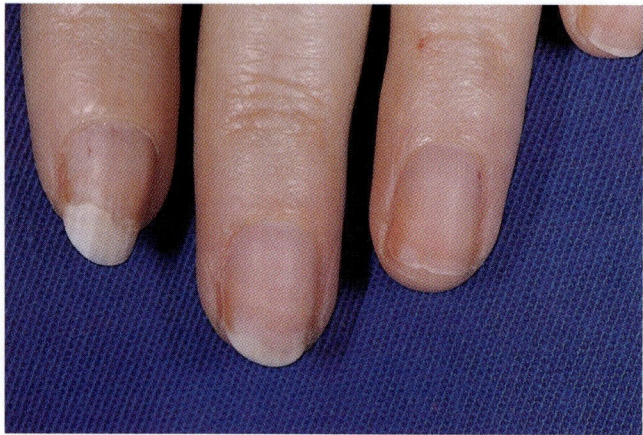

FIGURE 37–23 • The mild onycholysis demonstrated here is the most common side effect of nail prostheses.

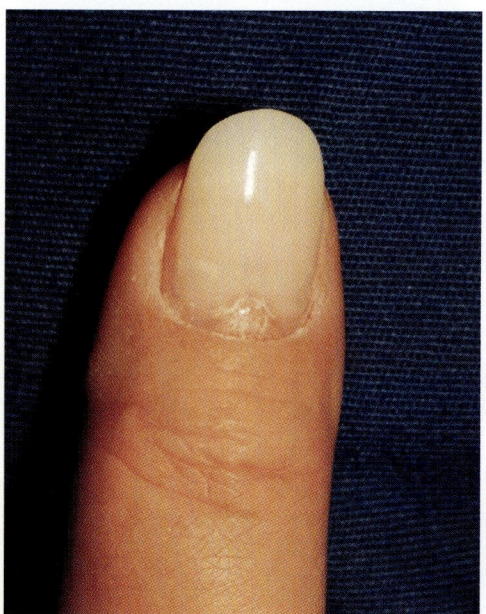

FIGURE 37–25 • A poorly trained nail sculpture artist can permanently damage the natural nail plate with aggressive use of a high-speed drill.

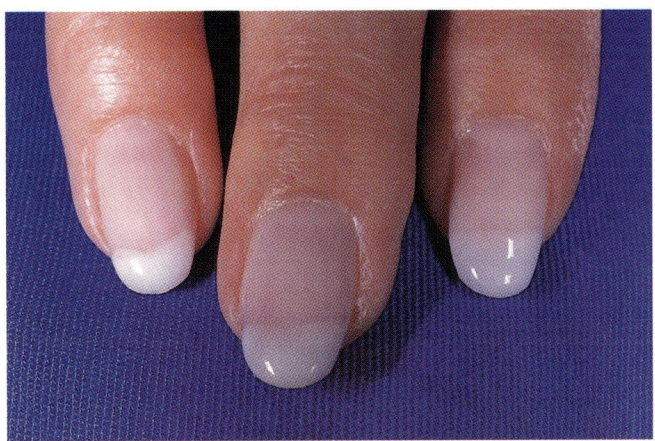

FIGURE 37–26 • Gel nails are hardened with ultraviolet light instead of air drying.

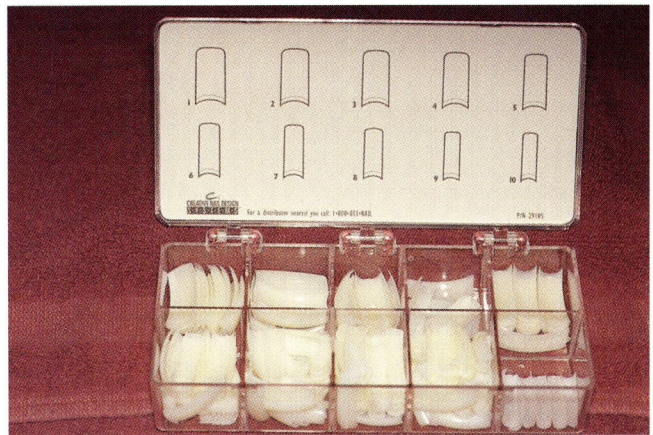

FIGURE 37–29 • Preformed nail tips come in a variety of sizes and shapes.

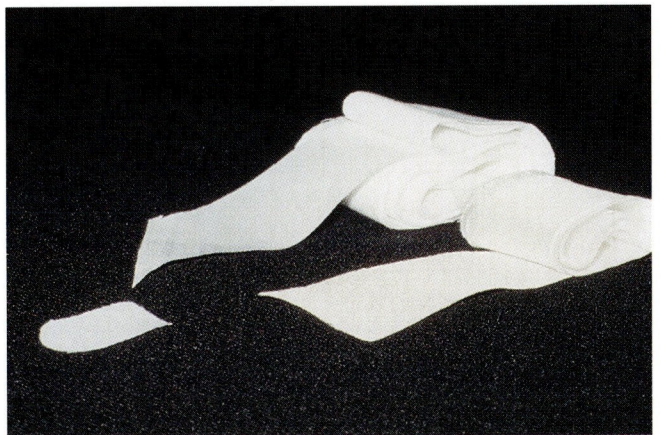

FIGURE 37–27 • Strips of linen or silk can be cut to the shape of the nail plate.

3. Photobonded Sculptured Nails

The sculptured nails previously described allow the acrylic to cure at room temperature. By contrast, photobonded nails utilize an acrylic that polymerizes under a magnesium light for 1 to 2 minutes. This technique is similar to restorative dental bonding (Fig. 37–26). Photo-onycholysis and paresthesias have been reported as a result of this procedure.[13]

4. Cloth Wraps

Additional strength can be achieved with nail sculptures by embedding silk or cotton cloth in the acrylic prior to hardening (Fig. 37–27). Several layers of liquid acrylic are then applied to seal the cloth. The cloth texture appears through the clear nail sculpture

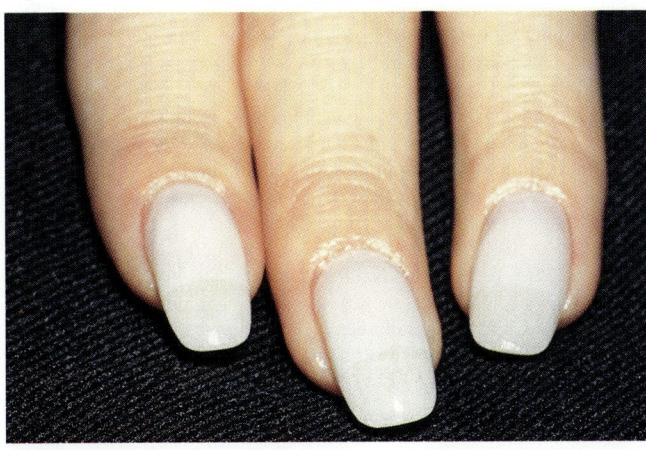

FIGURE 37–28 • Embedding linen in the final layers of polymer, as shown here, can strengthen the nail sculpture.

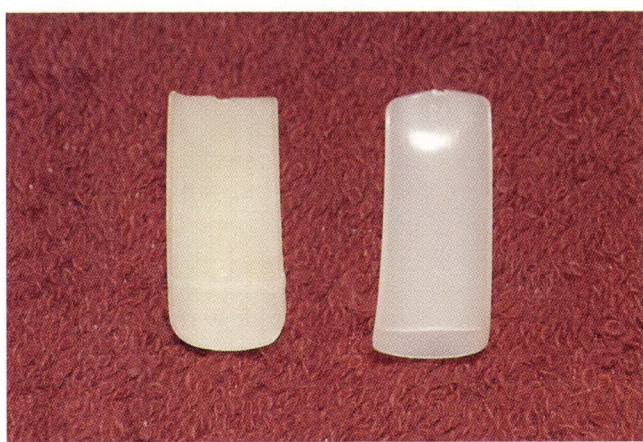

FIGURE 37–30 • The top surface of the preformed nail tip is smooth. However, the undersurface, shown here, is offset so that the natural nail plate can fit smoothly into the prosthesis.

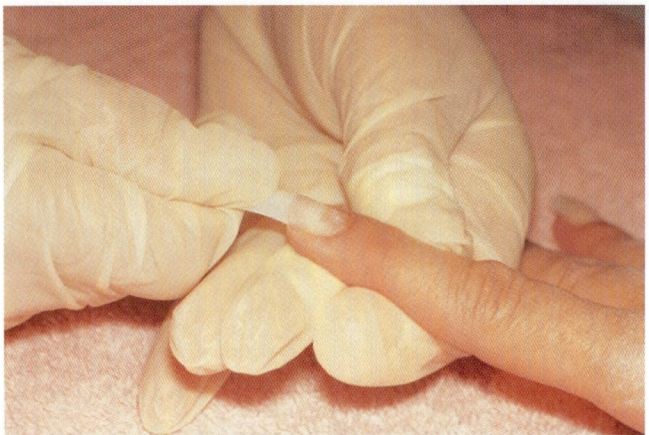

FIGURE 37–31 • The preformed nail tip is glued onto the natural nail plate using a methacrylate-based adhesive.

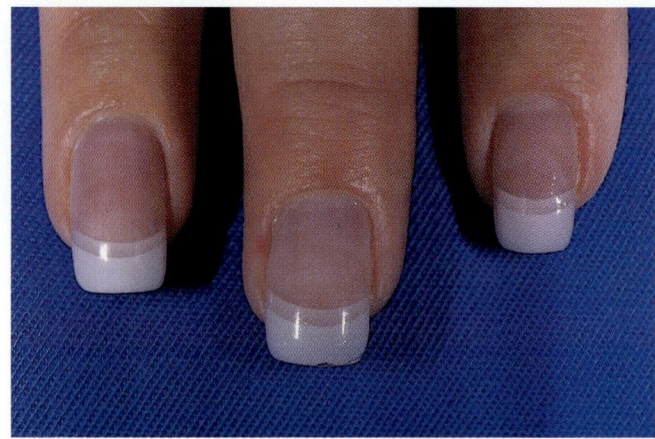

FIGURE 37–33 • Some preformed nail tips are available with designs.

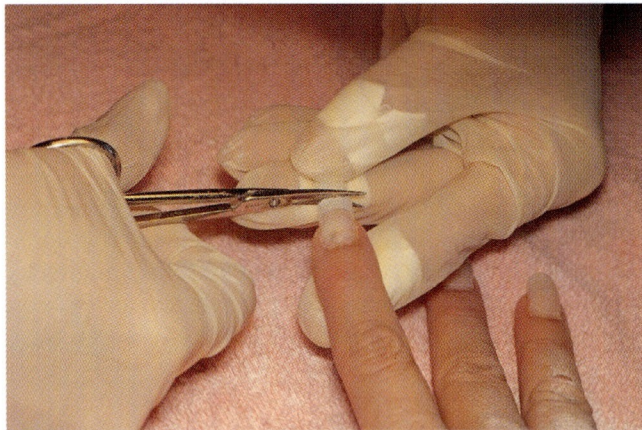

FIGURE 37–32 • The nail tip is trimmed to the desired length with scissors prior to application of the polymer.

(Fig. 37–28), so these nails are generally polished. Linen wraps provide greater nail strength than silk wraps.

5. Sculptures with Artificial Tips

Another technique of elongating nails is to combine custom-made nail sculptures with preformed artificial tips. The tips are available in a variety of sizes, shapes, lengths, and colors (Figs. 37–29 and 37–30). This technique involves gluing the premade tip to the distal nail and trimming it to the desired final length (Figs. 37–31 and 37–32). Once adhesion has occurred, the formable acrylic polymer, as dicussed previously, is applied to cover the portion of the natural nail plate not covered by the premade tip (Fig. 37–33). This is currently the most popular salon method of nail elongation. It is less time consuming than creating an entire nail sculpture from acrylic, and the price of a set of artificial nails is lower. The possibility of developing traumatic onycholysis is enhanced with this variation, as extremely long nails can be created.

REFERENCES

1. Brauer EW. Selected prostheses primarily of cosmetic interest. Cutis 6:521–524, 1970.
2. Lazar P. Reactions to nail hardeners. Arch Dermatol 94:446–448, 1966.
3. Viola LI. Fingernail elongators and accessory nail preparations. In Balsam MS, Sagarin E (eds.). Cosmetics, Science and Technology, 2nd ed. New York: Wiley-Interscience, 1972, pp. 543–552.
4. Barnett JM, Scher RK, Taylor SC. Nail cosmetics. Dermatol Clin 9:9–17, 1991.
5. Baden H. Cosmetics and the nail. In Diseases of the Hair and Nails. Chicago: Yearbook Publishers, 1987, pp. 99–102.
6. Marks JG, Bishop ME, Willis WF. Allergic contact dermatitis to sculptured nails. Arch Dermatol 115:100, 1979.
7. Fisher AA. Cross reactions between methyl methacrylate monomer and acrylic monomers presently used in acrylic nail preparations. Contact Dermatitis 6:345–347, 1980.
8. Goodwin P. Onycholysis due to acrylic nail applications. J Exp Dermatol 1:191–192, 1976.
9. Lane CW, Kost LB. Sensitivity to artificial nails. Arch Dermatol 74:671–672, 1956.
10. Fisher AA. Permanent loss of fingernails from sensitization and reaction to acrylic in a preparation designed to make artificial nails. J Dermatol Surg Oncol 6:70–71, 1980.
11. Fisher AA, Franks A, Glick H. Allergic sensitization of the skin and nails to acrylic plastic nails. J Allergy 28:84, 1957.
12. Baran R, RPR Dawber. The nail and cosmetics. In Samman PD, Fenton DA (eds.). The Nails in Disease, 4th ed. Chicago: Yearbook Publishers, 1986, p. 129.
13. Fisher AA. Adverse nail reactions and paresthesia from photobonded acrylate sculptured nails. Cutis 45:293–294, 1990.

INDEX

· · · · · · · · —

Note: Page numbers in *italics* indicate figures; those followed by t indicate tables.

ISBN 0-443-06548-9

90071